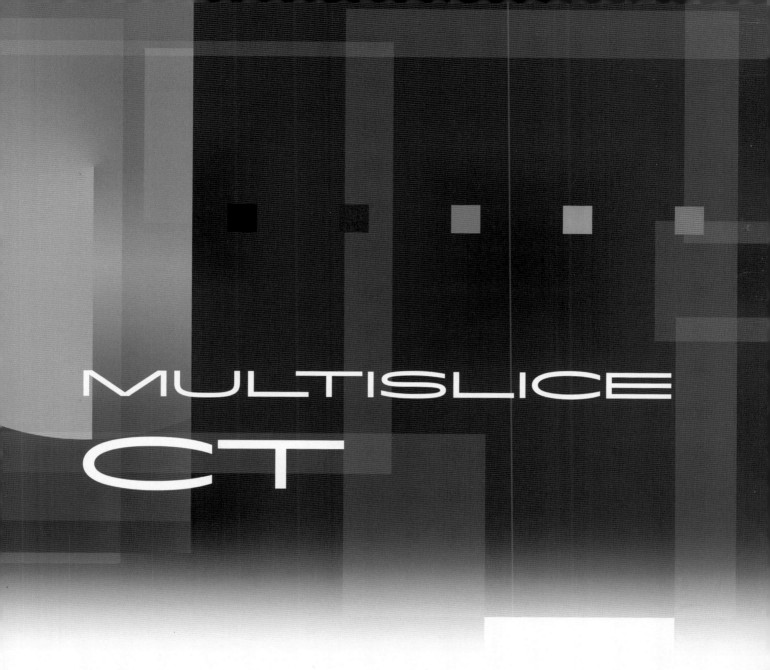

MULTISLICE CT

Principles and Protocols

Friedrich Knollmann, MD
Professor and Vice Chairman of Diagnostic Radiology
Klinikum der Georg-August-Universität
Göttingen, Germany

Fergus V. Coakley, MD
Associate Professor of Radiology
Chief, Abdominal Imaging Section
University of California, San Francisco
School of Medicine
San Francisco, California

MULTISLICE CT

Principles and Protocols

SAUNDERS

ELSEVIER

SAUNDERS
ELSEVIER

1600 John F. Kennedy Boulevard, Suite 1800
Philadelphia, PA 19103-2899

MULTISLICE CT: PRINCIPLES AND PROTOCOLS   ISBN-13: 978-1-4160-0268-0
First Edition   ISBN-10: 1-4160-0268-5
Copyright 2006, Elsevier, Inc. All rights reserved.

NOTICE

International Standardized Book Number
ISBN-13: 978-1-4160-0268-0
ISBN-10: 1-4160-0268-5
WN 206

Printed in China.

Last digit is the print number: 9 8 7 6 5 4 3 2 1

To the patients of the Charité whose health we have strived to improve with diagnostic imaging; to Professor Roland Felix, MD, PhD, Chairman of Radiology at the Charité, Campus Virchow-Klinikum, Berlin, Germany; and to my collaborators at the Charité's Virchow-Klinikum.

Friedrich Knollmann, MD

To my wonderful wife, Sara, and to my equally wonderful children, Declan and Fiona. I have learned more from them than I have ever taught to my residents and fellows.

Fergus V. Coakley, MD

Contributors

Bobby Bhartia, MRCP, FRCR

Consultant Radiologist, Department of Radiology, St James' University Hospital, Leeds, West Yorkshire, United Kingdom

Stefano Binaghi, MD

Department of Radiology, Interventional Neuroradiology Unit, University of Lausanne; Department of Radiology, Centre Hospitalier Universitaire Vaudois, Lausanne, Switzerland

Patrick Browaeys, MD

Resident, Department of Radiology, Centre Hospitalier Universitaire Vaudois, Lausanne, Switzerland

Fergus V. Coakley, MD

Associate Professor of Radiology, Radiology Department, University of California, San Francisco, San Francisco, California

Laure S. Fournier, MD

Professor, Rene Descartes University—Paris; Department of Radiology, Hospital European Georges Pompidou, Paris, France

Guy Frija, MD

Professor, Rene Descartes University—Paris; Department of Radiology, Hospital European Georges Pompidou, Paris, France

Donald P. Frush, MD

Chief, Division of Pediatric Radiology, Department of Radiology, Duke Medical Center; Faculty, Medical Physics Program, Duke University, Durham, North Carolina

Michael Galanski, MD

Department of Diagnostic Radiology, Hannover Medical School, Hannover, Germany

Franco Iafrate, MD

Fellow, Department of Radiological Sciences, University of Rome "La Sapienza," Rome, Italy

Ella A. Kazerooni, MD, MS

Professor, Department of Radiology, Division of Thoracic Radiology, University of Michigan Medical School; Radiologist, Department of Radiology, University of Michigan Health System, Ann Arbor, Michigan

Friedrich Knollmann, MD

Professor and Vice Chairman of Diagnostic Radiology, Klinikum der Georg-August-Universität, Göttingen, Germany

Andrea Laghi, MD

Researcher, Assistant Professor, Department of Radiological Sciences, University of Rome "La Sapienza," Rome, Italy

Valérie Laurent, MD

Service de Radiologie Brabois Adultes, Centre Hospitalier Universitaire, Nancy, France

Catherine Lefort, MD

Professor, Rene Descartes University—Paris; Department of Radiology, Hospital European Georges Pompidou, Paris, France

Stéphane Lenoir, MD

Départment d'Imagerie, Institut Mutualiste Montsouris, Paris, France

Martin G. Mack, MD, PhD

Department of Diagnostic and Interventional Radiology, University Hospital of Frankfurt, Frankfurt, Germany

Yvonne K. Maratos, MD

Department of Radiology, Hospital European Georges Pompidou; Rene Descartes University, Paris, France

Reto A. Meuli, MD

Associate Professor, Department of Radiology, University of Lausanne, Centre Hospitalier Universitaire Vaudois, Lausanne, Switzerland

Lionel Meyer-Bisch, MD

Service de Radiologie Brabois Adultes, Centre Hospitalier Universitaire, Nancy, France

Smita Patel, MBBS, MRCP, FRCR

Assistant Professor, Staff Physician, Department of Radiology, University of Michigan Medical Center, Taubman Center, Ann Arbor, Michigan

Roberto Passariello, MD

Professor and Chairman, Department of Radiological Sciences, University of Rome "La Sapienza," Rome, Italy

Denis Regent, MD

Service de Radiologie Brabois Adultes, Centre Hospitalier Universitaire, Nancy, France

Marie-Pierre Revel, MD

Department of Radiology, Hospital European Georges Pompidou; Rene Descartes University, Paris, France

Michael Rieger, MD

Clinical Department of Diagnostic Radiology, Innsbruck Medical University, Innsbruck, Austria

Patrik Rogalla, MD

Department of Radiology, Charité Hospital, Universitätsmedizin Berlin, Berlin, Germany

Georg Stamm, MD

Abteilung Diagnostische Radiologie, Medizinische Hochschule Hannover, Hannover, Germany

Afia Umber, MD

University of California—San Francisco; Alameda County Medical Center, Internal Medicine, Oakland, California

Thomas J. Vogl, MD, PhD

Department of Diagnostic and Interventional Radiology, University Hospital of Frankfurt, Frankfurt, Germany

Benjamin M. Yeh, MD

Assistant Professor, Abdominal Imaging, Department of Radiology, University of California, San Francisco, San Francisco, California

Marc Zins, MD

Chief, Department of Radiology, Saint Joseph Hospital, Paris, France

Preface

Strictly, multislice computed tomography (MSCT) is already over 10 years old, since the Elscint CT Twin scanner used a dual array of two side-by-side detector rows that represented an early version of multislice technology and was first introduced in 1992. However, the most recent advances in CT scanner technology offer unprecedented advances in clinical and technical capabilities that significantly exceed previous specifications and can be considered revolutionary rather than simply evolutionary with respect to current and future developments. The emergence of 4-row MSCT in 1998 was a major technological breakthrough that dramatically changed the practice of CT. The temporal resolution of MSCT is now comparable to MRI, and both the spatial resolution and extent of coverage exceeds MRI.

MSCT may appear to be simply an incremental improvement in spiral CT technology. This view of MSCT is incomplete because the remarkable capability to rapidly acquire numerous thin sections in multiple phases of enhancement provides both great challenges for image handling and storage, as well as great opportunities for three-dimensional postprocessing and display. Three-dimensional data sets, narrow collimation, and multiphasic imaging provide improved lesion detection, multiplanar capability, and the ability to perform high-quality CT angiography.

With this new technology, which continues to evolve, come significant new challenges, particularly with respect to managing the vast quantity of image data that are generated. This remains an unsolved problem that will require the development of innovative image processing and viewing strategies. The traditional paradigm of reviewing tomographic slices may well be replaced by a primarily volumetric approach. The rapidity with which body cavities can be imaged with MSCT also requires new thinking with respect to the rate of intravenous contrast administration, contrast injection duration, contrast bolus volume, and scan delays.

Finally, the radiation dose is increased with MSCT (although some factors can be adjusted to limit this dose increase), which is compounded by multiphasic imaging. Careful attention must be paid to technical parameters during scanning, with tailoring of the dose and imaging protocol to the clinical question. With the introduction of 4-, 8-, 16-, and 64-row CT systems, early adopters have been wondering if the new technology renders older generations obsolete, and if so, if use of a multislice CT scanner offers so important advantages that they may define a new standard of care.

Notwithstanding the enthusiasm many researchers have demonstrated when welcoming the latest developments, this book tries to emphasize a clinical value perspective that seems timely in view of the recent changes in how health care is applied. Given these new challenges that are in many respects revolutionary rather than evolutionary, we felt it was appropriate for a text that specifically addresses the techniques and applications of MSCT.

Friedrich Knollmann, MD
Fergus V. Coakley, MD

Contents

MULTISLICE CT

Principles and Protocols

1

Multislice Computed Tomography in Acute Stroke

Patrick Browaeys
Stefano Binaghi
Reto A. Meuli

EPIDEMIOLOGY AND ETIOLOGY

According to the most recent World Health Organization (WHO) statistics (2002), stroke was the fourth leading cause of death worldwide, with nearly 5.5 million cases, and the third leading cause in Western countries, accounting for nearly 10% of all deaths.[1] It is the leading cause of major disability in adults, and its total costs (both direct and indirect) are estimated for 2004 at $53.6 billion in the United States alone.[2,3]

Accounting for 70% of cases, ischemic stroke is the most frequent subtype,[4] and no proven successful therapy was available until the trial of the National Institute of Neurological Disorders and Stroke in 1995, using recombinant tissue-type plasminogen activator.[5]

Ischemic stroke itself has several subtypes. The most common classification includes five subtypes: cardioembolism, large-artery atherosclerosis, small-vessel occlusion, stroke of other determined etiology, and stroke of undetermined etiology.[6] Except for stroke of undetermined etiology, cardioembolism is, without dispute, the most prominent subtype. Large-artery atherosclerosis accounts for the second or the third largest percentage, depending on American or European population studies, respectively.[7,8]

PHYSIOPATHOLOGY

The brain consumes the most energy of any organ. Although it occupies just 2% of total body weight, approximately 20% of the body's resources are allocated to it.[9] Still, cerebral parenchyma cannot stock glucose. Instead, high and stable blood perfusion is required to maintain correct functionality. Normal values of cerebral blood flow (CBF) are about 50 ml/100 g/min. These can vary with cerebral activity (maxima and minima, respectively, with seizure and coma) and differ between gray and white matter, with the first requiring up to three times the needs of the second.[10] To ensure high and constant irrigation without variation in cerebral perfusion pressure, complex mechanisms of CBF autoregulation must be active. The increase in oxygen extraction fraction (OEF) is the second mechanism able to protect from reduced irrigation.[11]

Nevertheless, many pathological conditions go beyond these regulations or OEF capabilities and can provoke significant alteration of brain perfusion. When hypoperfusion is moderate, neuronal life is not threatened. Positron emission tomography (PET) studies provide the best accuracy, in absolute values, for calculating ischemic thresholds. They show that when blood supply falls under 12 to 22 ml/100 g/min, electrical activity stops in affected neurons. This is the electrophysiological definition of the ischemic penumbra first described 25 years ago.[12] At present, we know that neurons probably respond to distinct blood flow thresholds specific to distinct functions.[13] Another way to define penumbra is to say that it corresponds to threatened viable parenchyma, which natural evolution leads to infarct if ischemia persists.[14] However, neurons can recover if perfusion is enhanced, depending on the duration and severity of ischemic penumbra.[15] When blood flow is less than approximately 12 ml/100 g/min, ischemic parenchyma usually results in cell death with no chance of recuperation, even if blood flow is restored.[16-18] The reason is that such a low level of perfusion leads to neuronal morphological alteration (membrane failure), which cannot be repaired after it occurs.[19-21] Because of this time-severity relation, penumbra usually has a centrifugal extension from the infarct core(s) (Figure 1-1).

TREATMENT PRINCIPLES

Current efficient treatments face the problem of patient selection, according to clinical status and common imaging methods, considering that the native computed tomography (CT) findings are unreliable.[22] Initial guidelines that recommended thrombolysis to a range up to 3 hours have now increased to 6 hours after stroke onset.[5,23] As PET and magnetic resonance imaging (MRI) provide evidence that the therapeutic window is potentially wider than the criteria in use, precise determination of the ischemic penumbra should be the key to free clinicians from rigid, time-based thrombolysis protocols.[24,25] Knowledge of the exact penumbra/infarct size ratio could prevent the risky use of thrombolysis, which ultimately might not be beneficial. Effectively, intracranial hemorrhage is the major secondary effect of thrombolysis and, although it is sometimes independent of thrombolysis, it should always be taken into account by the clinician.[26]

When stroke occurs, perfusion CT can help us to discriminate penumbra and infarct in ischemic lesions.

MULTISLICE COMPUTED TOMOGRAPHY PROTOCOL

Our complete MSCT protocol for acute ischemic stroke is based on four steps (Table 1-1), in the following order: native head CT, perfusion CT, CT angiography (CTA) of neck vessels up to the Circle of Willis, and post-contrast head CT. Our exams are conducted on a 16-detector array MSCT (Lightspeed CT; General Electric, Milwaukee, Wisconsin).

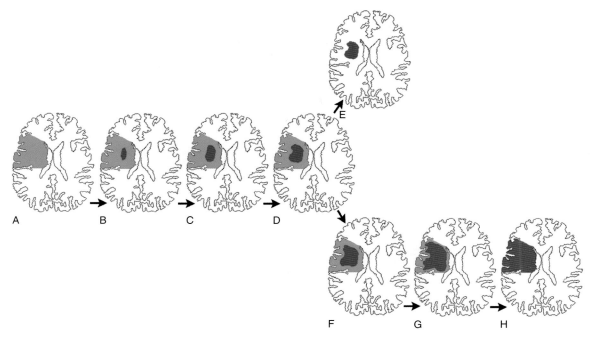

Fig. 1-1 Concepts of infarct progression and ischemic penumbra. A, At stroke onset, parenchymal blood supply falls and compromises viability of a fairly large region. **B,** The initial core of infarct *(red)* appears rapidly where ischemia is major and occupies first a reduced fraction of the global ischemic lesion while penumbra, still salvageable, is fairly large *(green)*. **C, D,** Without any therapeutic intervention or spontaneous reperfusion, parenchyma located in penumbra turns progressively into infarct. **F,** Ischemic lesion with recovery potential (penumbra) turns into infarct, if no spontaneous reperfusion occurred, with minutes and hours **(G)** progression ("time is brain"); the entire ischemic area is transformed into infarct **(H). E,** If reperfusion occurs, whether it is spontaneous (very inconsistent) or medically provoked, penumbra can be saved with the hope of morbidity reduction.

Native and Post-Contrast Head CT

Native and post-contrast head CT are required because of other sources than ischemic stroke in acute neurological disorders (e.g., hemorrhage, neoplasms). Native head CT also aids in determining adequate slices for perfusion CT. We conduct this part, in axial mode, by joint 10- and 5-mm slices in the supratentorial and infratentorial brain, respectively. The post-contrast head CT is performed after the perfusion CT and the CTA, with no further injection of contrast agent.

Perfusion CT

Our perfusion CT scanning sequence includes two 40-second acquisitions, each one composed of one image per second in cine mode at two adjacent levels, due to MSCT aptitude. These two acquisi-

tions, separated from one another by 3 minutes, are performed 7 seconds after initiation of 50 ml iohexol injection (300 mg/ml of iodine; Accupaque 300, Amersham Health, Little Chalfont, UK) in an antecubital vein, at a rate of 5 ml/s with power pump. The delay between the two injections is sufficient to avoid interference of the first contrast media residue. In addition, our experience indicates that this injection rate is the highest one bearable by patients when a peripheral vein is used. Furthermore, higher flow rates do not modify time-concentration curves, whereas lower ones seem to overestimate cerebral blood flow.[27-29]

With a slice thickness of 10 mm, we are thus able to cover brain parenchyma on 40 mm. Particular attention is provided for slice selection. In nearly all cases, they are chosen to go through basal nuclei for the caudal slice with eviction of lenses. Exceptionally, the gantry is a little more tilted to offer better coverage of the posterior fossa and the occipital

Table 1-1 Complete MSCT protocol for acute ischemic stroke in our institution

	Acquisition mode	Acquisition parameters	Collimation	Contrast	Injection rate	Delay after injection before acquisition	Acquisition course	Acquisition duration
1. Native head CT	Sequential		10mm supratentorial 5mm infratentorial	No	/	/	Skull base to vertex	
2. Perfusion CT First series	Sequential; cine mode	80 kVp 100 mA	2 slices of 10 mm	50 ml Iohexol	5 ml/s	7 sec	40 stationary rotations	40 seconds
			Selection of perfusion slices					
			Delay: 3 min					
Second series	Sequential; cine mode	80 kVp 100 mA	2 slices of 10 mm	50 ml Iohexol	5 ml/s	7 sec	40 stationary rotations	40 seconds
3. CTA of neck vessels and circle of Willis	Helicoïdal	120 kVp 430 mA	1.25 mm pitch: 1.75	50 ml Iohexol	5 ml/s	Defined by perfusion sequence	Aortic arch to circle of Willis	
4. Post-contrast head CT	Sequential		10mm supratentorial 5mm infratentorial	No	/	/	Skull base to vertex	

lobes when strong evidence of ischemia is suspected (i.e., hypodensity on native CT).

The technical parameters of the acquisitions are 100 mA and 80 kVp, since Wintermark et al.[30] demonstrated that 80 kVp used in place of 120 kVp provides better contrast enhancement and white-gray matter contrast without significantly increasing noise, as well as a global reduction in patient dose by a 2.8-fold factor.

In the post-processing of perfusion CT, major choices are required for effective computing of data acquisition. The first key of computation is the selection of arterial input function or the arterial reference time-concentration curve, used in our central volume deconvolution method. The reference artery should be the one with the earliest and biggest enhancement. It should have a caliber that allows us to select the region of interest (ROI). Pixels of this reference artery must offer a high amplitude time-concentration curve and the most regular appearance (Figure 1-2). The second key of computation is the determination of the venous function, used for the CBV calculation. Here, the ROI must provide the highest peak value, with a regular curve shape. The vertical portion of the superior longitudinal sinus best fits these conditions. Careful attention should be paid to avoid any

partial volume effect with close calvarian or intra-sinusal septations (see Figure 1-2). Partial volume effect on the venous output function is a major source of error in the calculation of CBV and thus CBF. The use of a small ROI in the vertical portion of the superior longitudinal sinus, looking to the highest peak value, will guarantee correct CBV values. For selection of input and output function, it is interesting to note that, in a same vessel, the size of ROI can influence curve appearance, which delineates principally the subtle but real partial volume effect between two "apparently equivalent" pixels (see Figure 1-2).

Computed Tomography Angiography of Neck Vessels and the Circle of Willis

After the second perfusion acquisition and another delay of 3 minutes, we proceed with the CTA from the aortic arch to the circle of Willis. Acquisition starts after a third and final injection of 50 ml iohexol, with precise timing established by the previous perfusion sequence and injection rate at 5 ml/s. The technical parameters of the acquisition are 120 kVp and 430 mA, with a 1.25 mm nominal detector collimation, and a pitch of 1.75. Reconstructed slices of 1.25 mm every 1 mm are achieved, and radiologist-computed maximum intensity projection (MIP) or three-dimensional (3-D) rendering images are subsequently obtained.

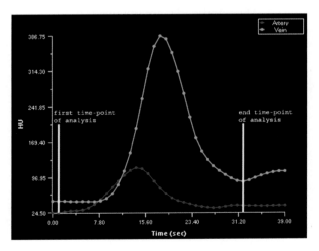

Fig. 1-2 Selection of the arterial and venous functions for perfusion processing. Arterial and venous reference pixels should be selected to produce ample, smooth, and regular enhancement curves. In particular, venous curve should have the maximal amplitude to avoid overestimation of rCBV. The interval of analysis should be chosen from its beginning at the first point before arterial enhancement. It should be chosen to its end when the venous curve has returned to baseline values.

PERFUSION MULTISLICE COMPUTED TOMOGRAPHY

A Powerful Tool for Studying Parenchyma Viability

Despite more than 20 years of theoretical description, perfusion MSCT's accession into clinical use was possible only with the development of multi-array CT detectors and their great rapidity in slice acquisition.[31-36] Moreover, MSCT allows us to cover more than one slice in a stationary acquisition.

After an iodinated contrast media injection, enhancement of both cerebral vessels and brain parenchyma is obtained. The latter is a misleading notion, because iodinated contrast medium is supposed to stay completely intravascular, at least at the first pass. The theoretical model that provides the best predictions for our injection rates and the most robust results, relating to its few basic assumptions (no extract at first pass being the main one), is based on the central volume principle.[37] It considers each regional capillary network as an isolated unit with one arterial input and one venous output. Also, every vascular fraction of contrast entering in one unit is ultimately supposed to leave it. MSCT permits one to consider every pixel of parenchyma as such a unit, with a customized enhancement curve for each one. Because the curve enhancement of a unit ($C_u(t)$) can be described as the convolution product of the time-concentration curve in the entry of the system (or the arterial input function chosen as reference = $C_a(t)$) by an impulse function ($h(t)$):

$$C_u(t) = C_a(t) \otimes h(t) = \int_{s=0}^{t} C_a(t-s)*h(s)*ds$$

Reverse operation, or deconvolution, allows us to extract the impulse function $h(t)$ if $C_u(t)$ and $C_a(t)$ are known, which can be done precisely with a stationary scan of a brain area. This deconvolution operation can be computed by a parametric or non-parametric pathway. Because non-parametrical processes do not require, in contrast to many other mathematical processes of this type, additions of hypothesis (e.g., structure of the isolated unit), it showed better and stronger results than other approaches.[38] Next, we use the least-mean square method to perform the deconvolution instead of singular value decomposition; the latter is the preferred approach for MR perfusion algorithms, but it is more complex and therefore more difficult to implement here and provides no particular benefit.[39,40]

Finally, since the central volume model does not take account of contrast media recirculation possibilities, we need to correct the time-concentration curves through a gamma-variate fitting.

In a second step, mean transit time *(MTT)* is deduced by an integration of impulse function:

$$MTT = \int_{t=0}^{\infty} h(t)*t*dt$$

MTT represents the mean time needed for a unitary contrast bolus to cross the capillary network.

The last step consists of *rCBV* calculation. An iodinated contrast medium is strictly limited at the vascular compartment in healthy parenchyma. Apparent enhancement of parenchyma is, in fact, due to a partial volume effect with the capillary contained in it.[41-44] Therefore, vascular volume in parenchyma can be deduced from a comparison between a parenchymal enhancement curve and another one of an exclusive vascular volume; the latter is believed to be devoid of partial volume effect. The sole vascular segment fulfilling these properties, assuming that it has to be reproductively and easily selected by an operator, is the superior sagittal sinus.

The equation is rather simple:

$$rCBV = \frac{\int_{a}^{b} C_u(t)dt}{\int_{a}^{b} C_v(t)dt}$$

where the numerator represents the area under the parenchymal enhancement curve, and the denominator represents the area under the superior sagittal sinus enhancement curve ($C_v(t)$). Nevertheless, a correction must be provided in regards to the difference between capillary and venous sinus hematocrit, since vascular distribution of contrast media is purely limited to plasma fraction, which differs from a ratio approaching 0.85 between the first and the second.[45,46] A second correction has been described in cases of contrast extravascular leaking, but it has no real interest in routine practice of acute stroke, because blood-brain barrier disruption is a later phenomenon.[47]

After *MTT* and *rCBV* are obtained, *rCBF* simply follows as:

$$rCBF = \frac{rCBV}{MIT}$$

rCBF data achieved with perfusion CT analysis were demonstrated to strongly correlate with results obtained from microsphere methods and stable xenon-CT calculation, which are standards of reference. However, this *rCBV* estimate approach, using the partial averaging effect, has the consequence of overestimating *rCBV* for parenchymal pixels situated near arterial vessels.[37,48] Because absolute CBV and CBF values can vary in healthy people with technical conditions[49] and usually decrease with the age of patients,[50] we compare CBF values of the two hemispheres. The ill hemisphere is established by clinical examination. The global ischemic area is defined by all the pixels showing more than 34% decrease in rCBF compared with the contralateral homologus one, considered to be healthy. In this ischemic area, infarct tissue coexists with penumbra. The definition of penumbra, which is described as the viable parenchyma that is destined for death if no reperfusion occurs, allows us to retrospectively determine it with DWI imaging. Effectively, if no thrombolytic therapy or spontaneous reperfusion is realized, delayed DWI imaging will show an abnormal signal in all the initially ischemic area, entirely turned into infarct. So, we choose an empiric 34% decrease threshold because the map of ischemic area created with it best matched the final area infarct obtained with DWI imaging (in the same patient, of course). The other method of characterizing penumbra (i.e. the loss of electrophysiological capabilities) is far more abstract for clinical use.

Inside the ischemic area, we discriminate penumbra from infarct by an *rCBV* threshold of 2.5 ml/100 g/min. When cerebral perfusion pressure (CPP) drops, vasodilation of the vessels of the affected area is one mechanism that can be used to autoregulate cerebral blood flow. Nevertheless, when CPP is too weak and provokes cellular death, parenchyma involved loses vasodilatation regulation.[51] *rCBV* is the reflection of this vasodilation process, and the threshold we use has been confirmed as a good limit for detecting high-risk infarct regions[11, 52-55] (Table 1-2).

Interpretation of all data is discussed in Table 1-3, and normal perfusion maps are seen in Figure 1-3.

Perfusion Computed Tomography versus Native Head Computed Tomography

Native head CT is used as the first investigational step for strokes in most hospitals. However, the four "classical" native head CT signs in ischemic stroke (focal brain swelling, localized hypodensity, obscuration of the basal ganglia, and hyperdensity of the middle cerebral artery [MCA]) are frequently absent in up to 50% of cases in the first 6 hours after the stroke onset.[22] These limitations in early detection are a major drawback, because crucial decisions about therapy have to be made before this time. Among these limitations, native CT scans cannot give us any information about the severity of ischemia, nor can they then discriminate penumbra from infarct. Finally, native head CT offers very little information about thrombolysis prognosis. Rather, it only indicates that hypoattenuating areas greater than one third of the MCA territory are at a higher risk of hemorrhage, whereas small hypodensities seem to lead to a better outcome with regards to native CT with no visible alteration.[56] On the other hand, perfusion CT detects ischemia as rapidly as MRI (because perfusion-weighted image [PWI] uses the same basic principles) a few minutes after onset.[54,57]

Perfusion Computed Tomography versus PWI/DWI MR

On MRI, determination of penumbra has been commonly accepted as the mismatch between PWI and diffusion-weighted image (DWI) abnormalities, with the latter believed to be irreversible infarct parenchyma.[58-62] However, examples of recovering parenchyma with DWI alteration exist, and studies have confirmed this.[63] Also, most peripheral zones of PWI abnormalities seem to have a mild reduced

Table 1-2 CBF/CBV Ratios Cut off for Differentiation of Ischemia Level in Acute Stroke Perfusion CT

	No ischemia	Penumbra	Infarct
Ratio ill/healthy contralateral homologous areas	rCBF > 66%	rCBF < 66% rCBV > 2.5 ml/100 g	rCBF < 66% rCBV < 2.5 ml/100 g

Table 1-3 Alterations of rMTT, rCBV, and rCBF in Cases of Ischemia (Comparison with Contralateral Homologous Region)

	rMTT	rCBV	rCBF
Healthy parenchyma	=	=	=
Penumbra	↑	↑	↓
Infarct	↑	↓	↓

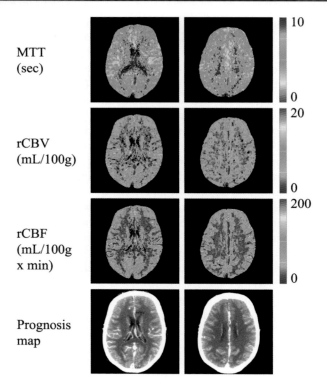

MTT (sec)

rCBV (mL/100g)

rCBF (mL/100g x min)

Prognosis map

10

0

20

0

200

0

Fig. 1-3 **Normal perfusion maps.** Mean transit time *(MTT)*, regional cerebral blood volume *(rCBV)*, regional cerebral blood flow *(rCBF)*, and prognostic map obtained in a patient without stroke. We see symmetrical values of MTT, rCBV, rCBF, and, of course, a perfusion-computed map without penumbra or infarct. In healthy people, mean CBF values are above 50 ml/100 g/min) with a gray/white matter ratio between 2 and 3. This ratio is, up to now, not well demonstrated by perfusion CT values. Moreover, because normal values of CBF are variable among individuals and cerebral activity, interpretation of MTT, CBV, CBF, and prognosis are accomplished by comparing homologous contralateral areas. For the creation of a prognosis map, a decrease of more than 34% CBF values, compared with contralateral hemisphere, determines ischemia. CBV values of more than 2.5 ml/100 g/min indicate penumbra. CBV values of less than 2.5 ml/100 g/min indicate infarct.

flow with no compromised survival.[64,65] These facts are evidence that infarct and penumbra patterns on MRI are not as simple as previously thought.

In addition, perfusion CT is able to describe, as precisely as MRI, infarct parenchyma determined on DWI-MR sequences by a quantitative evaluation of simultaneous decreasing *rCBF* and *rCBV* values (Figure 1-4). Equivalent characterization of penumbra is performed when *rCBF* drops and *rCBV* rises (Figure 1-4), with the best correlation being obtained with MR *MTT* abnormality.[66,67]

At this time, perfusion CT brain coverage is incomplete because of the limited size of the detector. Nevertheless, several approaches, including modifying the sampling rate of enhancement, are explored to compensate for this weak point.[68] We will see later that CTA sometimes can be used in a way that surpasses this aspect.

MSCT Emergency Supremacy

Numerous pathologic characterizations can be made by a CT scanner. These include almost every life-threatening emergency (e.g., pulmonary embolism, aortic dissection or rupture, acute abdomen), all types of trauma, weapons injuries, and certain stages of strokes. In the particular case of early ischemic stroke, DWI-PWI MR has been shown to provide better detection results than native CT and is actually a neuroimaging reference.[69] Also, for acute spine compression, which is harmful although rarely life threatening, tomodensitometry gives poor diagnostic results and MRI will absolutely be needed. On the other hand, MR is markedly unable to detect pulmonary embolisms and air in the peritoneum and would be inconvenient for global screening in bone fractures. In addition, anamnesis for MRI safety (e.g., old pacemakers, ear implants) can be problematic when patients are aphasic or unconscious, whereas no such limits exist for a CT scanner, except possibly with pregnant patients. Organization of reanimation support is also far easier when no MRI investigations are required. All theses facts compromised MRI examination, and recent studies show that more than 90% of ischemic stroke patients are eligible for CT whereas less than 60% are eligible for MRI.[70] MRI access is also restrained in contrast to CT scanners, which are much more common and are even found at small medical facilities.

The use of perfusion CT for the acute management of ischemic stroke instead of DWI-PWI MR may allow CT to cover nearly all emergency pathological conditions and is the unique investment needed for it. Only acute spine compression could be transferred, which is uncommon (Table 1-4).

Since we know that *time is brain*, rapidity must be considered as a key point for the management of patients who have suffered an acute ischemic stroke. In our institution, our complete dedicated protocol, including patient positioning and removal of the CT table, lasts on average less than 20 minutes, whereas a specific perfusion procedure

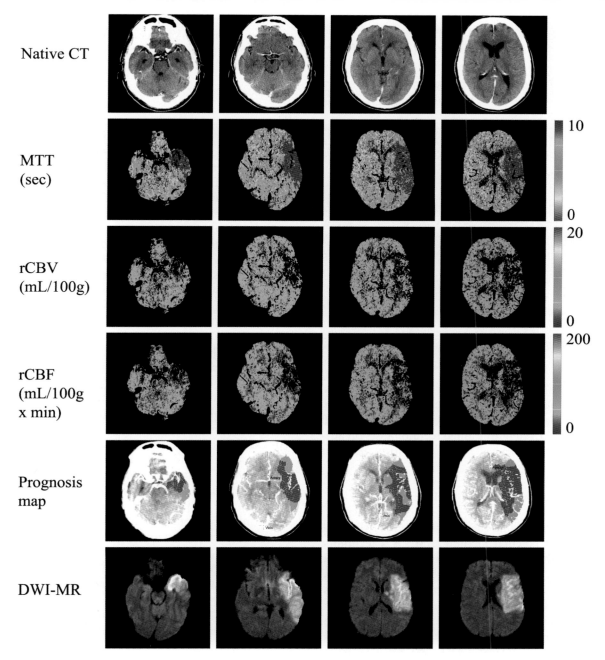

Fig. 1-4 Demonstration of infarction by perfusion CT in early stroke. A 70-year-old patient hospitalized 2 hours after developing acute right hemiplegia and hypoesthesia, fluent aphasia, and right hemianopsia. On the initial native head CT, performed immediately after the patient's arrival, no signs of ischemia are detectable with native acquisition (first line). On the contrary, perfusion CT protocol shows extended ischemia on nearly all of the left MCA territory, with a great proportion of supposed infarct (*red*, fifth line) in comparison with penumbra (*green*, fifth line). In areas with prolonged MTT (second line) and reduced rCBF (fourth line), these two patterns are differentiated by the rCBV value, which increases during the autoregulation blood-flow process, when parenchyma is still viable (penumbra) until neuronal death (infarcts) stops it and provokes a dramatic decrease of rCBV. Nevertheless, thrombolysis was attempted 2 hours and 45 minutes after the onset of symptoms. As we anticipated with perfusion CT results, there was a very slight recuperation. Delayed DWI-MR confirmed a large infarct area in the left MCA territory (sixth line).

Table 1-4 Modality Approach in Major Emergencies Needing Imagery

Indicative frequencies of suspicion in our general hospital	MRI	MSCT scanner
++		Body trauma
++		Acute abdomen
++		Pulmonary embolism
+		Weapon injury
+−		Aortic pathology
+++		Head trauma
−	Acute spine compression	
+−		Intracranial aneurysm research
++		Intracranial bleeding
++		Acute ischemic stroke →→?

lasts only about 9 minutes for the two sequences. This is comparable with other groups, who can reach an acquisition velocity up to less than 10 minutes.[71,72] Even with trained technologists on adequate MR sequences, such "performance" is unbeatable at this time.

Semi-Quantitative Aspect of PWI

Two perfusion techniques are used with MRI. The arterial spin labeling method (ASL) is a technique using presaturated and electromagnetically inverted extracranial protons. They interact with extravascular brain water and alter its magnetic properties. These properties are proportional to perfusion.[73] The second technique relies on the same theoretical baseline as perfusion CT and is called *dynamic susceptibility contrast (DSC)*. DSC imaging is based on the principle that a paramagnetic contrast medium has to decrease relaxation in areas adjacent to it. Perturbations are proportional to perfusion.[74-76]

However, the DSC method rests on a reliable MR arterial input function (AIF), which at this time is frequently not the case. Lots of unquantifiable variables, such as the amount of contrast entering and leaving a given region with regards to time, prevent its determination, and MR-PWI imaging still provides only relative MTT, CBV, and CBF values. Even with recent efforts to suppress artifacts created

by the arterial tissue delay enhancement, in the most commonly used SVD-deconvolution method, the problem is not entirely resolved.[39]

Clinical Implications

The decision to use therapeutic thrombolysis still depends on time windows, without concern for multiple and various evolutions of ischemia in every ill patient. Only a few imagery data are widely used to infer this protocol: intracranial bleeding, impairment of more than a third of MCA territory, or evidence of another underlying pathological condition, such as neoplasm.

Several studies demonstrate the efficacy of early thrombolysis on clinical improvement.[5,77-80] Others correlate theses neurological recoveries with the salvation of penumbra parenchyma.[81,82]

The goal then is to determine penumbra in a rapid, efficient, reliable, and broadly accessible way. We explained previously that perfusion CT was as good as MRI for precise determination of the ischemic area. In addition, maps of ischemic parenchyma obtained with perfusion CT correlate with the National Institute of Neurological Disorders and Stroke (NIHSS) score on patient admission, which definitely confirms this technique's reliability. An example of successful thrombolysis realized to a patient with extended penumbra demonstrated by perfusion CT is given in Figure 1-5.

The Lausanne Stroke Index (LSI) was defined as the quotient of penumbra area by total ischemic area (infarct + penumbra). Because the LSI is significantly correlated with NIHSS score improvement in cases of arterial recanalization, it has a good potential recuperation ratio (PRR) and allows the establishment of a prognosis if reperfusion occurs.[66] According to this type of index, the arbitrary time window used today could be adapted to each individual patient to provide the best treatment.

CT ANGIOGRAPHY OF NECK VESSELS AND THE CIRCLE OF WILLIS

State-of-the-Art CTA in Acute Stroke Imaging Protocols

Although it is not widely used for the evaluation of acute ischemic stroke, CTA provides critical data

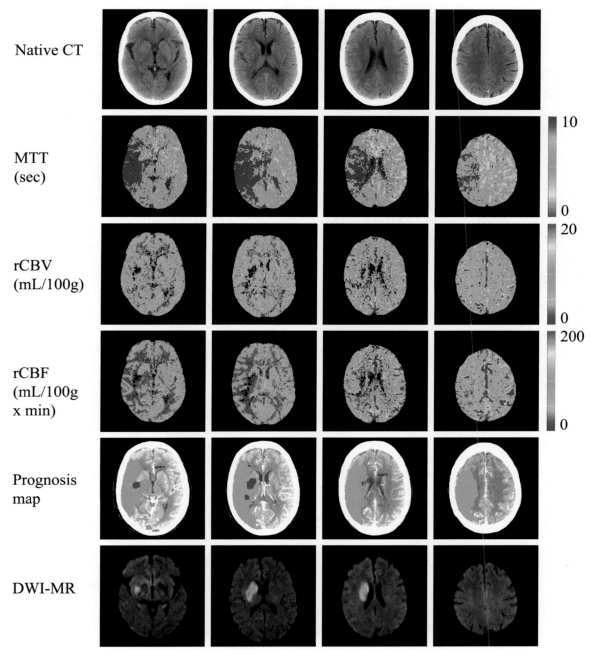

Native CT

MTT
(sec)

10

0

rCBV
(mL/100g)

20

0

rCBF
(mL/100g
x min)

200

0

Prognosis
map

DWI-MR

Fig. 1-5 Salvation of penumbra after thrombolysis. A 68-year-old patient hospitalized 4 hours and 30 minutes after developing acute left hemiplegia and hypoesthesia, dysarthry, and left hemianopsia, left heminegligence. As seen in the preceding patient, no signs of ischemia are present on the initial head-CT native sequences (first line). However, perfusion CT demonstrates rising of MTT and fall of rCBF in right MCA territory, attesting large ischemia, with extended penumbra *(green)* and infarct *(red)* localized in lenticulostriate area (fifth line). Contrast in rCBV values in ischemic parenchyma is particularly well emphasized with pronounced elevation in superficial left MCA territory instead of sinking in deep one. Thrombolysis was performed at 5 hours and 15 minutes after the onset of symptoms. A large amount of threatened parenchyma was rescued, as we can see in the delayed DWI-MR, where the only deep lesion as previously shown by perfusion CT still persists. Dysarthry, hemianopsy, and heminegligence recovered, but severe left hemisyndrome persisted because of corticospinal tractus lesions.

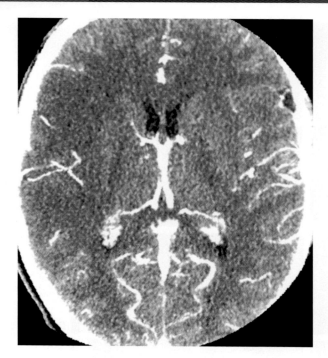

Fig. 1-6 MIP reconstruction of CTA source image. Enhancement and vessel quantity of insular right parenchyma is markedly reduced when compared with heterolateral hemisphere. This method can be another clue in detecting hypoperfused parenchyma.

for its management. Besides the evaluation of immediate and delayed prognosis, a knowledge of thrombus localization or morphology and the extent/type of intracranial or extracranial cerebrovascular disease is needed when a thrombolytic therapy is planned.[83] Such information can also be obtained by MR angiography (MRA) or conventional angiography, but the noninvasive aspects and rapidity of acquisition associated with MSCT make it very competitive.

We must indicate that some centers use CTA in a slightly different way for determining infarct and penumbra. When hypoperfusion area is defined by the extension of CBV and CBF abnormalities, the infarct core is distinguished by the region of unenhanced brain tissue in the CTA source image covering it.[70] An example of this use is given in Figure 1-6.

With perfusion CT, CTA provides MSCT with a complete solution for acute ischemic stroke imaging.

Technical Aspects of CTA Data Analysis

The actual performance of image postprocessing is made possible with multi-slice helicoïdal CT. Effec-

tively, helicoïdal techniques are needed for high isotropic resolution, when maximum speed provided by multislice conformation allows acquisition in the arterial phase contrast of all the vessels explored.

We analyze images from acquisition in two different ways. First, axial study of slices allows us to determine focal anomalies in vessels, which have a common pattern, like atheromatosis, calcifications, or enhancement interruption in arterial trunks. However, patterns can be difficult to specify without another point of view, so we process a second analysis with 3-D (or assimilated) applications. Arterial tortuosity and global vascular anatomy benefit from an MIP reconstruction, which permits multiplanar reconstruction with thickness modulation to view vessels (Figure 1-7, B-C [normal vascular anatomy]). On the opposite scale, density of very small vessels cannot be appreciated correctly in the axial mode, whereas MIP has great sensitivity for this and is used in such cases (Figure 1-7, A [detection of occlusion by MIP]).

Multiple vasculitis lesions, like successions of widening and stenoses, can be missed in the axial view if they are small or distant from each other, but they are easier to associate with a complete one-screen view of the vessel. This could be accomplished with MIP. The best, but more time-consuming, approach is volume rendering (VR) reconstruction. We usually only perform VR when studying vessels where MIP cannot correctly suffice without fastidious manipulations of osseous structures. Vertebrobasilar segments particularly benefit from this tool, since they are nearly always close to the skull. Even though VR is the most powerful tool for studying 3-D aspects of vascular structures, source image analysis is still needed because of potential information loss with 3-D imaging.[84]

Use of CT Angiography

At this time, angioplasty is generally performed when intracranial stenoses are symptomatic or when maximal medical treatment has been conducted without the expected results. Examples include the persistence of transient ischemic attack or an ischemic stroke event under anticoagulant/anti-aggregant molecules.[85] However, associated lesions discovered with CTA performed during stroke management could help with planning for preventive interventional acts in patients at risk for recurrence in other cerebrovascular sites.

Intracranial vascular anatomy, combined with the location of arterial occlusion, determines to a

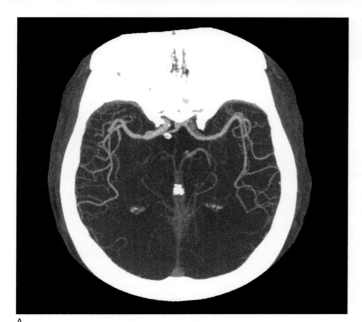

A

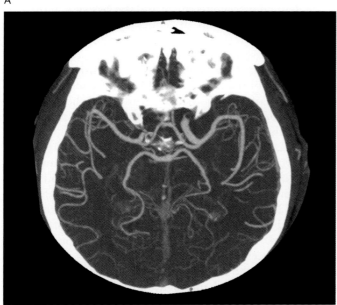

B

Fig. 1-7 MSCT MIP imaging of the circle of Willis and basilar circulation in a pathologic case and a normal one. MIP images (A) obtained with MSCT CTA show occlusion of the right posterior cerebral artery. On another patient normal features of the circle of Willis and basilar circulation in (B) and (C) can be seen.

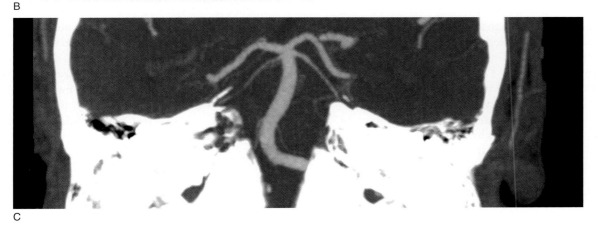

C

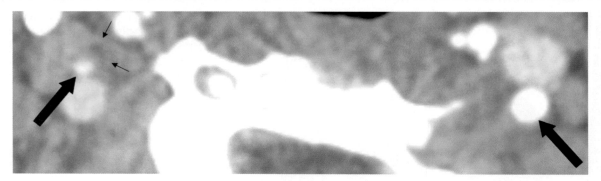

Fig. 1-8 Example of internal carotid artery dissection. This flamelike sign could be inconsistent and difference with thrombus difficult on MIP reconstructions. Analysis of axial slices is still necessary. Narrowed lumen in a right internal carotid artery dissection *(large arrows)*. The residual lumen is eccentric, with slight visible enhancement of the original wall vessel *(small arrows)*.

tremendous degree the outcome of an embolic event and the result of an emergency treatment. The initial CT angiography can help the clinician determine the chance of success and the length of time available for therapy. Indeed, some ischemic lesions may need therapy within minutes, whereas others can wait many hours or days. It is well known that the status of the lenticulostriate perforators determines the outcome and length of time for rescue[86,87] before therapy will no longer be effective and at which point it may become dangerous. This explains why it is of paramount importance to know the location of the occlusion, justifying the use of CT angiography when dealing with acute stroke. In the occlusion of the origin of the internal carotid artery (ICA), clinical symptoms are caused mainly by an embolus to the intracranial circulation from the stagnant ICA. If there is no intracranial embolic migration, the status of the circle of Willis will determine the clinical symptoms. In this case, the threatened watershed area is usually Wernicke's area with sensory and motor cortex. The time for rescue can be prolonged as long as no deep perforators are occluded, and therapy usually is not necessary if there is no intracranial embolus. The prognosis is usually good, depending on the ongoing emboli.[88] In the occlusion of the ICA bifurcation, the so-called T lesion, the thrombus extends from the ICA into the MCA and anterior cerebral artery (ACA). This type of occlusion has been shown to carry the worst prognosis among all types of carotid occlusions.[89,90] Indeed, this pattern of occlusion on one side can directly interrupt the supply to the lenticulostriate arteries; on the other side it usually interrupts the ICA supply to the ACA, which constitutes the primary source of collateral circulation to the MCA territory through the pial collaterals. The time for rescue in this case is limited, and the prognosis is usually poor and

totally dependent on the pial collateral supply. In the occlusion of the M1 segment of the MCA, all or part of the lenticulostriate arteries may be occluded. This type of occlusion has two main implications: the lack of collateralization in the lenticulostriate territory and the risk of hemorrhage from reperfusion of lenticulostriates after a relatively short period. Thus the time allowed for rescue is very short, and the prognosis is poor because of the limited time to reestablish perfusion in the territory of the perforators. One of the more common types of embolic occlusion involves the M1 bifurcation of the MCA; no lenticulostriate arteries are occluded (except those that rarely arise from the M2 segment), and the most threatened area is the proximal M2 territory. The prognosis of an occlusion of the M1 bifurcation can be good if the amount of retrograde pial collateral supply to distal M2 is intact. The analysis of the collaterals in the watershed area can be done with the use of the CTA axial raw images, by evaluating the contrast enhancement of the arterial branches located distally to the embolic occlusion. In an MCA stroke, the arterial enhancement of the branches located in the sylvian fissure is compared with the distal cortical branches in the same territory.[91]

Another important point that can be evaluated by CTA during emergency imaging of an acute stroke is the presence of an ICA dissection (Figure 1-8).

The occlusion of a dissected vessel produces a cerebral infarction of embolic origin in more than 50% of cases and is accompanied by infarction more often than other vessel wall abnormalities. Moreover, the therapeutic management is very controversial concerning the use of thrombolysis and thus differs from the protocol used in atherosclerotic occlusions. The possibility of an intracranial dissection causing subarachnoid hemorrhage in more than 20% of patients[92] should be kept in mind when reading a CTA suspected of dissection. By using the axial raw images, it is often possible to recognize the double lumen aspect of the ICA or vertebral artery, characterized by the crescent shape of the ICA-enhanced lumen. The embolic event can also be related to a chronic course of spontaneous dissection of the ICA with a stenosis or a cervical aneurysm.[93] CTA can disclose high-risk situations such as thrombus inside the dissecting aneurysm, which could be the origin of an acute embolic stroke, or the combination of a tight stenosis associated with a poor intracranial collateral supply, which could increase the risk of a hemodynamic stroke. Moreover, CTA could be very helpful in the choice of treatment for these specific chronic cervical ICA dissections, such as maximal antithrombotic treatment or a carotid stenting to enlarge the diameter of the ICA and to protect against clot migration from the sac.[94]

CTA should always be performed during the investigation of the earliest crucial stages of an ischemic insult when decisions regarding thrombolytic therapy are made. Indeed, Nabavi et al[95] developed the Multimodal Stroke Assessment Using CT (MOSAIC), a score system based on multidetector row CT technology that takes into account the three main CT modalities (noncontrast CT, CTA, and perfusion CT) to predict infarction size in emergency settings, as well as the clinical outcome in hyperacute stroke. The actual CT protocols offer new insights into the pathophysiology of acute ischemic stroke. CT is used not only as an exclusion criterion for thrombolysis, but also provides individual inclusion and exclusion criteria based on tissue physiology. CT in this setting has become very helpful in selecting patients who are eligible for thrombolysis. It is possible to predict whether a particular occlusion can be successfully revascularized, the individual patient prognosis, the outcome after revascularization, and, in particular, the development of intracranial hemorrhage after treatment, which reflects reperfusion of necrotic tissue. At our institution, thrombolysis is considered when perfusion CT indicates that the infarct size is not more than 30% of the total surface of the MCA territory. In the time interval between 0 to 3 hours from the onset of symptoms, an intravenous systemic thrombolysis is performed, whereas in the time interval between 3 to 6 hours the possibility of an intraarterial (IA) local thrombolysis is considered. IA thrombolysis has been used most successfully in patients with acute MCA occlusion. Other potential indications to IA thrombolysis include patients with extracranial ICA occlusion, intracra-

nial ICA "T occlusion," or basilar artery occlusion.[96] If an IA thrombolysis is considered, CTA can depict, in addition to the vascular lesion, concomitant pathologies, such as tandem stenosis, anatomic variations, and even significant aortic arch disease. This helps the interventional neuroradiologist in the selection of the proper strategy of angiographic material choice and microcatheter navigation.

At this point, exclusion criteria for thrombolysis need to be reemphasized[96]:
1. Any type of intracranial hemorrhage.
2. A significant mass effect with a midline shift related to a large infarct.
3. Acute hypodense parenchymal lesion or effacement of the cerebral sulci in more than one third of the MCA territory or suspected stroke region.
4. Intracranial tumor (except a small incidental meningioma).
5. Suspected carotid arterial dissection.
6. Any nonatherosclerotic arteriopathy (e.g., vasculitis)
7. The presence of an intracranial aneurysm.

IA thrombolysis provides an alternative to IV thrombolysis in selected patients with acute ischemic stroke. There is no clear rationale for IV versus IA fibrinolytic therapy, and the choice of the modality is already debated. Indeed, when we compare the main studies, which evaluated the use of IV recombinant tissue plasminogen activator (r-tPA) for acute stroke (the National Institute of Neurological Disorders and Stroke [NINDS],[5] the European Cooperative Acute Stroke Study [ECASS I and II],[78,80] and the Alteplase Thrombolysis for Acute Noninterventional Therapy [ATLANTIS][97]) with the IA trials (the Prolyse in Acute Cerebral Thromboembolism Trial [PROACT I[77] and II][79] and the Emergency Management of Stroke EMS Bridging Trial[98]), it appears that no clear guidelines are actually defined. The real limitation of IA local thrombolysis consists of the additional time required to begin treatment compared with peripheral IV thrombolysis. In summary, CTA in association with perfusion CT can yield crucial information concerning the site of arterial occlusion, the capacity of the collaterals of the circle of Willis and of the leptomeningeal territory, the differentiation between atherosclerotic thromboembolism and arterial dissection, and the associated lesions that can modify the indications for thrombolysis, such as intracranial aneurysm. CTA is a useful tool for helping in the selection of the modality and type of treatment for an acute stroke. Moreover, the anatomical vascular depiction allows the planning of successive interventional procedures, such as carotid or vertebral stent angioplasties.

CONCLUSION

With its poor sensitivity in the first hours following acute stroke, the time of the isolated use of isolated native head CT is past in the management of acute ischemic stroke.

The advent of the helicoïdal principle and multi-array development make it possible for CT to compete with MRI.

Between the two emerging techniques in acute stroke imaging, DWI-PWI MR and perfusion CT, the latter seems able to efficiently provide the most important clinical information, which is the size of the penumbra to be saved.

Based on CBF, CBV, and MTT interpretation, the distinction between infarct core and penumbra is reliable. Additional preliminary results suggest that acute ischemic stroke thrombolysis patient selection with perfusion CT would show equivalent clinical outcomes as patient selection completed by DWI-PWI MR. This should be the final step for definitively validating perfusion CT.

In addition, feasibility with perfusion CT is higher than that with MR, and the procedure costs are minimal in terms of the amount of time for patient management. Also, the current limitation in terms of brain coverage soon will be overcome by the newest technologies, such as plane detectors.

When we add the capabilities of CTA in terms of thrombolytic therapy, MSCT seems the most appropriate choice for acute stroke imaging, because it provides the most data and gives clinicians the best options for making therapeutic decisions. No more other time-consuming or invasive investigations are needed, and access to MSCT is easy in most institutions.

Acknowledgments

We sincerely thank Mr. Micah Murray for his help in editing this manuscript.

REFERENCES

1. World Health Organization: The world health report 2003, Geneva, WHO, 2003.
2. Caro JJ, Huybrechts KF: Stroke treatment economic model (STEM): predicting long-term costs from functional status, *Stroke* 30:2574-2579, 1999.
3. American Heart Association: Heart Disease and Stroke Statistics, 2004 Update, 2004.
4. Feigin VL, Lawes CM, Bennett DA, et al: Stroke epidemiology: a review of population-based studies of incidence, prevalence, and case-fatality in the late 20th century, *Lancet Neurol* 2:43-53, 2003.
5. National Institute of Neurological Disorders and Stroke rt-PA Stroke Study Group: Tissue plasminogen activator for acute ischemic stroke, *N Engl J Med* 333:1581-1587, 1995.
6. Adams HP Jr., Bendixen BH, Kappelle LJ, et al: Classification of subtype of acute ischemic stroke. Definitions for use in a multicenter clinical trial. TOAST. Trial of Org 10172 in Acute Stroke Treatment, *Stroke* 24:35-41, 1993.
7. Petty GW, Brown RD Jr., Whisnant JP, et al: Ischemic stroke subtypes: a population-based study of incidence and risk factors, *Stroke* 30:2513-2516, 1999.
8. Kolominsky-Rabas PL, Weber M, Gefeller O, et al: Epidemiology of ischemic stroke subtypes according to TOAST criteria: incidence, recurrence, and long-term survival in ischemic stroke subtypes: a population-based study, *Stroke* 32:2735-2740, 2001.
9. Nehlig A. Metabolism of the central nervous system. In Mraovitch S, editor. *Neurophysiological basis of cerebral blood flow control: an introduction*, London, 1996, John Libby, pp 177-196.
10. Lassen N: Cerebral blood flow and oxygen consumption in man, *Physiol Revue* 39:183-238, 1959.
11. Harper AM: Autoregulation of cerebral blood flow: influence of the arterial blood pressure on the blood flow through the cerebral cortex, *J Neurol Neurosurg Psychiatry* 29:398-403, 1966.
12. Astrup J, Siesjo BK, Symon L: Thresholds in cerebral ischemia—the ischemic penumbra, *Stroke* 12:723-725, 1981.
13. Hossmann KA: Viability thresholds and the penumbra of focal ischemia, *Ann Neurol* 36:557-565, 1994.
14. Hakim A, Evans A, Berger L, et al: The effect of nimodipine on the evolution of human cerebral infarction studied by PET, *J Cereb Blood Flow Metab* 9:523-534, 1989.
15. Heiss W, Rosner G: Functional recovery of cortical neurons as related to degree and duration of ischemia, *Ann Neurol* 14:294-301, 1983.
16. Baron JC, Rougemont D, Soussaline F, et al: Local interrelationships of cerebral oxygen consumption and glucose utilization in normal subjects and in ischemic stroke patients: a positron tomography study, *J Cereb Blood Flow Metab* 4:140-149, 1984.
17. Powers WJ, Grubb RL Jr, Darriet D, et al: Cerebral blood flow and cerebral metabolic rate of oxygen requirements for cerebral function and viability in humans, *J Cereb Blood Flow Metab* 5:600-608, 1985.
18. Heiss WD, Kracht L, Grond M, et al: Early [(11)C]Flumazenil/H(2)O positron emission tomography predicts irreversible ischemic cortical damage in stroke patients receiving acute thrombolytic therapy, *Stroke* 31:366-369, 2000.
19. Siesjo BK: Pathophysiology and treatment of focal cerebral ischemia. II. Mechanisms of damage and treatment, *J Neurosurg* 77:337-354, 1992.
20. Siesjo BK: Pathophysiology and treatment of focal cerebral ischemia. I. Pathophysiology, *J Neurosurg* 77:169-184, 1992.
21. Harris RJ, Symon L, Branston NM, et al: Changes in extracellular calcium activity in cerebral ischaemia, *J Cereb Blood Flow Metab* 1:203-209, 1981.

22. von Kummer R, Holle R, Gizyska U, et al: Interobserver agreement in assessing early CT signs of middle cerebral artery infarction, *AJNR Am J Neuroradiol* 17:1743-1748, 1996.

23. Rother J, Schellinger PD, Gass A, et al: Effect of intravenous thrombolysis on MRI parameters and functional outcome in acute stroke <6 hours, *Stroke* 33:2438-2445, 2002.

24. Baird AE, Benfield A, Schlaug G, et al: Enlargement of human cerebral ischemic lesion volumes measured by diffusion-weighted magnetic resonance imaging, *Ann Neurol* 41:581-589, 1997.

25. Marchal G, Beaudouin V, Rioux P, et al: Prolonged persistence of substantial volumes of potentially viable brain tissue after stroke: a correlative PET-CT study with voxel-based data analysis, *Stroke* 27:599-606, 1996.

26. Levy DE, Brott TG, Haley EC Jr, et al: Factors related to intracranial hematoma formation in patients receiving tissue-type plasminogen activator for acute ischemic stroke, *Stroke* 25:291-297, 1994.

27. Wintermark M, Meuli R: Le scanner de perfusion revisité avec la technologie multibarrette: accès direct à la viabilité du parenchyme cérébral. In Blum A, editor: *Scanographie volumique multicoupe*, Paris, 2002, Masson, pp 203-217.

28. Reiser UJ: Study of bolus geometry after intravenous contrast medium injection: dynamic and quantitative measurements (chronogram) using an X-ray CT device, *J Comput Assist Tomogr* 8:251-262, 1984.

29. Claussen CD, Banzer D, Pfretzschner C, et al: Bolus geometry and dynamics after intravenous contrast medium injection, *Radiology* 153:365-368, 1984.

30. Wintermark M, Maeder P, Verdun FR, et al: Using 80 kVp versus 120 kVp in perfusion CT measurement of regional cerebral blood flow, *AJNR Am J Neuroradiol* 21:1881-1884, 2000.

31. Ladurner G, Zilkha E, Sager WD, et al: Measurement of regional cerebral blood volume using the EMI 1010 scanner, *Br J Radiol* 52:371-374, 1979.

32. Zilkha E, Ladurner G, Iliff LD, et al: Computer subtraction in regional cerebral blood-volume measurements using the EMI-Scanner, *Br J Radiol* 49:330-334, 1976.

33. Ladurner G, Zilkha E, Iliff D, et al: Measurement of regional cerebral blood volume by computerized axial tomography, *J Neurol Neurosurg Psychiatry* 39:152-158, 1976.

34. Axel L: Cerebral blood flow determination by rapid-sequence computed tomography: theoretical analysis, *Radiology* 137:679-686, 1980.

35. Axel L: A method of calculating brain blood flow with a CT dynamic scanner, *Adv Neurol* 30:67-71, 1981.

36. Axel L: Tissue mean transit time from dynamic computed tomography by a simple deconvolution technique, *Invest Radiol* 18:94-99, 1983.

37. Wintermark M, Maeder P, Thiran JP, et al: Quantitative assessment of regional cerebral blood flows by perfusion CT studies at low injection rates: a critical review of the underlying theoretical models, *Eur Radiol* 11:1220-1230, 2001.

38. Ostergaard L, Weisskoff RM, Chesler DA, et al: High resolution measurement of cerebral blood flow using intravascular tracer bolus passages. I. Mathematical approach and statistical analysis, *Magn Reson Med* 36:715-725, 1996.

39. Smith MR, Lu H, Trochet S, et al: Removing the effect of SVD algorithmic artifacts present in quantitative MR perfusion studies, *Magn Reson Med* 51:631-634, 2004.

40. Ostergaard L, Sorensen AG, Kwong KK, et al: High resolution measurement of cerebral blood flow using intravascular tracer bolus passages. II. Experimental comparison and preliminary results, *Magn Reson Med* 36:726-736, 1996.

41. Newhouse JH: Fluid compartment distribution of intravenous iothalamate in the dog, *Invest Radiol* 12:364-367, 1977.

42. Phelps ME, Kuhl DE: Pitfalls in the measurement of cerebral blood volume with computed tomography, *Radiology* 121:375-377, 1976.

43. Gado MH, Phelps ME, Coleman RE: An extravascular component of contrast enhancement in cranial computed tomography. I. The tissue-blood ratio of contrast enhancement, *Radiology* 117:589-593, 1975.

44. Gado MH, Phelps ME, Coleman RE: An extravascular component of contrast enhancement in cranial computed tomography. II. Contrast enhancement and the blood-tissue barrier, *Radiology* 117:595-597, 1975.

45. Sakai F, Nakazawa K, Tazaki Y, et al: Regional cerebral blood volume and hematocrit measured in normal human volunteers by single-photon emission computed tomography, *J Cereb Blood Flow Metab* 5:207-213, 1985.

46. Larsen OA, Lassen NA: Cerebral hematocrit in normal man, *J Appl Physiol* 19:571-574, 1964.

47. St Lawrence KS, Lee TY: An adiabatic approximation to the tissue homogeneity model for water exchange in the brain. I. Theoretical derivation, *J Cereb Blood Flow Metab* 18:1365-1377, 1998.

48. Cenic A, Nabavi DG, Craen RA, et al: Dynamic CT measurement of cerebral blood flow: a validation study, *AJNR Am J Neuroradiol* 20:63-73, 1999.

49. Fiorella D, Heiserman J, Prenger E, et al: Assessment of the reproducibility of postprocessing dynamic CT perfusion data, *AJNR Am J Neuroradiol* 25:97-107, 2004.

50. Leenders KL, Perani D, Lammertsma AA, et al: Cerebral blood flow, blood volume and oxygen utilization. Normal values and effect of age, *Brain* 113(1):27-47, 1990.

51. Markus HS: Cerebral perfusion and stroke, *J Neurol Neurosurg Psychiatry* 75:353-361, 2004.

52. Lee KH, Cho SJ, Byun HS, et al: Triphasic perfusion computed tomography in acute middle cerebral artery stroke: a correlation with angiographic findings, *Arch Neurol* 57:990-999, 2000.

53. Mayer TE, Hamann GF, Baranczyk J, et al: Dynamic CT perfusion imaging of acute stroke, *AJNR Am J Neuroradiol* 21:1441-1449, 2000.

54. Hunter GJ, Hamberg LM, Ponzo JA, et al: Assessment of cerebral perfusion and arterial anatomy in hyperacute stroke with three-dimensional functional CT: early clinical results, *AJNR Am J Neuroradiol* 19:29-37, 1998.

55. Hossmann KA: Neuronal survival and revival during and after cerebral ischemia, *Am J Emerg Med* 1:191-197, 1983.

56. von Kummer R, Allen KL, Holle R, et al: Acute stroke: usefulness of early CT findings before thrombolytic therapy, *Radiology* 205:327-333, 1997.

57. Koenig M, Klotz E, Luka B, et al: Perfusion CT of the brain: diagnostic approach for early detection of ischemic stroke, *Radiology* 209:85-93, 1998.

58. Oppenheim C, Samson Y, Manai R, et al: Prediction of malignant middle cerebral artery infarction by diffusion-weighted imaging, *Stroke* 31:2175-2181, 2000.

59. Lythgoe MF, Thomas DL, Calamante F, et al: Acute changes in MRI diffusion, perfusion, T(1), and T(2) in a rat model of oligemia produced by partial occlusion of the middle cerebral artery, *Magn Reson Med* 44:706-712, 2000.

60. Kluytmans M, van Everdingen KJ, Kappelle LJ, et al: Prognostic value of perfusion- and diffusion-weighted MR imaging in first 3 days of stroke, *Eur Radiol* 10:1434-1441, 2000.

61. Kim JH, Lee SJ, Shin T, et al: Correlative assessment of hemodynamic parameters obtained with T2-weighted perfusion MR imaging and SPECT in symptomatic carotid artery occlusion, *AJNR Am J Neuroradiol* 21:1450-1456, 2000.

62. Gonzalez RG, Schaefer PW, Buonanno FS, et al: Diffusion-weighted MR imaging: diagnostic accuracy in patients imaged within 6 hours of stroke symptom onset, *Radiology* 210:155-162, 1999.

63. Kidwell CS, Saver JL, Mattiello J, et al: Thrombolytic reversal of acute human cerebral ischemic injury shown by diffusion/perfusion magnetic resonance imaging, *Ann Neurol* 47:462-469, 2000.

64. Davis SM, Donnan GA: Advances in penumbra imaging with MR, *Cerebrovasc Dis* 17 (suppl) 3:23-27, 2004.

65. Parsons MW, Yang Q, Barber PA, et al: Perfusion magnetic resonance imaging maps in hyperacute stroke: relative cerebral blood flow most accurately identifies tissue destined to infarct, *Stroke* 32:1581-1587, 2001.

66. Wintermark M, Reichhart M, Thiran JP, et al: Prognostic accuracy of cerebral blood flow measurement by perfusion computed tomography, at the time of emergency room admission, in acute stroke patients, *Ann Neurol* 51:417-432, 2002.

67. Wintermark M, Reichhart M, Cuisenaire O, et al: Comparison of admission perfusion computed tomography and qualitative diffusion- and perfusion-weighted magnetic resonance imaging in acute stroke patients, *Stroke* 33:2025-2031, 2002.

68. Wintermark M, Smith WS, Ko NU, et al: Dynamic perfusion CT: optimizing the temporal resolution and contrast volume for calculation of perfusion CT parameters in stroke patients, *AJNR Am J Neuroradiol* 25:720-729, 2004.

69. Fiebach JB, Schellinger PD, Jansen O, et al: CT and diffusion-weighted MR imaging in randomized order: diffusion-weighted imaging results in higher accuracy and lower interrater variability in the diagnosis of hyperacute ischemic stroke, *Stroke* 33:2206-2210, 2002.

70. Schramm P, Schellinger PD, Klotz E, et al: Comparison of perfusion computed tomography and computed tomography angiography source images with perfusion-weighted imaging and diffusion-weighted imaging in patients with acute stroke of less than 6 hours' duration, *Stroke* 35:1652-1658, 2004.

71. Meuli RA: Imaging viable brain tissue with CT scan during acute stroke, *Cerebrovasc Dis* 17 (suppl) 3:28-34, 2004.

72. Lev MH, Segal AZ, Farkas J, et al: Utility of perfusion-weighted CT imaging in acute middle cerebral artery stroke treated with intra-arterial thrombolysis: prediction of final infarct volume and clinical outcome, *Stroke* 32:2021-2028, 2001.

73. Lia TQ, Guang Chen Z, Ostergaard L, et al: Quantification of cerebral blood flow by bolus tracking and artery spin tagging methods, *Magn Reson Imaging* 18:503-512, 2000.

74. Rother J, Guckel F, Neff W, et al: Assessment of regional cerebral blood volume in acute human stroke by use of single-slice dynamic susceptibility contrast-enhanced magnetic resonance imaging, *Stroke* 27:1088-1093, 1996.

75. Rosen BR, Belliveau JW, Vevea JM, et al: Perfusion imaging with NMR contrast agents, *Magn Reson Med* 14:249-265, 1990.

76. Edelman RR, Mattle HP, Atkinson DJ, et al: Cerebral blood flow: assessment with dynamic contrast-enhanced T2-weighted MR imaging at 1.5 T, *Radiology* 176:211-220, 1990.

77. del Zoppo GJ, Higashida RT, Furlan AJ, et al: PROACT: a phase II randomized trial of recombinant pro-urokinase by direct arterial delivery in acute middle cerebral artery stroke. PROACT investigators. Prolyse in Acute Cerebral Thromboembolism, *Stroke* 29:4-11, 1998.

78. Hacke W, Bluhmki E, Steiner T, et al: Dichotomized efficacy end points and global end-point analysis applied to the ECASS intention-to-treat data set: post hoc analysis of ECASS I, *Stroke* 29:2073-2075, 1998.

79. Furlan A, Higashida R, Wechsler L, et al: Intra-arterial prourokinase for acute ischemic stroke. The PROACT II study: a randomized controlled trial. Prolyse in Acute Cerebral Thromboembolism, *JAMA* 282:2003-2011, 1999.

80. Hacke W, Kaste M, Fieschi C, et al: Randomised double-blind placebo-controlled trial of thrombolytic therapy with intravenous alteplase in acute ischaemic stroke (ECASS II). Second European-Australasian Acute Stroke Study Investigators, *Lancet* 352:1245-1251, 1998.

81. Parsons MW, Barber PA, Chalk J, et al: Diffusion- and perfusion-weighted MRI response to thrombolysis in stroke, *Ann Neurol* 51:28-37, 2002.

82. Klotz E, Konig M: Perfusion measurements of the brain: using dynamic CT for the quantitative assessment of cerebral ischemia in acute stroke, *Eur J Radiol* 30:170-184, 1999.

83. Wildermuth S, Knauth M, Brandt T, et al: Role of CT angiography in patient selection for thrombolytic therapy in acute hemispheric stroke, *Stroke* 29:935-938, 1998.

84. Tomandl BF, Hastreiter P, Iserhardt-Bauer S, et al: Standardized evaluation of CT angiography with remote generation of 3D video sequences for the detection of intracranial aneurysms, *Radiographics* 23:e12, 2003.

85. Schumacher HC, Khaw AV, Meyers PM, et al: Intracranial angioplasty and stent placement for cerebral atherosclerosis, *J Vasc Interv Radiol* 15:S123-132, 2004.

86. Theron J, Coskun O, Huet H, et al: Local intraarterial thrombolysis in the carotid territory, *Interven Neuroradiol* 2:111-126, 1996.

87. Theron J, Courtheoux P, Casasco A, et al: Local intraarterial fibrinolysis in the carotid territory, *AJNR* 10:753-765, 1989.

88. Furlan AJ: Natural history of atherothrombotic occlusion of cerebral arteries: carotid versus vertebrobasilar territories. In Hacke W, editor: *Thrombolytic therapy in acute ischemic stroke*, Heidelberg, 1991, Springer-Verlag.

89. Toni D, Fiorelli M, Gentile M, et al: Progressing neurological deficit secondary to acute ischemic stroke: a study on predictability, pathogenesis, and prognosis, *Arch Neurol* 52:670-675, 1995.

90. Kucinski T, Koch K, Grzyska U, et al: The predictive value of early CT and angiography for fatal hemispheric swelling in acute stroke, *AJNR* 19:839-846, 1998.

91. Knauth M, Kummer RV, Jansen O, et al: Potential of CT angiography in acute ischemic stroke, *AJNR* 18:1001-1010, 1997.

92. Pelkonen O, Tikkakoski T, Pyhtinen J, et al: Cerebral CT and MRI findings in cervicocephalic artery dissection, *Acta Radiol* 45(3):259-265, 2004.

93. Schievink WI: Spontaneous dissection of the carotid and vertebral arteries, *N Engl J Med* 344:898-906, 2001.

94. Binaghi S, Chapot R, Rogopoulos A, et al: Carotid stenting of chronic cervical dissecting aneurysm: a report of two cases, *Neurology* 59:935-937, 2002.

95. Nabavi DG, Kloska SP, Nam EM, et al: MOSAIC: Multimodal stroke assessment using computed tomography. Novel diagnostic approach for the prediction of infarction size and clinical outcome, *Stroke* 33:2819-2826, 2002.

96. Higashida RT, Furlan AJ: Trial design and reporting standards for intra-arterial cerebral thrombolysis for acute ischemic stroke, *Stroke* 34:e109-e137, 2003.

97. Clark WM, Wissman S, Albers GW, et al: Recombinant tissue-type plasminogen activator (alteplase) for ischemic stroke 3 to 5 hours after symptom onset: the ATLANTIS study: a randomized controlled trial: alteplase thrombolysis for acute noninterventional therapy in ischemic stroke, *JAMA* 282:2019-2026, 1999.

98. Lewandowski C, Frankel M, Tomsick T: Combined intravenous and intra-arterial rt-PA versus intra-arterial therapy of acute ischemic stroke: Emergency Management of Stroke (EMS) Bridging Trial, *Stroke* 30:2598-2605, 1999.

CHAPTER 2.

Multislice Computed Tomography of the Head and Neck

Martin G. Mack
Thomas J. Vogl

Imaging of the head and neck has changed completely during the past decade. Computed tomography (CT) and magnetic resonance imaging (MRI) have become more important in head and neck imaging. With the improvement of CT imaging techniques, shorter examination times, thinner sections, and higher resolution are now possible without losing image quality.[1-4] Even CT angiography has a definite place as an add-on modality in head and neck imaging.[5-7]

Mirror examination and endoscopy are the methods of choice in screening for laryngeal and hypopharyngeal tumors. Since the predominant tumor type is squamous cell carcinoma, these mucosal lesions can be directly visualized and biopsied. The limitations of clinical examination combined with laryngoscopy are well described. The purpose is to describe the role of current scan protocols for multislice CT (MSCT) imaging of the head and neck region and to define results and clinical impact. MSCT is extremely helpful in the evaluation of the head and neck, especially if multiplanar reconstructions (MPRs) are used.

Depending on the clinical question, different CT protocols are presented for imaging of the head and neck. The appearance of different pathological findings on imaging studies and how adapted scan protocols help to improve differential diagnosis will be discussed. Particular focus will be put on imaging of the skull base, the nasopharynx, the oropharynx, the hypopharynx, and the larynx.[8,9] A work flow for the differential diagnosis of benign and malignant tumors and malformations as well as variations will be provided.

The role of imaging modalities such as CT and MRI is to assess the infiltration depth and to detect submucosal tumor spread. Pretreatment CT measurement of tumor volume has been reported to permit stratification of patients with laryngeal squamous cell carcinoma treated with definitive radiotherapy into groups in which local control is more likely and less likely. For voice conservation surgery, precise knowledge of tumor extent is crucial. The short examination times, if MSCT is performed, even allow the clinician to use the functional information (e.g., E-phonation during scanning) for optimal diagnostic workup.

This chapter will focus on normal anatomy, benign and malignant tumors, congenital variations and malformations, and the differential diagnosis.

SKULL BASE

MSCT provides better delineation of the bony structures of the skull base and face than conventional radiography. Its superior resolution and absence of superimposed structures offer significant advantages for the evaluation of neoplastic and traumatic lesions, with the result that CT has largely supplanted conventional motion-controlled tomography in the head and neck region. CT is also excellent for demonstrating sites of bone destruction and lymph node enlargement (e.g., malignant lymphomas, metastases). Another advantage of CT is its ability to characterize tissue structures by densitometry. Bony structures have attenuation values as high as 100 Hounsfield units (HU) (metal), whereas water has an attenuation of 0 HU and air is assigned a value of −1000 HU. Thus various soft tissues such as muscle, glands, connective tissue, and tumors have positive attenuation values, whereas fatty tissue has negative attenuation values. By selecting a bone or soft-tissue "window," the examiner can highlight CT image details that are relevant to a particular inquiry.

A routine examination scan protocol is shown in Table 2-1. Studies evaluating for inner ear pathol-

Table 2-1	Scan Protocol for the Skull Base
Indication	Patient with skull base trauma or middle and/or inner ear disease
Protocol designed for	Sensation 16 or volume zoom
Patient preparation	No special requirements
Oral contrast	Not necessary
IV contrast administration	Not necessary
Tube settings	kV 120 mAs 220
Collimation	16 × 0.6 mm or 2 × 0.5 mm
Slice thickness	0.6 or 0.5 mm
Increment	0.2 mm
Anatomical coverage	Skull base
Recon kernel	Bone window, soft tissue window
Breath hold	Not necessary
Window settings	Standard
Postprocessing	MPR reconstructions in coronal plane
In case of tumorous lesions, repeat the protocol described above after administration of contrast medium	
Contrast medium	Iomeprol, 400 mg I/ml
Injection protocol	100 ml @ 2 ml/sec
Start delay	50 seconds

ogy (e.g., otosclerosis) should use high-resolution CT scanning (HRCT) with a slice thickness of less than 1 mm. This technique can define the ossicular chain, the semicircular canals, the foramen ovale, and the tympanic membrane. CT evaluations for neoplastic lesions often require the intravenous injection of an iodinated contrast agent to heighten the contrast of the tumor with its surroundings and to improve vascular delineation. A scan protocol for CT angiography is shown in Table 2-2.

The anterior skull base forms a bony boundary separating the nasopharynx from the frontal lobes of the brain. As such, it poses a special challenge to clinical and radiological diagnosis. A number of primary osseous lesions can arise in this region, but more commonly the anterior skull base is infiltrated by lesions that have a nasopharyngeal or intracranial origin.

The clinical examination is based largely on inspection, palpation, biopsy, and function tests of

Table 2-2	Scan Protocol for CT Angiography
Indication	Vascular disease (e.g., aneurysm, stenosis, dissection) as add-on modality or primary imaging modality
Protocol designed for	Sensation 16 or volume zoom
Patient preparation	No special requirements
Oral contrast	Not necessary
IV contrast administration	In most cases, no plain scans necessary
Contrast medium	Iomeprol, 400 mg I/ml
Injection protocol	100 ml @ 4-5 ml/sec
Start delay	Care bolus (bolus tracking) at the aortic arch
Scan direction	Caudocranial
Tube settings	kV 120 mAs 100
Collimation	16 × 0.75 mm or 4 × 1.0 mm
Slice thickness	0.75 or 1.0 mm
Increment	0.5 mm
Anatomical coverage	Aortic arch to skull base
Recon kernel	Soft tissue window
Breath hold	Quiet breathing
Window settings	Standard
Postprocessing	MPR reconstructions in coronal and sagittal planes MIP reconstructions

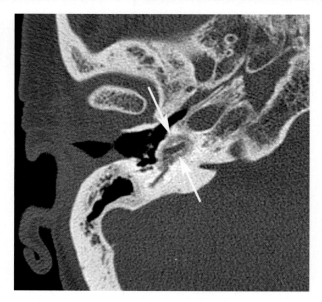

Fig. 2-1 Otosclerosis (transverse image, bone window).

the cranial nerves that supply this region. Because the anterior skull base is clinically inaccessible, lesions in this area are usually advanced when diagnosed and require accurate imaging evaluation to direct further treatment planning. An understanding of the complex anatomy of this region is essential for the optimum application of imaging procedures and the interpretation of differential diagnostic criteria.

It is convenient for imaging purposes to subdivide the middle skull base into the middle ear, temporal bone, jugular fossa, internal auditory canal, and cerebellopontine angle. With its ability to define bony details, CT has become the primary imaging modality for evaluating diseases of the external and middle ear. The two broad categories in the differential diagnosis of hearing disorders are conductive hearing loss due to middle ear pathology and sensorineural hearing loss caused by inner ear pathology.

Clinical Symptoms

Acute hearing loss:

- Conductive hearing loss
- Sensorineural hearing loss
- Traumatic hearing loss

Chronic hearing loss:

- Tinnitus
- Fluctuant hearing loss
- Pediatric hearing loss

The cardinal symptom of middle ear anomalies and variations is conductive hearing loss.

Otosclerosis is a primary focal disease of the labyrinthine capsule. The most common site of a focus is in the labyrinthine capsule just anterior to the oval window. This focus tends to extend posteriorly to fix the stapes footplate and at times invades and thickens the footplate. Similar foci occur in other areas of the labyrinthine capsule, particularly in the cochlea (Figure 2-1).

Furthermore, multiple inflammatory lesions (Figure 2-2), benign and malignant tumors, and congenital malformations and variations could be diagnosed in the skull base region (Table 2-3).

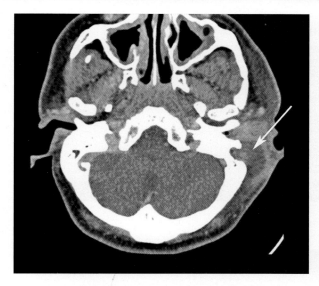

Fig. 2-2 Mastoiditis on the left side (transverse contrast-enhanced image, soft tissue window).

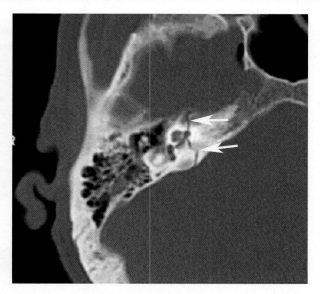

Fig. 2-3 Transverse temporal bone fracture *(arrows)*. Slight signs of a longitudinal temporal bone fracture are also present (transverse image, bone window).

Table 2-3	Common lesions of the skull base
Congenital variations and malformations	Encephalocele Pneumosinus dilatans Fibrous dysplasia Paget's disease
Inflammatory lesions	Mucocele Abscess Neuritis Labyrinthitis Osteomyelitis Granuloma Meningitis Otitis Mastoiditis Sarcoidosis
Benign tumors	Neurinoma Meningioma Glomus tumor, paraganglioma Cholesteatoma Adenoma Hemangioma Lipoma Chordoma
Malignant tumors	Carcinoma Metastases Sarcoma Lymphoma Esthesioneuroblastoma

In trauma patients with suspected skull base injury, MSCT is the method of choice for the evaluation of temporal bone fractures, which are subdivided into longitudinal fractures, transverse fractures, and combined (longitudinal and transverse) fractures (Figure 2-3). In patients with a temporal bone fracture, a careful evaluation of the inner ear, the facial nerve, and the ossicles is necessary because of the high number of related injuries (Table 2-4).[10]

FACE AND PARANASAL SINUSES

With the advent of modern therapeutic procedures such as functional sinus surgery (FSS), sectional imaging modalities have assumed major importance in diagnosis as well as treatment planning, especially in patients with chronic inflammatory diseases such as maxillary, ethmoid, and frontal sinusitis. Today it is common practice to precede planned interventions with a CT examination, which affords maximum spatial resolution for defining key bony structures and aerated spaces. Several pathological entities including inflammatory

Table 2-4 Findings in temporal bone fractures

Finding	Longitudinal	Transverse
Frequency	80%	20%
Hearing loss	Conductive (60%)	Sensorineural (95%)
Facial nerve injury	Geniculate ganglion (10-20%)	Horizontal portion (40%)
Tympanic membrane perforation	Yes	No
Inner ear	Spared	Involved
External auditory canal involvement	Often	Rare
Blow	Temporal/parietal	Occipital
Fracture line	Parallel to long axis	Perpendicular to long axis
Ossicular disruption	Common, especially incus	Rare

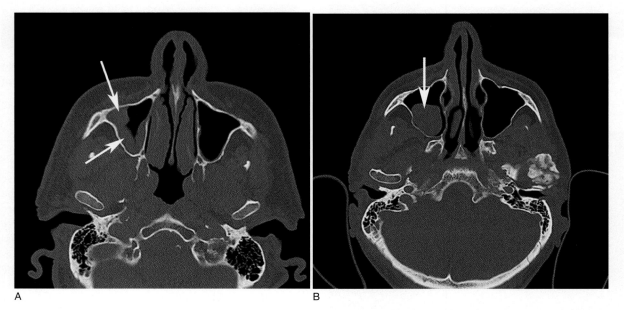

A   B

Fig. 2-4 A, Chronic sinusitis with diffuse mucosa thickening in the right maxillary sinus (transverse image, bone window). **B,** Polyp in the right maxillary sinus (transverse image, bone window).

processes and benign or malignant tumors lead to the unspecific symptom of nasal obstruction. In general, disturbances of the epithelium in acute and chronic sinusitis (Figure 2-4) lead to mucus retention and possible superinfection. In problem cases such as chronic inflammation or complete paranasal sinus obstruction, MRI makes an excellent adjunct for differentiating inflammatory and neoplastic processes.[11-14]

Orbital abscesses or mucoceles should be considered, which are possible complications of sinusitis (Figure 2-5). The differential diagnosis includes mycotic and granulomatous infections. Benign or malignant space-occupying lesions involving the paranasal sinuses are rare findings compared to these inflammatory processes. Benign tumors include inverted papilloma (Figure 2-6), juvenile angiofibroma, and osteoma; malignant tumors include mostly squamous cell carcinoma (Figure 2-7), non-Hodgkin's lymphoma, or metastases. Esthesioneuroblastoma, sarcoma, or bone-associated tumors are additional differential diagnoses (Table 2-5).

When evaluating sinonasal pathology, the examiner must remember that development of the paranasal sinuses and nasal cavity is not completed

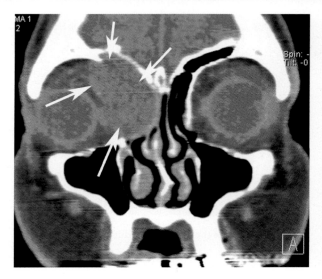

Fig. 2-5 Mucoceles *(arrows)* of the right frontal sinus with affection of the right orbit (coronal MPR image, contrast enhanced, soft tissue window).

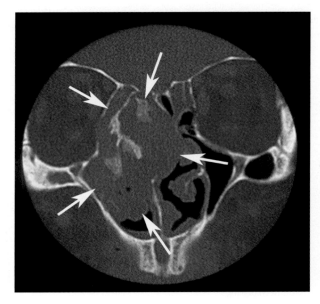

Fig. 2-6 Inverted papilloma with some calcifications in the right nasal cavity and right maxillary sinus (coronal MPR, bone window).

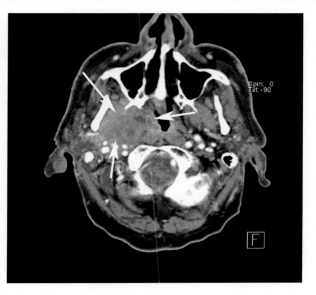

Fig. 2-7 Nasopharyngeal carcinoma on the right side with infiltration of the prestyoid compartment of the parapharyngeal space, the masticator space, and the carotid space (transverse contrast enhanced image, soft tissue window).

Table 2-5 Paranasal sinuses

Congenital variations and malformations	Choanal atresia
	Choanal stenosis
	Dermoid cyst
	Cleft palate
Inflammatory lesions	Acute sinusitis
	Chronic sinusitis
	Mucocele
	Pyocele
	Specific inflammation (syphilis, tuberculosis, sarcoidosis)
Benign tumors	Osteoma
	Papilloma
	Fibroma
	Chondroma
	Lipoma
	Myxoma
	Hemangioma
	Lymphoma
Malignant tumors	Squamous cell carcinoma
	Adenoid cystic carcinoma
	Adenocarcinoma
	Osteosarcoma
	Malignant lymphoma
	Metastases

until puberty. A precise knowledge of the various developmental stages of the paranasal sinuses will help to avoid errors of interpretation, especially on conventional radiographs. In infants younger than 1 year of age, it is normal for x-ray films to show clouding or incomplete development of the paranasal sinuses. Thus clinical significance cannot be attributed to sinus opacification in this age

Table 2-6	Scan Protocol for Facial Trauma
Indication	Patient with facial trauma
Protocol designed for	Sensation 16 or volume zoom
Patient preparation	No special requirements
Oral contrast	Not necessary
IV contrast administration	Not necessary
Tube settings	kV 120
	mAs 140
Collimation	16 × 0.75 mm or 4 × 1.0 mm
Slice thickness	0.75 or 1.0 mm
Increment	0.5 mm
Anatomical coverage	Skull base to mandible
Recon kernel	Bone window, soft tissue window
Breath hold	Not necessary
Window settings	Standard
Slice orientation	Transversal
Postprocessing	MPR reconstructions in coronal and sagittal planes

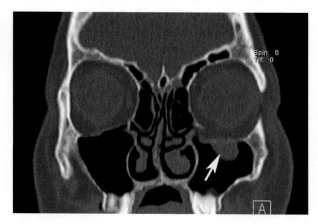

Fig. 2-8 Fracture of the floor of the orbita on the left side with fatty prolapse.

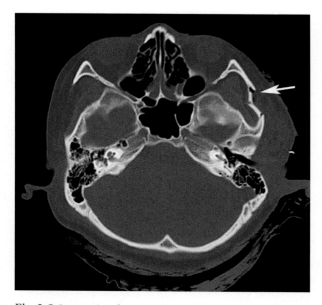

Fig. 2-9 Impression fracture of the zygomatic arch with soft-tissue hematoma.

group, and radiological evaluation of the paranasal sinuses for inflammatory changes should be avoided. In children older than 3 years, paranasal sinus opacification or air-fluid levels are considered a reliable indicator of inflammatory sinus disease. In children between 1 and 3 years of age, radiological studies should be interpreted with caution because of the limitations just described.

Traumatic lesions of the head and neck are usually fractures, which can be best diagnosed using high resolution MSCT imaging in combination with MPR reconstructions in sagittal and coronal slice orientation (Table 2-6) (Figures 2-8 to 2-11).[15,16] All scans are done in transverse slice orientation. Primary coronal scanning is no longer recommended because of the excellent image quality obtained with axial scanning and coronal and sagittal MPR reconstruction. The main advantages of this technique are superior patient comfort during the examination and the fact that dental beam hardening artifacts no longer influence the image quality for the evaluation of facial structures compared with primary coronal scanning.

However, many traumatic lesions cause additional injury to nerves and soft tissues. In these cases, plain and contrast-enhanced MRI can detect the traumatic lesion better than any other imaging modality.

In about 40% of patients with facial trauma, the zygomaticomaxillary complex is involved and should be evaluated carefully (Table 2-7).

In all cases, except trauma cases, the CT study should be done primarily with intravenous contrast (Table 2-8). Images without contrast are not necessary in almost all patients.

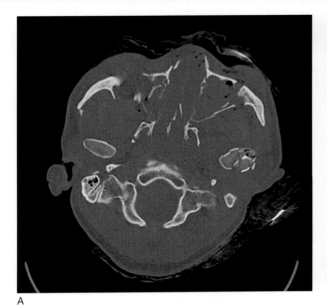

A

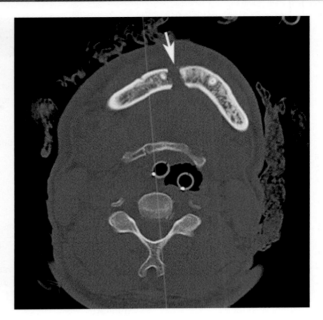

Fig. 2-11 Fracture of the mandible.

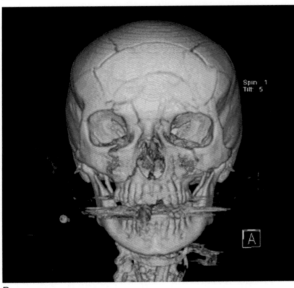

B

Fig. 2-10 A, Smash fracture of the face (transverse image, bone window) with multiple fractures of the bony structures of the face including the temporomandibular joint on the left side. B, Volume-rendered image of a smash fracture of the face.

Table 2-7	Facial fractures
Fracture type	**Prevalence**
Zygomaticomaxillary complex (tripod fracture)	40%
LeFort I	15%
LeFort II	10%
LeFort III	10%
Zygomatic arch	10%
Alveolar process of maxilla	5%
Smash fractures	5%
Other	5%

NASOPHARYNX AND RELATED SPACES

The nasopharynx forms an important boundary zone between the anterior and middle skull base and the parapharyngeal space. Diagnostic imaging is used in this region for the morphological evaluation, localization, and staging of primary lesions of the nasopharynx and nasal cavity. Because the clinical examination is limited to inspection by direct or fiberoptic techniques, supplemented in some cases by the sampling of biopsy material, radiological procedures have a major role in the detection, diagnosis, and differential diagnosis of clinically occult disease.

Given the wide availability of CT scanners, conventional radiographs of the nasopharynx are of minor importance today, and conventional tomography has become obsolete. A typical scan protocol was shown in Table 2-8. The scan region should

Table 2-8	Scan Protocol for Head and Neck Tumors (Except Laryngeal Cancer)
Indication	Patient with tumors in the nasopharynx, oropharynx, hypopharynx, parapharyngeal space, masticator space, parotid space, soft tissues of the neck
Protocol designed for	Sensation 16 or volume zoom
Patient preparation	No special requirements
Oral contrast	Not necessary
IV contrast administration	In most cases, no plain scans necessary
Contrast medium	Iomeprol, 400 mg I/ml
Injection protocol	100 ml @ 2 ml/sec
Start delay	50 seconds
Tube settings	kV 120
	mAs 200
Collimation	16 × 0.75 mm or 4 × 1.0 mm
Slice thickness	0.75 or 1.0 mm
Increment	0.5 mm
Anatomical coverage	Skull base to upper mediastinum
Recon kernel	Bone window, soft tissue window
Breath hold	Quiet breathing
Window settings	Standard
Postprocessing	MPR reconstructions in coronal and sagittal planes

cover the whole area between the skull base and the upper mediastinum. This is especially important because nasopharyngeal carcinomas often present with lymph node metastases.

The nasopharynx forms the upper portion of the pharynx and is continuous anteriorly with the nasal cavity. The roof of the nasopharynx is formed by the sphenoid bone, whereas its floor and junction with the oropharynx are at the level of the soft palate. These anatomical relationships are readily appreciated on sagittal and coronal sections. The pharyngeal recess (Rosenmüller fossa) is a pouch-like recess in the lateral wall of the nasopharynx directed toward the parapharyngeal space and lying directly adjacent to the eustachian tube orifice. This region is a common site of origination for nasopharyngeal malignancies. The torus tubarius is the posterior part of the cartilaginous eustachian tube. Lateral to the torus tubarius is the levator veli palatini muscle. The pharyngobasilar fascia, which runs between this muscle and the tensor veli palatini, combines with the levator veli palatini to define the boundary of the parapharyngeal space. The pharyngobasilar fascia is a tough connective-tissue structure that unites the pharynx with the skull base and is perforated bilaterally for passage of the eustachian tube. Infiltration of this fascia signifies the presence of an aggressive nasopharyngeal tumor.

Superficial structures like the pharyngeal recess and torus tubarius are readily identified on CT images, as are the pterygoid muscles. Because the mucosa shows greater enhancement on post-contrast images than the surrounding tissues, contrast-enhanced CT scans are excellent for visualizing the levator and tensor veli palatini muscles, the pharyngobasilar fascia, the tubal orifices, and the pharyngeal recess.

Approximately 5% of all malignant tumors of the head and neck originate in the nasopharynx, and more than 90% of these are carcinomas. The most common nasopharyngeal malignancies in adults are squamous cell carcinoma and lymphoepithelial neoplasms. Lymphomas and rhabdomyosarcomas are more common in children and tend to undergo early, extensive lymphogenous spread.

Given the variety of cell types that occur normally in the nasopharyngeal region, many different lesions may originate in the nasopharynx, ranging from embryological malformations to benign and malignant tumors. Carcinomas and lymphoepithelial tumors (Figure 2-12) account for about 75% of all nasopharyngeal neoplasms in adults.

Benign nasopharyngeal tumors are rare—the most common is juvenile nasopharyngeal fibroma (skull base angioma). Although nasopharyngeal

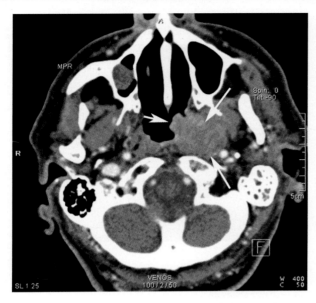

Fig. 2-12 Lymphoepitheloid carcinoma of the nasopharynx with infiltration of the parapharyngeal space on the left side.

Table 2-9	Common lesions of the nasopharynx
Congenital variations and malformations	Lymphatic hyperplasia Internal or external carotid aneurysm
Inflammatory lesions	Nasopharyngeal abscess Lymphoepithelial cyst Phlegmonous inflammation
Benign tumors	Tornwaldt cyst Dermoid cyst
Malignant tumors	Lymphoepithelial carcinoma Squamous cell carcinoma

Table 2-10	Parapharyngeal space
Congenital variations and malformations	Branchial cleft cyst (rare)
Inflammatory lesions	Cellulitis Abscess
Benign tumors	Paraganglioma Neurogenic tumors Meningioma
Malignant tumors	Adenoid cystic carcinoma Mucoepidermoid Malignant mixed tumors of salivary gland rests Lymphoma Direct spread of squamous cell carcinoma

fibroma is histologically benign, it tends to show malignant clinical characteristics because of its expansile, locally aggressive growth.

Mesenchymal tumors are the most common benign tumors of the nose and paranasal sinuses. This group includes papillomas, hemangiomas, fibromas, and other rare tumors.

Malignant tumors of the nasal cavity and paranasal sinuses account for less than 1% of all malignant neoplasms. The histological types are anaplastic carcinoma (59%), lymphoepithelial carcinoma (30%), squamous cell carcinoma, and mesenchymal tumors.

Two well-known congenital variants and malformations of the nasopharynx are the Tornwaldt cyst and hyperplasia of the torus tubarius. They are often detected incidentally on MR images. A Tornwaldt cyst is readily identifiable as a midline cystic mass.

An overview of the different inflammatory lesions, benign and malignant tumors, and congenital malformations and variations is presented in Tables 2-9 and 2-10.

The parapharyngeal space has irregular boundaries and is filled principally by fat. It extends from the skull base to the hyoid bone and has roughly the shape of an inverted pyramid. The inferior boundary of the parapharyngeal space is formed by the attachment of the posterior belly of the digas-

tric muscle to the greater cornua of the hyoid bone. At the level of the skull base, the parapharyngeal space is bound by the portion of the sphenoid bone around the foramen lacerum, medial to the foramen ovale, and the inferior surface of the petrous bone near the carotid canal and jugular fossa. The medial boundary of the parapharyngeal space is formed superiorly by the tensor veli palatini muscle and its fascia, the pharyngobasilar fascia, the levator veli palatini muscle, the superior pharyngeal constrictor muscle, and the jugular fossa. The lateral boundary of the space is the medial wall of the masticator space. The medial pterygoid muscle and interpterygoid fascia form the medial boundary of the masticator space, separating it from the parapharyngeal space.

The parapharyngeal space can be divided into a prestyloid compartment and a poststyloid (retrostyloid) compartment. The posterior compartment contains the neurovascular sheath. The masticator space is a separate fascial compartment enclosed by the superficial layer of the deep cervical fascia and contains the pterygoid muscles, masseter muscle, inferior temporalis muscle, and mandibular ramus.

MASTICATOR SPACE

The superficial layer of the deep cervical fascia splits along the inferior border of the mandible, creating a medial slip that runs along the pterygoid muscles and attaches to the skull base, and a lateral slip that runs over the superficial masseter muscle to the zygomatic arch and that continues cephalad over the temporalis muscle. Because there is no fascia separating the temporal area from the masticator space, this cephalad extension is also called the *suprazygomatic masticator space*.

The lateral pterygoid muscle arises by two heads from the infratemporal surface of the skull base and lateral sphenoid wing and inserts onto the medial aspect of the mandibular condyle. The medial pterygoid muscle arises in the fossa between the pterygoid plates and inserts onto the medial aspect of the angle of the mandible.

The temporalis muscle inserts onto the coronoid process of the mandible. The masseter muscle descends from its origin on the zygomatic arch to the lateral surface of the ramus, angle, and posterior body of the mandible.

By connecting the mandible with the skull base, the masticator space creates an avenue by which odontogenic infections and squamous carcinoma cells from the oropharynx can reach the skull base.

The mandibular division of the trigeminal nerve (V_3) runs along the skull base and exits through the foramen ovale to enter the masticator space. It transmits both sensory and motor fibers. The motor fibers are the masticator nerve—which supplies the masseter, temporalis, and medial and lateral pterygoid muscles—and the mylohyoid nerve, which supplies the mylohyoid muscle and the anterior belly of the digastric muscle in the region of the oral floor.

Common pathologies of the parapharyngeal space, masticator space, and retropharyngeal space are listed in Tables 2-10 to 2-12.

Table 2-11   Masticator space

Congenital variations and malformations	Hemangioma Lymphangioma
Inflammatory lesions	Odontogenic abscess Mandibular osteomyelitis
Benign tumors	Leiomyoma Osteoblastoma Neurogenic tumors
Malignant tumors	Soft tissue sarcoma Osteosarcoma Malignant schwannoma Metastases Minor salivary gland tumors

Table 2-12   Retropharyngeal space

Congenital variations and malformations	Lymphangioma Hemangioma
Inflammatory lesions	Cellulitis Abscess
Benign tumors	Lipoma
Malignant tumors	Lymph node metastases Non-Hodgkin's lymphoma Direct invasion from squamous cell carcinoma

OROPHARNYX AND ORAL CAVITY

The classification of malignant tumors of the oropharynx, oral cavity, and oral floor follows the TNM system of the UICC, which is based on the size of the tumor and the extent of its spread. Tumor size is classified as follows:

- Stage T1 tumors are smaller than 2 cm at their greatest diameter and are confined to their site of origin.
- Stage T2 tumors are between 2 cm and 4 cm in diameter.
- Stage T3 tumors are larger than 4 cm in diameter but have not invaded adjacent structures.
- Stage T4 tumors signify the invasion of adjacent structures.

Squamous cell carcinoma is the most common of all mass lesions of the oropharynx, oral cavity, and oral floor (Figure 2-13).

Approximately 80% of oropharyngeal carcinomas are tonsillar. Smaller numbers originate from the palate (approximately 15%) and posterior pharyngeal wall (approximately 4%). The most common primary site for tonsillar cancers is the anterior pole of the tonsils (Figure 2-14), followed by the posterior pole and adjacent posterior pharyngeal wall. These tumors tend to spread upward into the soft palate; downward into the lateral pharyngeal wall and tongue base; and laterally into the parapharyngeal space, mandible, and vascular sheath.

In addition to invading the parapharyngeal space, small mucosal tumors will infiltrate the body of the tongue in more than 70% of cases. With an extensive lesion, 40% of cases will show invasion of the longus colli muscle with indentation of the pharyngeal wall. These tumors metastasize early to regional lymph nodes, and distant metastasis (to the lung, bone, or liver) is not uncommon.

Inflammatory Lesions

Most inflammatory lesions of this region (e.g., cheilitis, gingivostomatitis, aphthae, pharyngitis, tonsillitis) are diagnosed and treated clinically.

Common pathologies of the oropharynx are listed in Table 2-13.

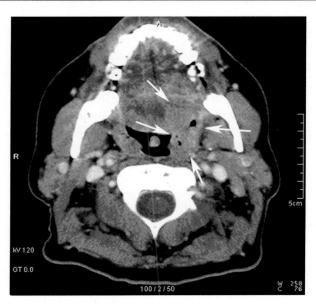

Fig. 2-14 Squamous cell carcinoma of the left tonsil with infiltration of the floor of the mouth.

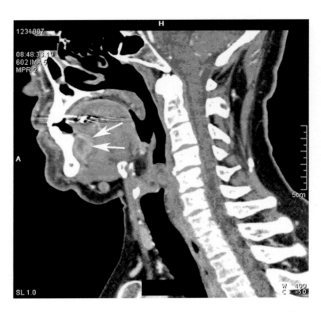

Fig. 2-13 Squamous cell carcinoma of the anterior part of the floor of the mouth with contact to the mandible. Note some artifacts due to dental filling.

Table 2-13	Oropharynx
Congenital variations and malformations	Hemangioma Lymphangioma Cystic hygroma Lingual thyroid tissue Thyroglossal duct cyst
Inflammatory lesions	Ludwig's angina secondary to abscess or cellulitis Gland inflammation Ranula Abscess
Benign tumors	Papilloma Pleomorphic adenoma Fibroma Lipoma Neuroma Osteoma Rhabdomyoma Myxoma
Malignant tumors	Squamous cell carcinoma Anaplastic carcinoma Malignant lymphoma Sarcoma

Lymph Nodes

Because nodal metastases are commonly found in patients who present with a primary tumor of the head and neck region and imply a life expectancy reduction of approximately 50%, it is essential that involved lymph nodes be accurately described and staged before initial treatment. Some reports indicate that 86% to 90% of all malignant tumors of the nasopharynx have already spread to the lymph nodes by the time of initial diagnosis.

Lymph node involvement is classified according to TNM system of the UICC:

- Stage N1 denotes involvement of a single ipsilateral node 3 cm or less in diameter.
- Stage N2a denotes involvement of a single ipsilateral node between 3 cm and 6 cm in diameter.
- Stage N2b denotes involvement of multiple ipsilateral nodes not more than 6 cm in diameter.
- Stage N2c denotes involvement of ipsilateral and contralateral nodes not more than 6 cm in diameter.
- Stage N3 denotes involvement of one or more nodes larger than 6 cm in diameter.

Affected lymph nodes may be described by groups or levels. The level terminology adopted by the American Joint Committee on Cancer (AJCC) is based on the fact that the extent and level of cervical nodal involvement by metastatic tumor seem to be an important prognostic indicator.

Level I   Submental and submandibular nodes
Level II   Upper jugular group (skull base to hyoid)
Level III Middle jugular group
Level IV   Lower jugular group (omohyoid muscle to clavicle)
Level V   Posterior triangle group
Level VI   Paralaryngeal and paratracheal group

Imaging Criteria and Their Differential Diagnosis

The following questions should be addressed when evaluating the oropharynx, oral cavity, and oral floor:

- What is the deep tissue extent of the lesion?
- What is the relation of the lesion to neurovascular structures?

- What is the stage of the lesion?
- In the oral cavity, has the tumor invaded the lingual septum, the mandible, or the tongue base?
- What is the lymph node status in the submental and submandibular spaces?

An analysis of the deep cervical lymph nodes is also essential. However, the differentiation between benign and malignant lymph nodes is difficult. An acceptable cutoff is 8 to 10 mm in the small axial axis. The visualization of a fatty hilus is an indication of a benign lymph node. The visualization of a central necrosis in the contrast-enhanced scans is a good indication of malignant lymph nodes.

HYPOPHARYNX AND LARYNX

The primary diagnostic evaluation of diseases of the hypopharynx and larynx is based on clinical procedures such as inspection and indirect examination, followed by endoscopic procedures such as microlaryngoscopy and other types of direct laryngoscopy with a self-supporting instrument. These procedures are adequate for evaluating the mucosae and taking tissue samples for histological examination. Phonetic studies and quantitative procedures such as stroboscopy and electromyography can yield valuable information about the mobility of the vocal cords. Deglutition can be evaluated with conventional oral contrast studies using barium or a water-soluble contrast medium, supplemented by video cinematography or high-speed cinematography.

The sectional imaging modalities of MSCT and MRI are mainly indicated for the evaluation of traumatic lesions, inflammatory masses, and tumor masses in these regions (Figure 2-15).

Normal Anatomy

The main subdivisions of the larynx are the supraglottis, glottis, and subglottis. The supraglottis extends from the ventricular folds (false vocal cords) above to the true vocal cords (vocal folds) below. It is bounded anteriorly by the thyroid cartilage and laterally and posteriorly by the aryepiglottic folds. The glottis includes the vocal cords, vocal muscles, and laryngeal ventricles (sinus

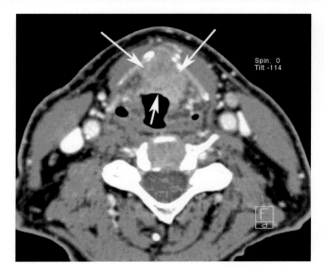

Spin: 0
Tilt -114

Fig. 2-15 Supraglottic laryngeal carcinoma.

Table 2-14	Scan Protocol for Laryngeal Cancer
Indication	Patient with laryngeal tumors
Protocol designed for	Sensation 16 or volume zoom
Patient preparation	No special requirements
Oral contrast	Not necessary
IV contrast administration	In most cases, no plain scans necessary
Contrast medium	Iomeprol, 400 mg I/ml
Injection protocol	100 ml @ 2 ml/sec
Start delay	50 seconds
Tube settings	kV 120 mAs 200
Collimation	16 × 0.75 mm or 4 × 1.0 mm
Slice thickness	0.75 or 1.0 mm
Increment	0.5 mm
Anatomical coverage	Skull base to upper mediastinum
Recon kernel	Bone window, soft tissue window
Breath hold	Quiet breathing
Window settings	Standard
Postprocessing	MPR reconstructions in coronal and sagittal planes

Note: This scan should be followed immediately by a second spiral scan focused on the larynx during E-phonation or a Valsalva maneuver. Before the examination, patients have to be trained intensively to perform the E-phonation or the Valsalva maneuver.

of Morgagni). The anterior and posterior attachments of the vocal cords are called the *anterior* and *posterior commissures*. The inferior borders of the thyroid and cricoid cartilages define the topographical boundaries of the subglottis, which is the laryngeal segment below the glottis and above the trachea.

MDCT is recommended with 0.75 to 1.0 mm collimation to allow the entire larynx to be acquired within a single breath hold. The data should be reconstructed in 1-mm thickness and with an overlapping reconstruction increment to enable optimal MPRs, which are recommended in angulated coronal and sagittal planes. Using this technique, the sensitivity and specificity of MDCT regarding the infiltration of the glottic region can reach 93% and 85%, respectively. Sensitivity and specificity of MDCT regarding the infiltration of the anterior part of the vocal cords in our series were 89% and 92%, respectively. The infiltration of the arytenoids was 83% and 96%, respectively. The scan protocol for the larynx is shown in Table 2-14. The vocal cords and vocal muscles display higher density on CT images, whereas the more superiorly placed ventricular folds show a lower density because of their fat content. (Coronal images are best for comparing these structures.) The mucosa lining the larynx is less than 1 mm thick, and diffuse or circumscribed thickening of the laryngeal mucosa is suggestive of disease. The preepiglottic and paralaryngeal spaces are occupied mostly by fat.

The medial preepiglottic space extends from the hyoid bone to the anterior commissure and is continuous laterally with the paralaryngeal space.

The hypopharynx extends from the oropharynx to the supraglottic portion of the larynx. It is bounded superiorly by the free margin of the epiglottis and the lateral pharyngoepiglottic folds that form the valleculae. Anterior to the epiglottis is the fat-filled preepiglottic space. The left and right piriform sinuses and the esophagus form the posterior boundaries of the hypopharynx. The aryepiglottic folds extend from the arytenoid cartilages to the epiglottis, forming a triangular airway. The apex of this triangle is formed by the anterior commissure; its basal angles are formed by the paired posterior commissures.

Soft Tissues of the Neck

The anatomical region of the neck is bounded above by the inferior border of the mandible and occipital bone and below by an imaginary plane between the suprasternal notch and the seventh cervical vertebra. Various fascial layers subdivide the neck into compartments that are important in the interpretation of transaxial images.

The visceral compartment is the most anterior of the fascia-defined spaces in the neck and contains the aerodigestive tract including the larynx, trachea, and esophagus. The thyroid gland and parathyroid glands are also located in this compartment. The normal thyroid gland appears on CT as a symmetric, homogeneous soft-tissue structure situated anterior and lateral to the trachea.

The posterior compartment contains the cervical vertebrae and associated flexor and extensor muscles including the scaleni, longus capitis, and longus colli. These muscle groups show CT densities comparable to those of the intrinsic tongue muscles.

The lateral compartment principally contains the neurovascular bundle about the common carotid artery. The carotid arteries and jugular veins are clearly distinguishable from surrounding fat or muscle tissue by higher density on contrast-enhanced CT images. Even small blood vessels can be identified on axial CT images. Coronal and sagittal MPRs are often added to the CT workup to provide a better demonstration of topographical relationships. The lateral compartment is particularly important for determining cervical lymph node status. Normal lymph nodes have more or less an oval shape. Sometimes a fatty hilus is detectable.

REFERENCES

1. Roos JE, Desbiolles LM, Willmann JK, et al: Multidetector-row helical CT: analysis of time management and workflow, *Eur Radiol* 12:680-685, 2002.

2. Imhof H, Czerny C, Dirisamer A: Head and neck imaging with MDCT, *Eur J Radiol* 45:S23-31, 2003.

3. Dammann F, Bode A, Heuschmid M, et al: Multislice spiral CT of the paranasal sinuses: first experiences using various parameters of radiation dosage, *Rofo Fortschr Geb Rontgenstr Neuen Bildgeb Verfahr* 172:701-706, 2000.

4. Baum U, Greess H, Lell M, et al: Imaging of head and neck tumors–methods: CT, spiral-CT, multislice-spiral-CT, *Eur J Radiol* 33:153-160, 2000.

5. Ertl-Wagner B, Hoffmann RT, Bruning R, et al: CT-angiographic evaluation of intracranial aneurysms—a review of the literature and first experiences with 4- and 16-slice multi detector CT scanners *Radiologe* 42:892-897, 2002.

6. Goodman D, Hoh B, Rabinov J, et al: CT angiography before embolization for hemorrhage in head and neck cancer, *Am J Neuroradiol* 24:140-142, 2003.

7. Yokoyama J: Usefulness of CT-angiography for superselective intra-arterial chemotherapy for advanced head and neck cancers, *Gan To Kagaku Ryoho* 29:2302-2306, 2002.

8. Keberle M, Tschammler A, Berning K, et al: Spiral CT of the neck: When do neck malignancies delineate best during contrast enhancement? *Eur Radiol* 11:1986-1990, 2001.

9. Keberle M, Tschammler A, Hahn D: Single-bolus technique for spiral CT of laryngopharyngeal squamous cell carcinoma: comparison of different contrast material volumes, flow rates, and start delays, *Radiology* 224:171-176, 2002.

10. Bell RS, Loop JW: The utility and futility of radiographic skull examination for trauma, *New Engl J Med* 284:236-239, 1971.

11. Jones N: CT of the paranasal sinuses: a review of the correlation with clinical, surgical and histopathological findings, *Clin Otolaryngol* 27:11-17, 2002.

12. Mudgil S, Wise S, Hopper K, et al: Correlation between presumed sinusitis-induced pain and paranasal sinus computed tomographic findings, *Ann Allergy Asthma Immunol* 88:223-226, 2002.

13. Eggesbo H, Sovik S, Dolvik S, et al: CT characterization of inflammatory paranasal sinus disease in cystic fibrosis, *Acta Radiol* 43:21-28, 2002.

14. Schwartz R, Pitkaranta A, Winther B: Computed tomography imaging of the maxillary and ethmoid sinuses in children with short-duration purulent rhinorrhea, *Otolaryngol Head Neck Surg* 124:160-163, 2001.

15. Philipp M, Funovics M, Mann F, et al: Four-channel multidetector CT in facial fractures: do we need 2 × 0.5 mm collimation? *Am J Roentgenol* 180:1707-1713, 2003.

16. Sun J, Le MD: Imaging of facial trauma, *Neuroimaging Clin N Am* 12:295-309, 2002.

CHAPTER 3

Lung Nodules

Marie Pierre Revel
Yvonne K. Maratos
Laure S. Fournier
Catherine Lefort
Stéphane Lenoir
Guy Frija

Computed tomography (CT) is the most sensitive imaging modality for detection of lung nodules. The lack of sensitivity of chest radiography for detecting nodules smaller than 2 cm has been clearly established.[1,2]

Helical CT is superior to conventional CT when the same slice thickness is used. Spiral acquisition during one single breath hold avoids potential misregistrations caused by inconsistent levels of inspiration[3] and reduces respiratory movement artifacts.[4] More recently, multislice technology has increased the diagnostic capabilities of CT scans in pulmonary nodule evaluation. Before the advent of MSCT, diagnosis of pulmonary nodules required at least two separate CT acquisitions. An initial CT acquisition with a slice thickness of 5 to 8 mm, depending on the equipment, was required to cover the entire thorax in a single apnea, to accurately detect lung nodules and to avoid respiratory misregistrations and the risk of undersampling the lung. A second acquisition was required, consisting of localized 1-mm thickness, high-resolution CT slices centered on the detected nodules, allowing a precise assessment of the periphery of the lesions[5] and of their density, for a purpose of characterization. As multislice CT scan dramatically reduces the acquisition time, this technology allows a high-resolution study of the entire thorax during a single apnea. Now a single MSCT acquisition is sufficient for detection and analysis of lung nodules.

In this overview, we will discuss the following questions:

- What kind of CT protocols, postprocessing methods, and reading mode are most efficient for detecting lung nodules?

- What kind of CT protocol should be used for the characterization of lung nodules?

- Which new tools are currently available with MSCT for lung nodule detection and characterization?

We will also discuss the specific problem of pulmonary nodules observed in patients with a known primary tumor.

We will finally address the specific problem of lung nodules found during lung cancer screening studies and discuss the controversy about lung cancer CT screening effectiveness.

LUNG NODULES

Definition and Prevalence

A solitary pulmonary nodule is defined as a unique focal, round, or oval area of increased opacity in the lung that is smaller than 3 cm in diameter.[6] Lesions larger than 3 cm in diameter are defined as focal masses and are very likely to be lung cancer. They should be assessed as soon as possible with bronchoscopic or percutaneous biopsy or by surgical resection, allowing a histopathological study.

The initial step in the assessment of a nodule is to confirm whether the abnormality, when discovered on a chest radiograph, truly corresponds to a pulmonary nodule. It has been shown that 20% of nodules seen on chest radiography were not confirmed as being a pulmonary nodule after CT examination.[7] Different entities can mimic a solitary pulmonary nodule, such as rib fractures, skin lesions, or pleural plaques (Figure 3-1). The second

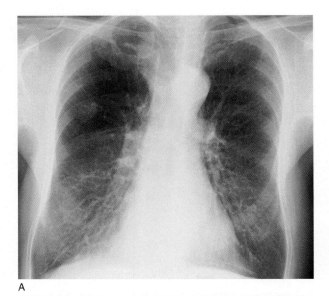

A

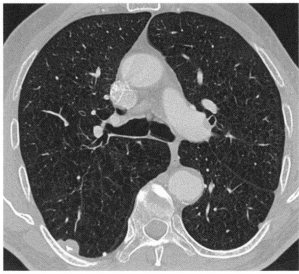

B

Fig. 3-1 **False nodule on chest radiography.** A posteroanterior chest radiograph demonstrates a rounded opacity in the right lung projecting on the posterior arch of the sixth rib (**A**) in a 64-year-old man. CT scan (**B**) shows that the nodular opacity is created by a partially calcified pleural plaque. Another smaller diffusely calcified plaque is demonstrated more medially in the right upper lobe. Contralateral noncalcified pleural plaque is also present.

step is to assess whether the detected nodule really is solitary, or if there are additional nodules that have not been visible on chest radiography. Multiple pulmonary nodules may suggest pulmonary metastasis, especially in patients with known prior malignancy.

Previous publications estimated that approximately 150,000 solitary pulmonary nodules are detected annually in the United States on chest radiography or conventional CT.[8] However, these data underestimate the real frequency of pulmonary nodules, because they do not consider the increased detection of pulmonary nodules by spiral CT scan. Lung cancer screening studies of high-risk patients with spiral CT discovered pulmonary nodules in 23% to 69% of patients.[9,10] MSCT, which allows thin-slice acquisition through the entire thorax and detection of nodules smaller than 5 mm of diameter, could make this percentage even higher.

Causes

The results of each study on the subject confirm that the vast majority of lung nodules are benign, even in high-risk patients.[9] There are numerous causes of pulmonary nodules, but the four most common, which account for 90% of these nodules, are primary lung cancer, pulmonary metastasis, granulomas, and hamartomas. The remaining 10% are caused by various entities.

Table 3-1 summarizes the main causes of pulmonary nodules.

Detection

Nodule detection depends largely on the acquisition technique and on postprocessing techniques used for image visualization. Examples of MSCT acquisition protocols are presented in Table 3-2.

Image Acquisition

Collimation

Collimation has been decreased from 10 mm used in conventional CT technique to 5 mm with single slice CT technique; it further decreases to 2.5 mm or 1.25 mm with 4-detector CT units. With a 0.5 to 0.8 second rotation time, 30 cm coverage along the z-axis with a 1.25 mm collimation acquisition only requires 5.5 to 9 seconds on 16-detector units compared with 20 to 30 seconds on 4-detector

Table 3-1	Benign and malignant causes of solitary pulmonary nodules
Tumors	
Malignant tumors	Lung carcinoma
	Pulmonary lymphoma
	Carcinoid tumor
	Solitary pulmonary metastasis
Benign tumors	Hamartochondroma, pulmonary cyst, leiomyoma, intrapulmonary bronchogenic cyst
Inflammatory or infectious	Granulomas (tuberculosis, histoplasmosis)
	Abscess
	Organizing pneumonia
	Plasmacytoma
	Pulmonary lymph node
	Round atelectasis
	Amyloidosis
Systemic disease	Rheumatoid arthritis
	Wegener granulomatosis
Vascular	Pulmonary artery aneurysm
	Arteriovenous fistula
	Pulmonary infarct
	Hematoma
Congenital	Bronchial atresia
	Sequestration
Other	Mucoid impaction

units (see Table 3-2). Thus high-resolution acquisition through the entire thorax during one single breath hold is obtained more easily on 16-detector units.

It has been shown that a narrow collimation enhances the sensitivity of CT scan for detection of lung nodules, especially for nodules less than 10 mm in diameter.

The use of 1.25-mm collimated thin slices allows detection of smaller pulmonary lung nodules than do 5 mm-slices. Fischbach et al. (2003)[11] showed that a thin slice thickness improved small nodule detection, confidence levels, and interobserver agreement. With 16-detector CT units, submillimetric slices can now be acquired. This should optimize lung nodule detection, even though no study has yet confirmed these data.

Table 3-2 Parameters used for thoracic MSCT acquisition*

CT parameters	4-Detector unit	16-Detector unit	
Slice thickness (mm)	1.25	1.25	0.625
Reconstruction interval[†] (mm)	1.25	1.25	0.625
Table speed[‡] (mm per rotation)	7.5	27.5	13.75
Pitch[‡] (collimation/table displacement)	1.5	1.375	1.375
Rotation time (sec)	0.5 to 0.8	0.5 to 0.8	0.5 to 0.8
Acquisition time for 30 cm length coverage (sec)	20 to 32 s	5.5 to 9	11 to 18
Number of native CT images per window for 30 cm length coverage	240	240	480
Reconstruction thickness (mm)	2.5 to 5	2.5 to 5	1.25 to 2.5
Field of view (cm)	25 to 35	25 to 35	
mAs	50 to 100	50 to 100	
kV	120	120	
Review mode	MIP mode and or cine viewing		

*Parameters indicated here are purely indicative and must be adapted to the MSCT equipment.
[†]To depict arterial type enhancement for slice thickness and reconstruction interval.
[‡]Other values can be selected.

Reconstruction Interval

The retrospective reconstruction of overlapping images reduces the problem of slice-to-slice volume averaging, and thus also enhances the detection of small lung nodules. Overlapping image reconstruction improves detection of pulmonary nodules smaller than the slice thickness in spiral CT-scan acquisition[12]; however, it has less impact when the slice thickness is already very thin.

Exposure Parameters

Several studies have compared standard and low-dose CT for detection of pulmonary nodules.[13-15] The definition of low-dose CT is not very precise nor consensual.

Low-dose CT acquisitions with 50 mAs and a 5 mm slice thickness detect as many nodules as CT scans performed with 200 mAs.[13] Other studies comparing 20 to 25 mAs acquisitions with standard dose acquisitions showed that the results were acceptable, even though detection of nodules was less accurate for nodules smaller than 5 mm and for nodules of different sizes using a pitch value of 2.[14,15]

Low-dose CT is required for CT screening studies, because the CT has to be repeated annually and focuses on nodule detection for which low-dose CT is as accurate as standard dose. For evaluating lung nodules, once detected, standard dose should be used, but there is no reason to exceed 100 mAs.

Ideally, the dose should correspond to the patient's weight in kilograms (e.g., 70 mAs for a patient who weighs 70 kg). A standard dose is required for an accurate evaluation of lung nodule attenuation values because the standard deviation of the measurements depends on the signal-to-noise ratio, which is better with standard dose. Standard dose is also needed for an optimal volumetric measurement of the nodule, achieved by segmentation, which separates the nodule from its environment. Standard dose is particularly required when the segmentation process is based on densitometric evaluation.

Image Review and Postprocessing

The main objective of postprocessing techniques is to improve differentiation between nodules and vessels.

Maximum Intensity Projection (MIP) Reconstruction

It has been shown that MIP reconstruction improves the detection rate of small high-density pulmonary nodules and increases the reader confidence level, compared with standard spiral CT images.[16] The optimal slab thickness required for pulmonary lung nodule detection is not clearly established. MIP reconstructions of single-slice CT acquisitions using a slab thickness of 15 mm are slightly superior to MIP reconstructions with a 30 mm slab thickness.[17] The slab thickness used for

MIP reconstruction of high-resolution multislice CT acquisitions is usually between 5 and 10 mm.

The main benefit of MIP reconstruction is a better delineation of pulmonary vessels (Figure 3-2) and a better differentiation between a true nodule and a vessel simulating a nodule on a single thin slice CT image. Another way to avoid this mistake is to perform cine viewing of the images, which helps to recognize "pseudo" nodules as part of a normal vascular structure. MIP reconstruction is also useful for the recognition of small arteriovenous fistulae mimicking a pulmonary nodule, by identifying a feeding artery and a draining vein in connection to the nodule. These two distinct vascular connections are strongly suggestive of arteriovenous fistulae (Figure 3-3).

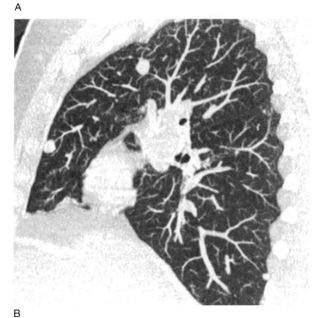

Fig. 3-2 MIP reconstruction for the detection of pulmonary nodules. Coronal (A) and sagittal (B) MIP reconstruction images are performed from a 16-detector CT acquisition. The nodules are clearly depicted and differentiated from vessels. Such MIP reconstructions reduce the number of images to be reviewed.

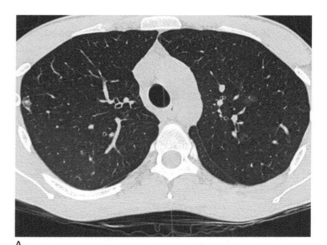

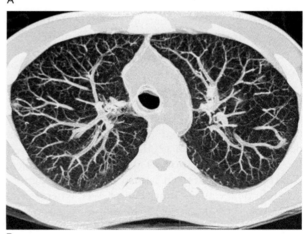

Fig. 3-3 MIP reconstruction of small pulmonary arteriovenous fistulas in a patient with Rendu-Osler-Weber disease. A MSCT scan demonstrates a part-solid subpleural nodule in the right upper lobe (A) in a 27-year-old man with Rendu-Osler-Weber disease. MIP reconstruction (B) shows connecting vessels corresponding to the feeding artery and draining vein. Note that focal ground glass opacity is visible in the left upper lobe in A and is also due to a small arteriovenous fistula, as shown on B. A third larger fistula is also detected within the left upper lobe on B.

The addition of MIP slabs significantly enhances reviewer detection of central nodules.[18]

The last advantage of MIP reconstruction is reduction of image numbers and of reading times.[17] When the entire thorax is scanned with a slice thickness of 1 mm, the number of images to be read routinely reaches several hundred.

Automated Vessel Subtraction

Other postprocessing techniques have been proposed to enhance pulmonary nodule detection. Automated vessel subtraction is one of them. This postprocessing technique improves detection of pulmonary nodules, especially central nodules, by suppressing the vessels that may mask small central nodules.[19] However, in clinical routine, MIP reconstruction is the most widely used postprocessing technique.

Cine Viewing

Cine viewing of helical CT scans of the chest improves the detection of pulmonary nodules,[20] especially for those that are smaller or equal to 5 mm in diameter.[21]

The advantages of cine viewing may be attributed to the ability to scroll through images, which allows an easy differentiation between vessels and nodules. Moreover, it reduces reading time.

Contrast Medium Injection

Contrast medium injection is not required for lung nodule detection. However, the study of contrast enhancement on serial delayed acquisitions as described by Swensen (2002)[22] has been proposed for the characterization of indeterminate nodules. Contrast administration is also useful for diagnosing pulmonary aneurysms (Figure 3-4), whereas the diagnosis of pulmonary arteriovenous fistula, which may also appear as a solitary pulmonary nodule, does not require contrast administration. In these cases, MIP or three-dimensional (3D) reconstructions allow identification of the connecting vessels.[23]

Characterization

Lung cancer screening studies[9,10,24,25] have shown that the vast majority of depicted nodules are benign in patients without prior malignancy. Thus invasive procedures should be avoided to assess the

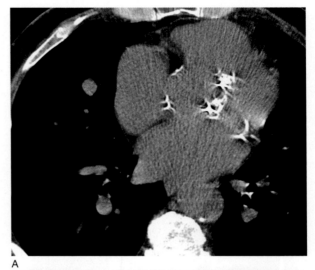

A

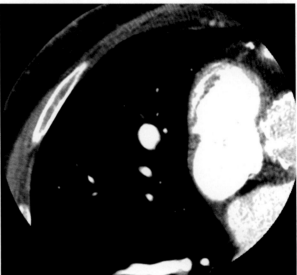

B

Fig. 3-4 Contrast-enhanced CT diagnosing a small pulmonary aneurysm. An unenhanced MSCT scan (**A**) shows a 14-mm-diameter round nodule in the middle lobe, in a 71-year-old man. Contrast-enhanced CT acquisition (**B**) performed 30 seconds after injection shows arterial type enhancement of the nodule. The patient history revealed previous Swan-Ganz catheterism for evaluating the pulmonary pressure, which had been complicated by the onset of hemoptysis. These data were not mentioned when the patient was referred 2 years later for solitary pulmonary nodule investigation.

This case raises the question whether immediate postinjection CT acquisition should be part of the CT enhancement study for characterizing a pulmonary nodule, which usually starts only 1 minute after injection.

nature of indeterminate nodules in these cases. Among the different noninvasive methods that have been developed in the last few years, many of them are exclusively based on CT, such as analysis of nodule morphology, study of contrast enhancement, and CT assessment of nodule growth. These methods are the most frequently used in the diagnostic workup of pulmonary nodules.

CT-Based Methods

Among the numerous benign causes of pulmonary nodules, some have a characteristic appearance on CT and are easy to recognize. This avoids the need for further investigation.

Four distinct entities should be recognized immediately: pulmonary aspergilloma, arteriovenous fistula, mucoid impaction, and rounded atelectasis. All four may have a nodular shape on CT.

Diagnosis of pulmonary aspergilloma is easily made, marked by a crescent air sign around a pulmonary nodule. The nodule corresponds to the fungus ball, and the crescent air sign is due to the fact that the fungus ball does not fill the entire pulmonary cavity in which it developed (Figure 3-5). The diagnosis of arteriovenous pulmonary fistula (AVPF) is made by identifying vascular connections

to a nodule, ideally on 3D CT reconstructions.[23] Approximately 65% of patients with AVPF have Rendu-Osler-Weber disease, whereas AVPF is found in 15% of patients with this disease.[26] Because of its high sensitivity for the detection of AVPF, CT is now systematically performed for patients with a family history of Rendu-Osler-Weber disease to prevent cerebral complications by treating detected fistula by embolization or by surgical resection. Diagnosis of mucoid impaction is easy when it is associated with bronchial enlargement. With cine view, the bronchus can be followed, leading to the mucoid impaction that could have been interpreted falsely as a pulmonary nodule. Diagnosis of rounded atelectasis (Figure 3-6) requires several criteria[27]: the round opacity has to be in contact with pleural thickening, bronchi and arteries must show a circular orientation caused by the rotation of the pulmonary parenchyma in the same territory, and the involved lobe must show a volume loss compared with the contralateral lung.

Other benign causes of pulmonary nodules (see Table 3-1) do not have a typical or specific CT appearance and require more detailed evaluation.

Morphological Evaluation with High-Resolution CT

High-resolution CT is mandatory for an accurate assessment of pulmonary nodules. A high-frequency reconstruction algorithm allows optimal detection of nodule borders, which is required for accurately evaluating the nodule shape and size. A low-frequency reconstruction algorithm is needed for evaluating nodule density.

Size and Shape

The likelihood of malignancy depends a lot on the size of the nodule in patients without prior malignancy. When the nodule is larger than 20 mm, the probability of malignancy reaches 80% to 85%. When it is smaller than 5 mm, the risk of malignancy is less than 1%.[9,28] This finding, combined with the fact that optimal diagnostic workup is not possible for such small nodules, led to the conclusion that noncalcified nodules smaller than 5 mm in diameter do not justify immediate workup, but only annual screenings to determine whether the nodule has grown. Indeterminate nodules are nodules between 5 and 20 mm in diameter, because nodules smaller than 5 mm are very likely to be benign, and

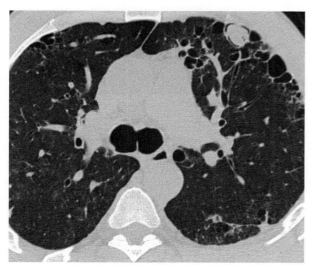

Fig. 3-5 **Pulmonary aspergilloma.** A view of the left upper lobe from a MSCT scan demonstrates a nodular opacity corresponding to a fungus ball within a peripheral subpleural cystic cavity due to honeycombing. This 44-year-old patient was referred for pulmonary fibrosis associated with collagenosis. The nodular opacity does not entirely fill up the cavity where it develops, which is usual in aspergillomas.

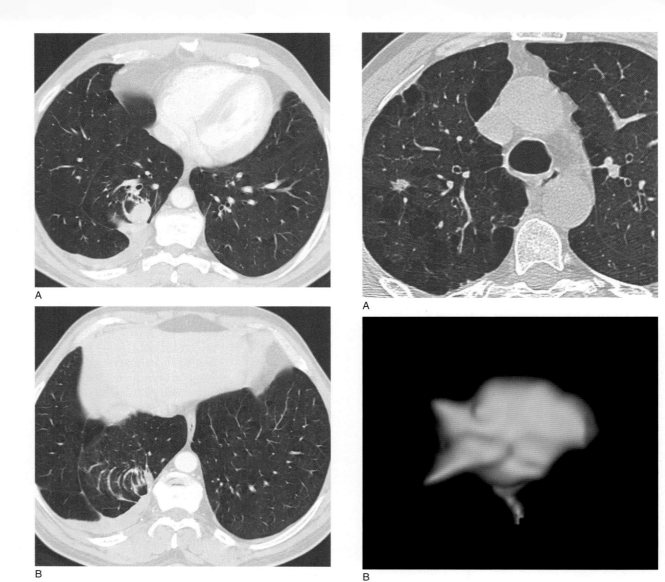

Fig. 3-6 Rounded atelectasis. MSCT scan through the right lower lobe demonstrates a rounded opacity, close to an area of pleural thickening (**A**), in a 51-year-old man. Right lower lobe shows volume loss, with posterior and medial displacement of the major fissure. Rotation of bronchovascular structures is well demonstrated (**B**).

Fig. 3-7 Malignant spiculated nodule. A view of the right upper lobe from an MSCT scan demonstrates a 12-mm–diameter spiculated nodule in a 57-year-old heavy smoker (**A**). Both upper lobes show subpleural and centrilobular emphysema. Three-dimensional surface rendering view (**B**) after segmentation of the nodule demonstrates the spiculations very well, although they were already obvious on native CT images.

nodules larger than 20 mm are likely to be malignant.

The Early Lung Cancer Action Project (ELCAP) baseline study (1999)[9] showed that 24% of the nodules between 6 and 10 mm were malignant; 33% of those between 11 and 20 mm were malignant.

Nodules with irregular borders, especially spiculated borders, are likely to be malignant (Figures 3-7 to 3-9). Spiculations, also described as the "corona radiate" sign, with fine linear strands extending outward from the nodule, indicate malignancy in 88% to 94% of cases.[28,29] Lobulated borders suggest asymmetric growth and are another predictive factor for malignancy[30] (Figure 3-10). However, lobulations occur in up to 25% of benign nodules,[31] especially in hamartomas that may show

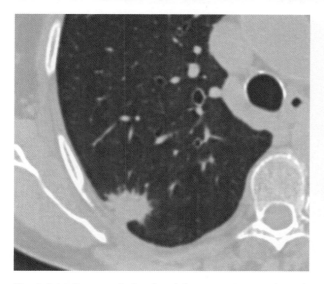

Fig. 3-8 Malignant spiculated nodule. An MSCT scan through the right upper lobe in an 81-year-old non-smoking woman demonstrates a 15-mm–diameter spiculated nodule. The diagnosis of stage I adenocarcinoma was proven at surgery.

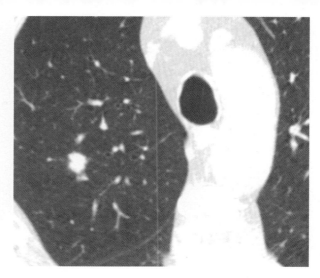

Fig. 3-10 Malignant lobulated nodule. An MSCT scan in a 65-year-old former smoker shows an 11-mm–diameter lobulated nodule in the right upper lobe. At right upper lobectomy, the nodule was shown to be an adenocarcinoma.

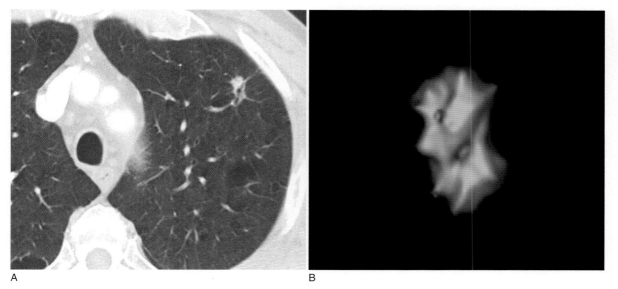

A   B

Fig. 3-9 Malignant spiculated nodule. A view of the left upper lobe from an MSCT scan demonstrates a 13-mm–diameter nodule in a 52-year-old former smoker (**A**). Air within the nodule is not due to cavitation but more likely is the result of underlying emphysema. Three-dimensional surface rendering view of the nodule (**B**) shows the spiculations more clearly. This case corresponded to squamous cell carcinoma on pathological examination.

slightly lobulated borders (see Figure 3-17). A smooth, nonlobulated border suggests a benign nodule but is also common in pulmonary metastasis. In patients with pulmonary embolism, pulmonary infarct may appear as a round, well-circumscribed nodule (Figure 3-11). Thus in oncology patients with pulmonary embolism and nodular opacity on CT, pulmonary infarct should be considered as a potential differential diagnosis of pulmonary metastasis.

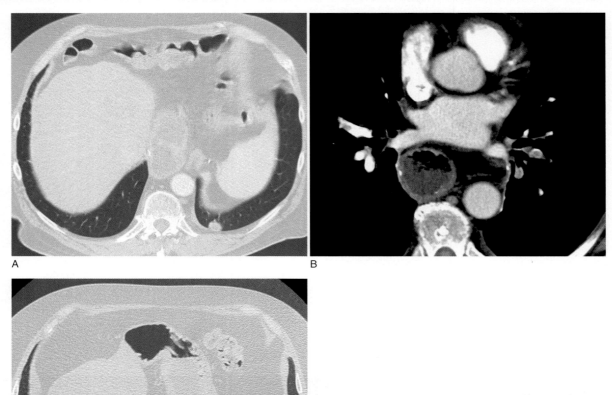

A

B

C

Fig. 3-11 Round nodule corresponding to pulmonary infarct. MSCT scan follow-up in a 66-year-old patient with esophageal carcinoma demonstrates a 17-mm–diameter left lower lobe nodule (**A**). Contrast CT also shows unexpected pulmonary embolism, with filling defects within the left lower lobe segmental arteries (**B**). Since previous CT scan did not show any radiological abnormality within the left lower lobe (**C**), the newly demonstrated nodule was interpreted as a potential metastasis. The patient underwent videothoracoscopic resection, leading to the diagnosis of round pulmonary infarct.

Number of Nodules

As discussed previously, some nodules that appear solitary on chest radiography may be associated with other nodules when viewed on CT. If the nodule remains solitary after CT, it may correspond to primary stage I lung carcinoma, but also to a unique lung metastasis or to a benign lesion. Numerous nodules are unlikely to represent primary lung carcinomas but may correspond to multiple lung metastasis, multiple granulomas, or bronchiolar nodules, in which case the typical tree-in-bud pattern is present.

Density Evaluation

Calcification

Thin-slice section CT is much more sensitive than standard radiography for the detection of calcifications within a nodule. Most of the time, visual analysis of CT images alone is sufficient to assess the presence of calcifications. In doubtful cases, quantitative measurements of attenuation values can be performed in order to confirm calcification of the nodule. Although the literature varies on this point, an attenuation value of 200 HU is advocated by many authors as a good discriminating factor between calcified and noncalcified nodules.[32]

The pattern of calcification in a solitary pulmonary nodule can help differentiate benign from malignant nodules. There are four benign patterns of calcification: central (Figure 3-12), diffuse (Figure 3-13), laminated, and "popcorn-like" (Figure 3-14). The first three patterns are typically seen in granulomatous infectious diseases, particularly histoplasmosis or tuberculosis. Popcorn-like

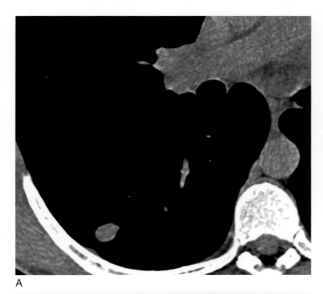

A

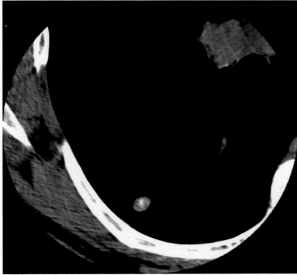

B

Fig. 3-12 Centrally calcified nodule. An MSCT scan through the right lower lobe demonstrates a noncalcified subpleural nodule (A) in a 35-year-old patient with HIV infection. The patient refused the proposed biopsy procedure. One year later (B), the nodule size had decreased, and central calcification had appeared, suggesting infectious granuloma as the cause of the nodule.

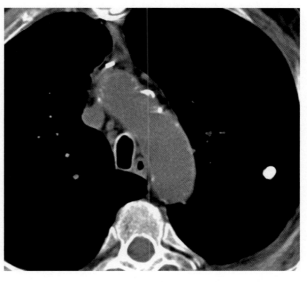

Fig. 3-13 Diffusely calcified nodule. Unenhanced MSCT image shows diffuse calcification of a left upper lobe nodule in a 60-year-old man. The nodule density is similar to that of atheromatous plaques that are seen on the thoracic aorta. Diffuse calcification of the nodule indicates its benign nature.

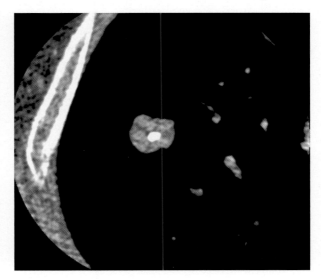

Fig. 3-14 Popcorn-like calcification. Detailed view of the right upper lobe from an MSCT scan demonstrates central, popcorn-like calcification in a non-homogeneous lobulated nodule in a 32-year-old man. This finding strongly suggests pulmonary hamartoma. The small areas of decreased attenuation may indicate a fatty component, but they were too small for an accurate attenuation value measurement.

calcification is characteristic of chondroid calcification in a hamartoma.

Calcification patterns that are stippled or eccentric have been associated with malignancy, and it is therefore important to differentiate these patterns from those associated with benign lesions. It may be especially difficult to distinguish between central and eccentric calcifications only on axial transverse CT sections. A calcification, which is closer to the top than to the bottom of a nodule, should not be considered as central, although it seems to be central on an axial transverse CT image. Such an error led to the misdiagnosis of a malignant nodule, in a case reported by Berlin (2003).[33]

The popcorn-like pattern may also be difficult to recognize. Diffuse calcification is thus the most reliable benign calcification pattern, except in a specific context such as osteosarcoma, where diffuse calcified lung metastasis may be observed. However, in these cases the primary lesion is usually known, which helps to establish a correct diagnosis.

Ground Glass Component

Even though the vast majority of noncalcified nodules are solid, totally obscuring the lung parenchyma, some noncalcified nodules present as focal ground glass opacity. They are called *non-solid nodules* (Figure 3-15). Others have a ground glass component coexisting with a solid component and are called *part-solid nodules* (Figure 3-16). These two categories represented 19% of the 233 nodules found during baseline screening of the ELCAP study.[34] They proved to be malignant in 34% of cases, whereas the malignancy rate of solid nodules was 7%. The malignancy rate for part-solid nodules was 63% (10/16), and the rate for non-solid nodules was 18% (5/28).[34] Another author reported that persistent focal ground glass opacities are associated with a high risk of malignancy, especially if lesions are larger or equal to 1 cm.[35]

Intranodular Fat

The presence of focal collections of fat within a nodule (Figures 3-17 and 3-18) with attenuation values ranging from −40 to −120 HU is a reliable indicator of a hamartoma, even though this sign is only present in 60% of the hamartomas in a study of 31 proved and 16 presumed tumors.[36] Presence of a focal area of fat proves that the nodule is benign. However, the attenuation value must be measured carefully to obviate partial volume

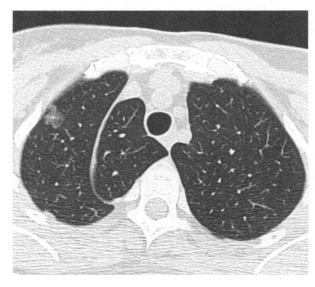

Fig. 3-15 Non-solid nodule. Lung cancer screening MSCT scan in a 53-year-old former smoker demonstrates a 16-mm–diameter, non-solid nodule in the right upper lobe. Azygos fissure is also demonstrated. The nodule remained unchanged on CT follow-up performed 1 month later, after the patient received antibiotics. At right upper lobectomy, the non-solid nodule was shown to represent a bronchioloalveolar carcinoma.

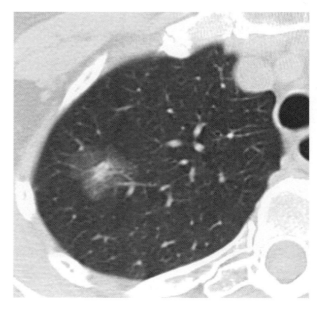

Fig. 3-16 Part-solid nodule. A view of the right upper lobe from an MSCT scan in a 58-year-old woman shows a central solid component within a 25-mm–diameter ground glass nodule. The diagnosis of adenocarcinoma was proven at surgery.

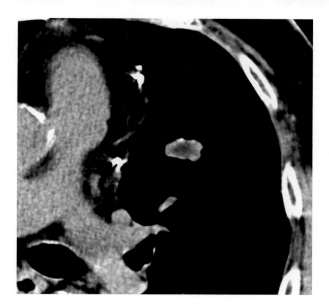

Fig. 3-17 **Intranodular fat component.** Unenhanced MSCT scan in a 74-year-old man demonstrates a 19-mm slightly lobulated nodule in the left upper lobe. Decreased attenuation is present in its central portion. The attenuation value is −60 HU, indicating a focal area of fat. This feature is diagnostic of pulmonary hamartoma.

averaging with pulmonary air at the periphery of the nodule.

Intranodular Aeric Component

There are three different patterns of intranodular aeric components, and all have a high predictive value for malignancy: cavitation with walls thicker than 5 mm (Figure 3-19), pseudocavitation (also called *bubble-like lucencies*) (Figure 3-20), and air bronchograms[32] (Figure 3-21). The latter two are more often encountered in adenocarcinomas and bronchioloalveolar carcinomas, whereas the former is more likely to be observed in squamous cell carcinomas. Air bronchograms can also be seen in pulmonary lymphoma and organized pneumonia, which may have a nodular shape.

Estimating the Probability of Malignancy on Morphological Criteria

Following morphological evaluation, lung nodules can be classified into three different categories: probably malignant, probably benign, or indeterminate nodules (Table 3-3). The last category represents the vast majority of lung nodules.[37] Probably malignant nodules are spiculated or lobulated nodules, nodules with a malignant pattern of

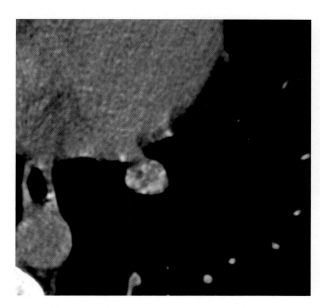

Fig. 3-18 **Intranodular fat component.** Detailed view from an MSCT scan through the left lower lobe demonstrates a retrocardiac solid noncalcified nodule, with a small area of decreased attenuation, in a 41-year-old woman. The measured attenuation value is −42 HU, indicating a focal area of fat.

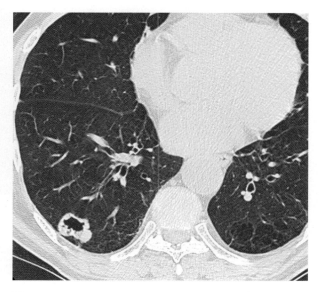

Fig. 3-19 **Cavitated nodule.** A view of the right lower lobe from an MSCT scan shows a 27-mm–diameter cavitated nodule in a 79-year-old man. The nodule walls measure up to 10 mm, which highly suggests malignancy. The diagnosis of squamous cell carcinoma was proved at surgery.

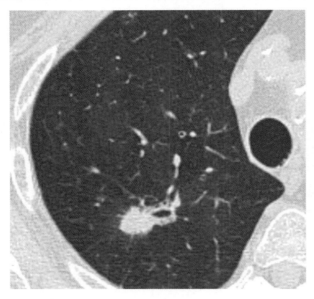

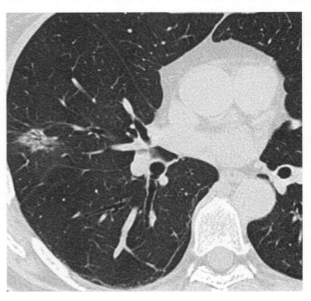

Fig. 3-20 **Bubble-like lucencies.** An MSCT scan in an 82-year-old woman shows a small focal air collection at the periphery of a right upper lobe spiculated nodule. These signs suggest malignancy. The diagnosis of adenocarcinoma was proved at surgery.

Fig. 3-21 **Air bronchogram.** An MSCT scan in a 50-year-old woman shows air bronchograms in a right upper lobe nodule. Anterior displacement of the right major fissure is also noted. These features strongly favor malignancy. At surgery, the nodule was shown to represent bronchioloalveolar carcinoma.

Table 3-3 Summary of the strongest predictive CT features for benign and malignant nodules

	Benign	Malignant
MORPHOLOGICAL CRITERIA		
Size*	Less than 5 mm (99%)†	More than 2 cm (85%)
Shape	—	Spiculated and lobulated
DENSITOMETRY		
	Fat component (100%) Global calcification (100%)	Part solid (63%)
Quantitative contrast enhancement	Less than 15 UH (98%)	—
CT estimated doubling time	More than 500 days	Less than 500 days

*In patients without prior malignancy.
† All percentages shown indicate the probability of benignity or of malignancy.

calcification, ground glass nodules larger than 1 cm, part-solid nodules, nodules with aeric components, and nodules growing in an interval under 2 years.

Probably benign nodules are those with a benign pattern of calcification and/or focal area of fat, small, grouped nodules with bronchiolar distribution and stable nodules over a 2-year period.

The 2-year stability criteria should be considered cautiously, because some slowly growing adenocarcinomas have been reported, especially in older adult patients. Bronchioalveolar and carcinoid tumors may also show slow growth patterns.

Functional Imaging with CT

Measurement of nodule enhancement and measurement of nodule growth with CT can be considered as functional imaging methods.

Lung Nodule Enhancement

Because there are differences in the vascularity of benign and malignant nodules, Swensen (2002)[22] made the hypothesis that the degree of contrast enhancement could differentiate benign from malignant lesions. He studied 356 nodules having a histological final diagnosis and found that malignant neoplasms enhanced significantly more than benign lesions. With 15 HU as a threshold value, the sensitivity was 98%. A lack of contrast enhancement had a strong predictive value for benignity. A positive test did not mean that the nodule was malignant, as the specificity of nodule enhancement was only 58%. To obtain these results, the CT acquisition and contrast medium administration protocol must follow strict criteria. A standard dose CT acquisition with a slice thickness that should not exceed half of the nodule dimension in the z-axis, and a 15-cm field of view, must be obtained 1, 2, 3, and 4 minutes after contrast agent injection (Figure 3-22 and Table 3-4). The dose of iodinated contrast

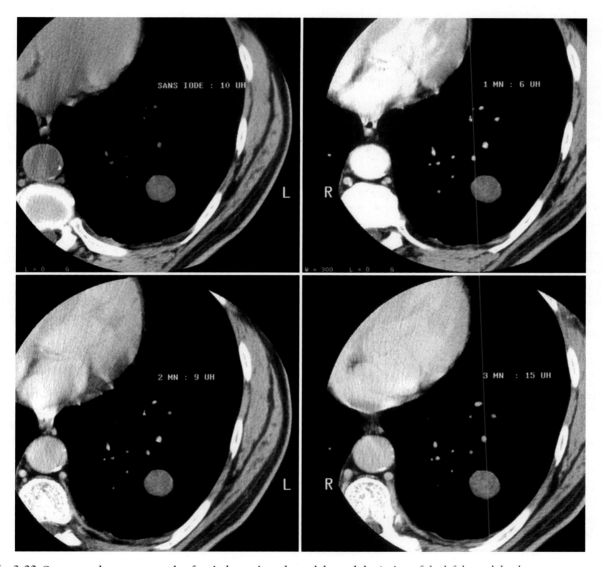

Fig. 3-22 Contrast enhancement study of an indeterminate lower lobe nodule. A view of the left lower lobe demonstrates a non-calcified 22-mm–diameter nodule with attenuation value of 10 HU on unenhanced MSCT scan. MSCT scan performed at the same level 1, 2, and 3 minutes after contrast administration shows attenuation values of 6, 9, and 15 HU, respectively. The post-contrast increase of attenuation value is less than 15 HU; therefore, the nodule can be considered benign with a 98% sensitivity. The patient was a 56-year-old woman.

Table 3-4 Parameters for contrast enhancement study

Amount of contrast	420 mg per kilogram
Delay	30 seconds,* 1 minute,[†] 2 minutes,[†] 3 minutes,[†] 4 minutes[†]
Flow velocity	2 ml/sec
mAs	Adapted to the patient's weight
kV	120 to 140
Field of view	15 cm
Slice thickness	6.25 or 1.25 (no more than half of the nodule diameter)
Reconstruction algorithm	Standard

*To depict arterial-type enhancement.
[†]Nodule enhancement less than 15 HU indicates a benign lesion (sensitivity is 98%); nodule enhancement more than 15 HU does not mean the nodule is malignant (specificity is only 58%).

medium needs to be adapted to the patient's weight and should be at least 420 mg/kg. Contrast must be injected at a rate of 2 ml/sec.

Lastly, this protocol has only been validated for relatively spherical nodules, which are homogeneous, measuring between 5 and 40 mm, without calcification or fat. Thus such a protocol is not applicable to all nodules.

Growth Assessment of Lung Nodules by CT

One way of characterizing indeterminate lung nodules is to perform CT follow-up in order to detect eventual growth of the nodules, which suggests malignancy. This monitoring is only justified for small, indeterminate lesions, especially for nodules less than 1 cm, for which other characterization methods are not easily applicable or validated. Indeed, the study of contrast enhancement and of fluorodeoxyglucose (FDG) uptake is mainly sensitive for nodules larger than 5 and 10 mm, respectively. On the other hand, nodules that are likely to be malignant, such as spiculated lesions, should not be followed up, because a histological examination should be obtained.

Monitoring indeterminate lung nodules by means of CT follow-up has proved to be efficient for lung cancer detection in the ELCAP study.[9] Nodules between 5 and 10 mm were followed up by CT scan at 3, 6, 12, and 24 months. A 2-year stability is widely recognized as a reliable indicator of benignity, even though some lung cancers may remain stable for a longer period. Data from chest radiography follow-up enabled the calculation of the approximate doubling times of lung cancer, which usually ranged between 30 and 500 days, with a mean of 100 days. However, longer doubling times have been reported for lung cancer in older adult patients, as well as for certain histological subtypes of lung cancer (e.g., slowly growing lung adenocarcinomas), where doubling times of 465 days or more can be observed.[38] Thus doubling times should not be estimated without considering the patient's age and the morphology of the nodules. In particular, ground glass nodules and nodules with air bronchograms may represent slowly growing bronchioloalveolar carcinomas or adenocarcinomas, which may have doubling times greater than 500 days. In one study estimating the mean doubling time values of confirmed lung carcinomas, values were 813 days, 457 days, and 149 days for ground glass nodules, part-solid nodules, and solid nodules, respectively.[39]

CT follow-up is mainly based on manual two-dimensional measurement of lung nodules, which has two major limitations. Some malignant nodules have asymmetric patterns of growth that 2D visualization methods may fail to identify.[40] The second and main limitation is that manual measurements are not reliable enough for an accurate detection of growth in small nodules. The repeatability of manual measurements has been found to be 1.3 mm for the best reader in one study evaluating 2D measurement repeatability.[41] This means that a 1-mm change in size, which would indicate a malignant rate of growth for a 10-mm nodule observed at a 3-month CT follow-up, may only be a result of measurement error and not to an actual change in size of the nodule. Thus manual measurement error can lead to an erroneous diagnosis of lung nodule malignancy. This is the reason why automated volumetric measurements have been developed for a more accurate estimation of lung nodule growth. These methods will be discussed later.

Other Methods of Lung Nodule Characterization

In a certain number of cases, all CT methods fail to characterize a lung nodule.

CT morphology of pulmonary nodules is often unable to differentiate benign and malignant lesions. Contrast enhancement studies are not applicable to all nodules because the low specificity of this technique does not allow nodules that show significant enhancement to be characterized as malignant.

CT follow-up is one way of managing indeterminate nodules with the risk that efficient treatment is delayed for undiagnosed malignant lesions. Therefore, a wait-and-watch strategy should not be adopted without first considering a patient's gender, age, and smoking history and how they affect the risk of malignancy. These clinical features have been combined with radiological characteristics for estimating the probability of malignancy using Bayesian analysis or other models. Another approach is to perform FDG–positron emission tomography (PET) imaging. The last option is to perform invasive procedures such as surgery or biopsy. In a small percentage of cases, even with appropriate management of indeterminate nodules, these invasive procedures will still be necessary for benign lesions.

Bayesian Analysis

Bayesian analysis uses likelihood ratios of different radiological findings (e.g., nodule size and shape) and clinical features (e.g., prior malignancy, smoking history) to estimate the probability of malignancy.[42] The likelihood ratio (LR) for a given characteristic is the ratio between the number of malignant nodules with the characteristic and the number of benign nodules with the same characteristic. A nondiscriminant characteristic has an LR of 1. An LR that is significantly greater than 1 is strongly suggestive of malignancy. An LR close to 0 strongly indicates benignity. For example, presence of hemoptysis in a patient with a solitary pulmonary nodule (SPN) has an LR value of 5.8, which is strongly suggestive of malignancy. On the other hand, the absence of hemoptysis has an LR ratio of 1, which is nondiscriminant.

In the odds-likelihood ratio form of Bayes theorem, the odds that an SPN is malignant (Odds ma) is the product of all likelihood ratios multiplied by the prior odds of malignancy (LR prior). The latter is subjectively estimated or based on the prevalence of malignancy in the patient population.

$$\text{Odds ma} = \text{LR prior} \times (\text{LR size} \times \text{LR shape} \times \text{LR smoking history})$$

The probability of malignancy is calculated as follows:

$$\text{Probability} = \text{Odds ma}/(\text{Odds ma} + 1).$$

Bayesian analysis for estimating the probability of malignancy for a given nodule can be conducted on Dr. J. Gurney's Web site at www.chestx-ray.com.

Programs for estimating the probability of nodule malignancy with Bayesian analysis are found there.

Other Probabilistic Models

Other models of pretest probability have been proposed. One such model uses logistic regression to identify six independent predictors of malignancy: age, smoking status, history of cancer, nodule diameter, spiculation, and upper lobe location.[43]

FDG-PET

PET can be considered as a functional imaging technique that uses metabolic substrates labeled with positron-emitting radioisotopes. 18-FDG, a glucose analog, is most commonly used. Increased glucose metabolism in tumors results in increased uptake and accumulation of FDG, permitting the differentiation of benign and malignant nodules.

Semiquantitative analysis can be performed using computation of standardized uptake values (SUVs) in addition to visual analysis.

FDG-PET as a single test predicts malignancy in SPNs more effectively than the standard criteria using Bayesian analysis.[44,45] FDG-PET also improves staging information of malignant nodules, especially for nodal staging and identification of unsuspected stage IV disease. The sensitivity for the diagnosis of malignant nodules is 96.8% in a meta-analysis published in 2001[46]; visual analysis seems slightly more sensitive than SUV analysis, but the difference is not statistically significant. PET-CT units that have been available recently offer the anatomical information provided by CT combined with the metabolic information provided by PET (both were acquired during a single examination and fused [Figure 3-23]). PET-CT offers the ability to accurately localize increased FDG activity. Small nodule size is one recognized limitation of PET sensitivity. SUV analysis has only an 80% sensitivity for detecting malignant nodules with a size equal or less than 1.5 cm.[47]

In fact, the sensitivity is mainly dependent on the metabolic activity. High-grade malignant subcentimetric nodules may be detected, whereas larger, low-grade malignant nodules may be missed. Ground glass and part-solid nodules corresponding to bronchioloalveolar or slowly growing adenocarcinomas may show negative PET results, as well as carcinoid tumors.[48]

Analyzing nodule CT morphology helps decide whether FDG-PET is a pertinent strategy and also helps analyze FDG-PET results. FDG-PET does not have a high negative predictive value for small nodules, ground glass, and part-solid nodules and thus should not be used to evaluate such nodules.

Invasive Procedures

When noninvasive methods fail to characterize indeterminate nodules, bronchoscopy, transthoracic needle aspiration[49] or core biopsy,[50] video-assisted thoracoscopic surgery (VATS), or thoracotomy may be performed. Bronchoscopy is often negative for peripheral nodules, except for cavitated lesions for which aspiration technique is more frequently contributive. Transthoracic needle aspiration and core biopsy (Figure 3-24) are optimally used in peripheral nodules. Both have a high accuracy in diagnosing malignancy,[51-53] reaching 96%. However, accuracy is lower (74%) for nodules smaller than 1.5 cm.[54] Core biopsy allows a histological study, which is more effective for diagnosing a specific benign entity.[55] Complications, most notably pneumothorax and hemorrhage, occur in approximately

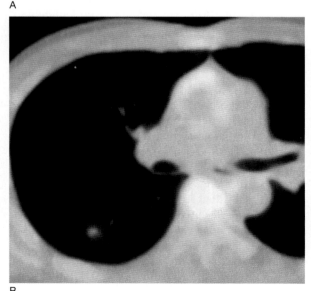

Fig. 3-23 PET-CT. CT scan through the upper segment of the right lower lobe demonstrates a 5-mm–diameter noncalcified nodule (**A**). PET-CT fused image (**B**) demonstrates FDG uptake of the nodule, which strongly favors malignancy. The patient was a 55-year-old man.

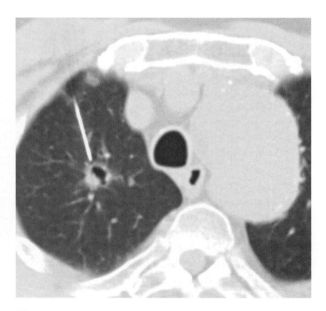

Fig. 3-24 Core biopsy of a cavitated pulmonary nodule. MSCT scan in a 68-year-old man shows a 19-gauge needle, accepting a 20-gauge semiautomatic cutting needle, placed at the periphery of a right upper lobe cavitated nodule. Several samples of the lesion can be obtained with coaxial needles. The nodule was proved to be an undifferentiated lung carcinoma.

5% to 30% of patients.[56,57] Hemorrhage is almost always self-limiting, and only about 15% of patients with pneumothoraces will eventually require chest tube placement.[56,57]

Video-assisted thoracic surgery is considered to be systematically diagnostic. The reported morbidity is 9.6%, and the mortality is 0.5%.[58] It is mainly indicated for peripheral lesions. For central lesions, there is a risk of conversion to thoracotomy.

Management Alternatives

Management alternatives for patients with nodules remaining indeterminate on CT include invasive procedures, FDG-PET, or watchfulness (Figure 3-25). Surgery is the diagnostic gold standard and the definitive treatment for resectable malignant nodules but should be avoided in patients with benign nodules. Biopsy often establishes a specific diagnosis, but it is also invasive and difficult to perform for small lesions, requiring highly experienced radiologists. Watchfulness avoids unnecessary invasive procedures but may delay diagnosis and treatment of malignant nodules. FDG-PET should be used predominantly when pretest probability and CT findings are discordant or in patients with intermediate pretest probability who are at high risk for surgical complications.[59] FDG-PET is less useful for small nodules. Their management

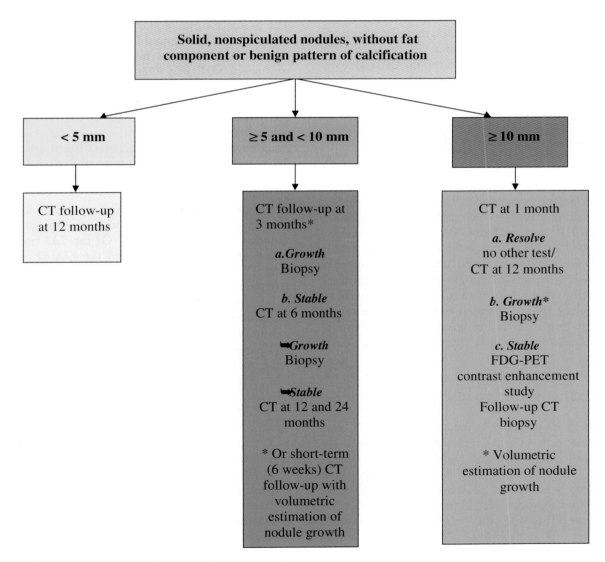

Fig. 3-25 Diagnostic algorithm (patients with no prior malignancy).

should be considered separately.[60] One possibility could be short-term observation of nodule growth by CT volumetry.

NEW TOOLS DEVELOPED WITH MSCT

Computer-Aided Diagnosis

A single CT examination on multislice CT produces a large quantity of image data. Therefore, computer-aided diagnosis (CAD) tools have been developed to automatically detect pulmonary nodules on CT images. MSCT has facilitated their development.[61] Their role is to help radiologists with the detection of pulmonary nodules; they may represent a valuable second opinion in a clinical setting for lung cancer screening. To be useful, CAD systems have to be sensitive and relatively specific. In other words, they need to detect nodules with an acceptable false-positive rate.

Using the CAD system has improved the board-certified radiologist's and resident's detection of pulmonary nodules at chest CT in the series of Awai et al. (2004).[62] In another study, the CAD system detected 12 nodules greater than or equal to 5 mm that were not mentioned in the radiologist's report, although they represented real nodules.[63] Armato et al. (2002)[64] applied their CAD system in a database of low-dose CT scans performed for lung cancer screening and found that 84% (32 of 38) of cancers that had been missed initially by radiologists were correctly detected by their CAD system, with an average of 1.0 false-positive detection per section.[64] Gurcan et al. (2002)[65] observed a comparable rate of false positive per slice (1.74) with another CAD system.

Software Evaluation of Doubling Time

By using the volumetric data from spiral CT, it is possible to develop computer programs that allow nodule segmentation and nodule volume measurement. For estimating lung nodule growth, these techniques have been proved to be more accurate and more reproducible[66,67] than manual 2D measurement. They are also more sensitive to small changes in volume (Figure 3-26), which are not as readily detectable at analysis of serial 2D images, because a change in diameter is only one third of the change in volume for spherical nodules. Because they are more reproducible and more sensitive, automated volumetric measurements should become the gold standard for nodule growth assessment. MSCT technique allowed the development of such volumetric measurements tools, which use a segmentation process based on threshold or gradient technique of segmentation, requiring thin slice to minimize volume averaging effects. Critical time to follow-up CT for nodules detected at baseline screening could be shortened from 3 months to 1 month for those with initial sizes between 5 and 10 mm.[67]

Pulmonary Nodules in Patients with a Known Primary Tumor

The presence of pulmonary nodules at chest CT in oncology patients should be considered separately.

Previous or current history of thoracic or extrathoracic malignancy increases the probability of malignancy of indeterminate lung nodules. The likelihood ratio of previous malignancy in Bayesian analysis is 4.95, nearly as high as the presence of hemoptysis, with size greater than 3 cm or spiculated borders, for which likelihood ratios are 5.08, 5.23, and 5.54, respectively.

Comparing the results among different series confirms these data.

In lung cancer screening studies, which exclude patients with prior malignancy, the vast majority of nodules found were benign.[9] Of the 233 nodules found at baseline screening in the ELCAP study, only 27 (12%) were proven to be malignant; the remaining 206 (88%) were benign. On the other hand, in the series of Quint et al. (2000)[68] that analyzed solitary pulmonary nodules in patients with extrapulmonary neoplasms, only 30 (19%) of the 161 patients with pulmonary nodules and extrathoracic malignancy had benign lesions; the remaining 131 patients (81%) had primary lung cancer (81/161, 50%) or metastasis (50/161, 31%). In this series, malignant lesions more frequently corresponded to non-small cell lung carcinoma than to metastasis, except in patients with melanoma, sarcoma, or testicular carcinoma.

However, surgical series generally overestimate the proportion of malignant lesions. In the series of Mery et al. (2004),[69] 68% of resected solitary pulmo-nary nodules were proved to be malignant, whereas benign lesions only represented 32% of the nodules. In this series, the proportion of malignant nodules was 63% in patients with no previous

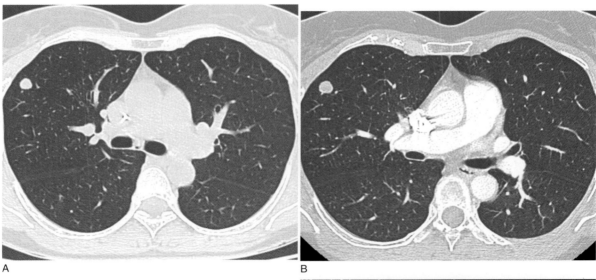

Fig. 3-26 Short-term assessment of nodule growth by volumetric software. An MSCT scan in a 60-year-old woman with an ovarian malignancy demonstrates a right upper lobe noncalcified nodule, with regular borders (**A**). CT follow-up 6 weeks later (**B**) showed no obvious change of the nodule size, based on visual assessment. The diameter increase was measured to be only 0.9 mm, which did not represent a significant change. Comparative volumetric measurements (**C**) revealed a 41% increase of the nodule volume, and the doubling time was estimated to be 114 days, which is typical for a malignant pulmonary nodule. At surgical excision, the nodule was proved to represent ovarian cancer metastasis, which is uncommon. This case illustrates that volumetric measurements are more sensitive for small changes in nodule size than diameter measurements.

cancer, 82% in those with a history of lung cancer, and 79% in patients with a history of extrapulmonary cancer. However, this series dealt with patients who had undergone surgical resection of their pulmonary nodules, which represents a strong bias.

Ginsberg et al. (1999)[70] analyzed the etiology of pulmonary nodules resected at video-assisted thoracoscopic surgery. The proportion of malignant lesions was 59% in patients with a known primary neoplasm. For nodules equal to or less than 5 mm, the proportion of malignancy was 42% in this series, compared with 32% in patients with no prior malignancy and nodules measuring 5 mm or less. This latter percentage is much higher than the percentage reported in the ELCAP study, where fewer than 1% of nodules measuring 5 mm or less were

found to be malignant. This discrepancy can again be explained by the fact that the series of Ginsberg is a surgical series, which introduces a bias, because not every patient with previous malignancy and nodules less than 5 mm is referred for VATS resection.

Nonsurgical series, which rely on follow-up, have a very different estimation of the proportion of malignant lesions among nodules found in patients with a known primary tumor.

Chalmers and Best (1991)[71] evaluated lung nodules detected on CT but not on chest radiography in patients with primary extrathoracic tumors. They found that in more than 80% of the cases, the nodules were benign. Keogan et al. (1993)[72] investigated small 4- to 12-mm nodules in patients with a primary lung cancer and found that 70% were benign, 11% were malignant, and the nature of the remaining 19% could not be determined.

In summary, previous history of malignancy is theoretically associated with an increased risk for malignancy in patients with indeterminate nodules. It is estimated at 59% overall and at 44% for nodules equal to or less than 5 mm, based on VATS resection series, which may have an overestimating bias. Series based on follow-up estimate the rate of malignancy of small nodules not to exceed 30%. However, these series may underestimate the malignancy rate, because malignant nodules can resolve or decrease after therapy or grow so slowly that they appear unchanged on follow-up CT.

For these reasons, it is not possible to propose a standardized diagnostic algorithm for nodules found in patients with a known primary tumor. To evaluate the probability of malignancy, the size of the nodule and the stage and type of the primary tumor have to be taken into account. It is also important to evaluate the impact of the therapeutic strategy of diagnosing the indeterminate nodules as malignant. For example, a nodule contralateral to the primary tumor in a patient with a resectable lung cancer should be assessed histologically first, before deciding whether to perform the surgical resection.

Lung Nodules and Lung Cancer Screening with CT

Lung cancer is now the most common cause of cancer-related death among men and women. However, patients with stage I surgical stage may have 10-year survival rates of up to 70%. This rationale is the basis for early detection programs using low-dose unenhanced CT scans. The first screening studies, with single slice CT technology, found two important results. CT screening detects lung cancer at early stages; for instance, 96% of the detected cancers in the ELCAP study were resectable. The second important result is that CT screening is positive in a great proportion of patients, showing lung nodules in 23% to 51% of the patients at baseline screening in the different series. Because MSCT allows the acquisition of thinner slices and the detection of smaller nodules, the proportion of positive CT scans could be even higher when MSCT is used.

Lung cancer screening studies also provided new information on lung nodules, such as the proportion of malignancy of part-solid nodules[34] and the malignancy rate of small nodules less than 5 mm,[9]

that were not previously known. Thus lung cancer screening helped the diagnostic workup of pulmonary nodules.

The benefit of lung cancer CT screening strategy has not yet been fully validated, as several biases have been described in the first single-arm CT screening studies. These biases have been described as lead-time bias, length bias, and overdiagnosis. They could lead to an overestimation of screening benefits.

Lead-time bias is observed when comparisons between screening and nonscreening cases are not adjusted for the timing of diagnosis. If CT screening detects lung cancer earlier, screened patients appear to have longer survival times than nonscreened patients, for whom diagnosis is made based on symptoms, even if death is not delayed in the screened group. The longer survival of screened patients is not due to delayed death but to earlier diagnosis during the preclinical phase.

Length bias refers to the tendency of screening to detect slow-growing cancers. Slow-growing cancers have a longer preclinical period, and are more likely to be detected by screening than are highly malignant lesions with short preclinical periods. Thus, screening tends to detect tumors of more indolent biology and of better prognosis.

Overdiagnosis bias refers to the detection of lung cancer that would have remained subclinical until death. All lung cancers are not necessarily lethal. This is supported by some autopsy studies that have found malignant pulmonary nodules in patients who have died of diseases other than lung cancer.[73]

Several randomized controlled trials have been initiated to circumvent these potential screening biases. Their aim is to establish whether the lung cancer–specific mortality is reduced in the screened patients, because lung cancer–specific mortality is the most appropriate measure of screening effectiveness.

If lung cancer screening is demonstrated to be effective, management of pulmonary nodules will represent a very important part in the routine radiological practice, because many nodules in many patients will require investigation.

CONCLUSION

The ability to detect pulmonary nodules, especially small nodules, has been increased by the introduction of MSCT technology, which allows thin-slice acquisition through the whole thorax within a short breath-hold time. The development of computer-aided diagnostic tools has been facilitated, and these tools may help the radiologist to accurately detect lung nodules by providing a second reading.

High-resolution MSCT also improves nodule characterization in accurately assessing nodule morphology and enhancement patterns. Finally, MSCT allows the use of volumetric software for a better estimation of short-term nodule growth. Estimation of doubling time in consecutive MSCT acquisitions offers a noninvasive way of characterizing indeterminate nodules. This method should prove useful especially for small nodules, for which other noninvasive characterization procedures cannot be used or fail.

Because of the increased detection with MSCT, accurate management of pulmonary nodules will become a major and challenging problem in clinical routine, especially if lung cancer CT screening is fully validated in the coming years.

REFERENCES

1. Muhm JR, Miller WE, Fontana RS, et al: Lung cancer detected during a screening program using 4-month chest radiographs, *Radiology* 148(3):609-615, 1983.
2. Austin JHM, Romney BM, Goldsmith LS: Missed bronchogenic carcinoma: radiographic findings in 27 patients with a potentially resectable lesion evident in retrospect, *Radiology* 182(1):115-122, 1992.
3. Friese SA, Rieber A, Fleiter T, et al: Pulmonary nodules in spiral volumetric and single slice computed tomography, *Eur J Radiol* 18(1):48-51, 1994.
4. Remy-Jardin M, Remy J, Giraud F, et al: Pulmonary nodules: detection with thick-section spiral CT versus conventional CT, *Radiology* 187(2):513-520, 1993.
5. Seemann MD, Staebler A, Beinert T, et al: Usefulness of morphological characteristics for the differentiation of benign from malignant solitary pulmonary lesions using HRCT, *Eur Radiol* 9(3):409-417, 1999.
6. Khouri NF, Meziane MA, Zerhouni EA, et al: The solitary pulmonary nodule: assessment, diagnosis, and management, *Chest* 91(1):128-133, 1987.
7. Erasmus JJ, Connolly JE, McAdams HP, et al: Solitary pulmonary nodules. I. Morphologic evaluation for differentiation of benign and malignant lesions, *Radiographics* 20(1):43-58, 2000.
8. Lillington GA: Management of solitary pulmonary nodules. How to decide when resection is required, *Postgrad Med* 101(3):145-150, 1997.
9. Henschke CI, McCauley DI, Yankelevitz DF, et al: Early Lung Cancer Action Project: overall design and findings from baseline screening, *Lancet* 354(9173):99-105, 1999.
10. Swensen SJ, Jett JR, Hartman TE, et al: Lung cancer screening with CT: Mayo Clinic experience, *Radiology* 226(3):756-761, 2003.
11. Fischbach F, Knollmann F, Griesshaber V, et al: Detection of pulmonary nodules by multislice computed tomography: improved detection rate with reduced slice thickness, *Eur Radiol* 13(10):2378-2383, 2003.
12. Diederich S, Lentschig MG, Winter F, et al: Detection of pulmonary nodules with overlapping vs. non-overlapping image reconstruction at spiral CT, *Eur Radiol* 9(2):281-286, 1999.
13. Karabulut N, Toru M, Gelebek V, et al: Comparison of low-dose and standard-dose helical CT in the evaluation of pulmonary nodules, *Eur Radiol* 12(11):2764-2769, 2002.
14. Diederich S, Lenzen H, Windmann R, et al: Pulmonary nodules: experimental and clinical studies at low-dose CT, *Radiology* 213(1):289-298, 1999.
15. Rusinek H, Naidich DP, McGuinness G, et al: Pulmonary nodule detection: low-dose versus conventional CT, *Radiology* 209(1):243-249, 1998.
16. Coakley FV, Cohen MD, Johnson MS, et al: Maximum intensity projection images in the detection of simulated pulmonary nodules by spiral CT, *Br J Radiol* 71(842):135-140, 1998.
17. Diederich S, Lentschig MG, Overbeck TR, et al: Detection of pulmonary nodules at spiral CT: comparison of maximum intensity projection sliding slabs and single-image reporting, *Eur Radiol* 11(8):1345-1350, 2001.
18. Gruden JF, Ouanounou S, Tigges S, et al: Incremental benefit of maximum-intensity-projection images on observer detection of small pulmonary nodules revealed by multidetector CT, *Am J Roentgenol* 179(1):149-157, 2002.
19. Croisille P, Souto M, Cova M, et al: Pulmonary nodules: improved detection with vascular segmentation and extraction with spiral CT. Work in progress, *Radiology* 197(2):397-401, 1995.
20. Seltzer SE, Judy PF, Adams DF, et al: Spiral CT of the chest: comparison of cine and film-based viewing, *Radiology* 197(1):73-78, 1995.
21. Tillich M, Kammerhuber F, Reittner P, et al: Detection of pulmonary nodules with helical CT: comparison of cine and film-based viewing, *Am J Roentgenol* 169(6):1611-1614, 1997.
22. Swensen SJ, Viggiano RW, Midthun DE, et al: Lung nodule enhancement at CT: multicenter study, *Radiology* 214(1):73-80, 2000.
23. Remy-Jardin M, Remy J: Spiral CT angiography of the pulmonary circulation, *Radiology* 212(3):615-636, 1999.
24. Diederich S, Wormanns D, Semik M, et al: Screening for early lung cancer with low-dose spiral CT: prevalence in 817 asymptomatic smokers, *Radiology* 222(3):773-781, 2002.
25. Sone S, Li F, Yang ZG, et al: Results of three-year mass screening programme for lung cancer using mobile low-dose spiral computed tomography scanner, *Br J Cancer* 84(1):25-32, 2001.
26. Pick A, Deschamps C, Stanson AW: Pulmonary arteriovenous fistula: presentation, diagnosis and treatment, *World J Surg* 23(11):1118-1122, 1999.
27. McHugh K, Blaquiere RM: CT features of rounded atelectasis, *Am J Roentgenol* 153(2):257-260, 1989.
28. Zerhouni EA, Stilik FP, Siegelman SS, et al: CT of the pulmonary nodule. A cooperative study, *Radiology* 160(2):319-327, 1986.
29. Henschke CI, Yankelevitz DF, et al: CT screening for lung cancer: suspiciousness of nodules according to size on baseline scans, *Radiology* 231(1):164-168, 2004.

30. Zwirewich CV, Vedal S, Miller RR, et al: Solitary pulmonary nodule: high-resolution CT and radiologic-pathologic correlation, *Radiology* 179(2):469-476, 1991.

31. Huston J, III, Muhm JR: Solitary pulmonary opacities: plain tomography, *Radiology* 163(2):481-485, 1987.

32. Kuriyama K, Tateishi R, Doi O, et al: Prevalence of air bronchograms in small peripheral carcinomas of the lung on thin-section CT: comparison with benign tumors, *Am J Roentgenol* 156(5):921-924, 1991.

33. Berlin L: Failure to diagnose lung cancer: anatomy of a malpractice trial, *Am J Roentgenol* 180(1):37-45, 2003.

34. Henschke CI, Yankelevitz DF, Mirtcheva R, et al: ELCAP Group: CT screening for lung cancer: frequency and significance of part-solid and nonsolid nodules, *Am J Roentgenol* 178(5):1053-1057, 2002.

35. Nakata M, Saeki H, Takata I, et al: Focal ground-glass opacity detected by low-dose helical CT, *Chest* 121(5):1464-1467, 2002.

36. Siegelman SS, Khouri NF, Scott WW, Jr, et al: Pulmonary hamartoma: CT findings, *Radiology* 160(2):313-317, 1986.

37. Ost D, Fein A: Evaluation and management of the solitary pulmonary nodule, *Am J Respir Crit Care Med* 162(3[1]):782-787, 2000.

38. Winer-Muram HT, Jennings SG, Tarver RD, et al: Volumetric growth rate of stage I lung cancer prior to treatment: serial CT scanning, *Radiology* 223(3):798-805, 2002.

39. Hasegawa M, Sone S, Takashima S, et al: Growth rate of small lung cancers detected on mass CT screening, *Br J Radiol* 73(876):1252-1259, 2000.

40. Yankelevitz DF, Reeves AP, Kostis WJ, et al: Small pulmonary nodules: volumetrically determined growth rates based on CT evaluation, *Radiology* 217(1):251-256, 2000.

41. Revel MP, Bissery A, Bienvenu M, et al: Are two-dimensional CT measurements of small noncalcified pulmonary nodules reliable? *Radiology* 231(2):453-458, 2004.

42. Gurney JW: Determining the likelihood of malignancy in solitary pulmonary nodules with Bayesian analysis. I. Theory, *Radiology* 186(2):405-413, 1993.

43. Swensen SJ, Silverstein MD, Ilstrup DM, et al: The probability of malignancy in solitary pulmonary nodules. Application to small radiologically indeterminate nodules, *Arch Intern Med* 157(8):849-855, 1997.

44. Gould MK, Lillington GA: Strategy and cost in investigating solitary pulmonary nodules, *Thorax* 53 (suppl)2:S32-37, 1998.

45. Dewan NA, Shehan CJ, Reeb SD, et al: Likelihood of malignancy in a solitary pulmonary nodule: comparison of Bayesian analysis and results of FDG-PET scan, *Chest* 112(2):416-422, 1997.

46. Gould MK, Maclean CC, Kuschner WG, et al: Accuracy of positron emission tomography for diagnosis of pulmonary nodules and mass lesions: a meta-analysis, *JAMA* 285(7):914-924, 2001.

47. Lowe VJ, Fletcher JW, Gobar L, et al: Prospective investigation of PET in lung nodules (PIOPILN), *J Clin Oncol* 16(3):1075-1084, 1998.

48. Libby DM, Smith JP, Altorki NK, et al: Managing the small pulmonary nodule discovered by CT, *Chest* 125(4):1522-1529, 2004.

49. Ohno Y, Hatabu H, Takenaka D, et al: CT-guided transthoracic needle aspiration biopsy of small (< or = 20 mm) solitary pulmonary nodules, *Am J Roentgenol* 180(6):1665-1669, 2003.

50. Lucidarme O, Howarth N, Finet JF, et al: Intrapulmonary lesions: percutaneous automated biopsy with a detachable, 18-gauge, coaxial cutting needle, *Radiology* 207(3):759-765, 1998.

51. Laurent F, Latrabe V, Vergier B, et al: Percutaneous CT-guided biopsy of the lung: comparison between aspiration and automated cutting needles using a coaxial technique, *Cardiovasc Intervent Radiol* 23(4):266-272, 2000.

52. Klein JS, Zarka MA: Thoracic needle biopsy: an overview, *J Thorac Imaging* 12(4):232-249, 1997.

53. Westcott JL, Rao N, Colly DP: Transthoracic needle biopsy of small pulmonary nodules, *Radiology* 202(1):97-103, 1997.

54. Li H, Boiselle PM, Shepard JO, et al: Diagnostic accuracy and safety of CT-guided percutaneous needle aspiration biopsy of the lung: comparison of small and large pulmonary nodules, *Am J Roentgenol* 167(1):105-109, 1996.

55. Klein JS, Salomon G, Stewart EA: Transthoracic needle biopsy with a coaxially placed 20-gauge automated cutting needle: results in 122 patients, *Radiology* 198(3):715-720, 1996.

56. Moore EH: Needle-aspiration lung biopsy: a comprehensive approach to complication reduction, *J Thorac Imaging* 12(4):259-271, 1997.

57. Miller JA, Pramanik BK, Lavenhar MA: Predicting the rates of success and complications of computed tomography-guided core-needle biopsies of the thorax from the findings of the preprocedure chest computed tomography scan, *J Thorac Imaging* 13(1):7-13, 1998.

58. Jimenez MF: Prospective study on video-assisted thoracoscopic surgery in the resection of pulmonary nodules: 209 cases from the Spanish Video-Assisted Thoracic Surgery Study Group, *Eur J Cardiothorac Surg* 19(5):562-565, 2001.

59. Gould MK, Sanders GD, Barnett PG, et al: Cost-effectiveness of alternative management strategies for patients with solitary pulmonary nodules, *Ann Intern Med* 138(9):724-735, 2003.

60. Libby DM, Smith JP, Altorki NK, et al: Managing the small pulmonary nodule discovered by CT, *Chest* 125(4):1522-1529, 2004.

61. Ko JP, Naidich DP: Lung nodule detection and characterization with multislice CT, *Radiol Clin North Am* 41(3):575-597, 2003.

62. Awai K, Murao K, Ozawa A, et al: Pulmonary nodules at chest CT: effect of computer-aided diagnosis on radiologists' detection performance, *Radiology* 230(2):347-352, 2004.

63. Wormanns D, Fiebich M, Saidi M, et al: Automatic detection of pulmonary nodules at spiral CT: clinical application of a computer-aided diagnosis system, *Eur Radiol* 12(5):1052-1057, 2002.

64. Armato SG, III, Li F, Giger ML, et al: Lung cancer: performance of automated lung nodule detection applied to cancers missed in a CT screening program, *Radiology* 225(3):685-692, 2002.

65. Gurcan MN, Sahiner B, Petrick N, et al: Lung nodule detection on thoracic computed tomography images: preliminary evaluation of a computer-aided diagnosis system, *Med Phys* 29(11):2552-2558, 2002.

66. Revel MP, Lefort C, Bissery A, et al: Pulmonary nodules: preliminary experience with three-dimensional evaluation, *Radiology* 231(2):459-466, 2004.

67. Wormanns D, Kohl G, Klotz E, et al: Volumetric measurements of pulmonary nodules at multi-row detector CT: in vivo reproducibility, *Eur Radiol* 14(1):86-92, 2004.

68. Quint LE, Park CH, Iannettoni MD: Solitary pulmonary nodules in patients with extrapulmonary neoplasms, *Radiology* 217(1):257-261, 2000.

69. Mery CM, Pappas AN, Bueno R, et al: Relationship between a history of antecedent cancer and the probability of malignancy for a solitary pulmonary nodule, *Chest* 125(6):2175-2181, 2004.

70. Ginsberg MS, Griff SK, Go BD, et al: Pulmonary nodules resected at video-assisted thoracoscopic surgery: etiology in 426 patients, *Radiology* 213(1):277-282, 1999.

71. Chalmers N, Best JJ: The significance of pulmonary nodules detected by CT but not by chest radiography in tumour staging, *Clin Radiol* 44(6):410-412, 1991.

72. Keogan MT, Tung KT, Kaplan DK, et al: The significance of pulmonary nodules detected on CT staging for lung cancer, *Clin Radiol* 48(2):94-96, 1993.

73. McFarlane MJ, Feinstein AR, Wells CK, et al: The "epidemiologic necropsy." Unexpected detections, demographic selections, and changing rates of lung cancer, *JAMA* 258(3):331-338, 1987.

4

Multislice Computed Tomography in the Investigation of Interstitial Lung Disease

Bobby Bhartia
Ella A. Kazerooni

The foundation for pulmonary high-resolution computed tomography (HRCT) was laid when Itoh et al. (1978)[1] demonstrated postmortem radiographs of lung thin sections, showing how they accurately depicted the anatomy of the secondary pulmonary lobule and the anatomic distribution of small pulmonary nodules. HRCT was initially used in the evaluation of the detailed, complex skull base anatomy.[2,3] Initial descriptions of HRCT in pulmonary disease are credited to Todo et al. (1982)[4] from Japan and appeared in the English literature with Nakata et al. (1985).[5] They demonstrated that HRCT was sensitive for the detection of diffuse peripheral lung disease and accurately correlated with the pathological findings.

The term *high resolution* encompasses techniques that combine the thinnest attainable beam collimation with reconstruction algorithms designed to produce high spatial resolution. The aim is to optimize the demonstration of the fine lung parenchymal anatomy. By analyzing the distribution of pathology relative to normal anatomy, potential etiologies can be determined. Before the advent of multislice CT (MSCT), HRCT techniques used incremental scanning to sample the lung parenchyma. In addition to supine inspiratory images, expiratory images may be obtained to look for air trapping and small airway disease, and prone images may be performed to reduce dependent opacities that may exaggerate the severity of disease or mimic its presence. MSCT allows large anatomical areas to be imaged rapidly using narrow slice collimation. Sixteen-row and greater MSCT allows isotropic imaging with voxels of equal dimensions in the x, y and z axes, thereby permitting distortion-free image reconstruction in any plane. Images obtained at thin beam collimation can be reconstructed into thin and thick images from the same data set. In this chapter we will review the anatomical and technical considerations for evaluating the lung parenchyma, review what is known about multislice HRCT, and suggest indications for which volumetric imaging may be superior to standard incremental HRCT studies.

ANATOMICAL CONSIDERATIONS

Axial incremental HRCT using a 1-mm beam collimation has a pixel size of 0.68 mm using a 35-cm scanning field of view (SFOV) and a 512 × 512 matrix. Despite this, objects as small as 0.1 mm in diameter can be identified if their attenuation is significantly different from surrounding structures. The smallest functional anatomical unit normally identified on HRCT, the secondary pulmonary lobule, measures 10 to 25 mm in diameter (Figure 4-1). The center of the lobule consists of a pulmonary arteriole and bronchiole supported by axial interstitial fibers that originate at the hilum and radiate outward along the airways.[6,7] The central bronchiole of the secondary pulmonary lobule measures 1 mm in diameter, with walls less than 0.1 mm thick. Airways less than 2 mm in diameter are not visible on HRCT because of the thin walls and partial volume averaging of air within and surrounding the bronchiole with the thin wall. However, arterioles as small as 0.2 mm in diameter are normally seen as branching structures extending to within 3 to 5 mm of the pleural surface. Visualization of the central arteriole is used to define the center of the secondary pulmonary lobule.[8] The periphery of the lobule includes pulmonary veins and lymphatics contained within the interlobular septa that extend from the visceral pleura of the

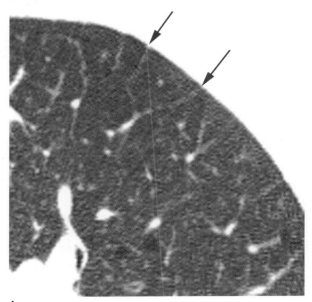

A

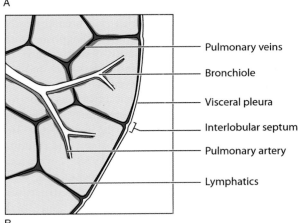

B

Fig. 4-1 The secondary pulmonary lobule as seen on volumetric HRCT (**A**) and a schematic diagram (**B**). The interlobular septa may occasionally be seen in normal subjects and denote the borders of the secondary pulmonary lobule *(arrows)*. The opacity at the center of the lobule represents the central arteriole. Note that the peripheral airways are not visible. (Reproduced courtesy of E.A. Kazerooni and the American Journal of Radiology.)

lung. The interlobular septa are 0.1 mm thick and 1.25 cm long. Occasionally they are visible in normal lungs when oriented orthogonally to the scan plane as nontapering linear opacities extending from the periphery of the lung. They are best seen in the nondependent anterior and lateral portions of the middle and upper lobes. Within the lobule are terminal bronchioles and alveoli, supported by a network of intralobular septa; the latter are very small and can be visualized only when they are abnormal.

INCREMENTAL HRCT TECHNIQUES

Early clinical studies convincingly demonstrated that HRCT is more sensitive than both conventional thick section CT and chest radiography for the detection and characterization of interstitial lung disease.[5,9,10] For example, in one study of 118 patients with various interstitial lung diseases (predominantly usual interstitial pneumonia, silicosis, sarcoidosis, and lymphangitis), the correct first-choice diagnosis was made in 57% of chest radiographs compared with 76% of HRCT examinations.[11] In addition, there is a greater degree of confidence in the first-choice diagnosis with HRCT than chest radiography. Comparisons of HRCT to conventional CT show that both modalities are equivalent for assessment of large parenchymal abnormalities, but that HRCT is superior for demonstrating fine abnormalities, including pleural thickening and irregularity, small cystic airspaces, ground-glass opacities, fibrosis, and traction bronchiectasis.[10] Murata et al. (1988)[12] evaluated the optimal collimation for HRCT techniques. With both 1.5- and 3-mm thick images, linear structures, such as normal and thickened septa and small bronchi, were equally visualized. However, abnormalities that result in a subtle increase or decrease in attenuation, such as ground-glass opacity or emphysema, were better identified on narrower collimation images (Figure 4-2). High spatial reconstruction algorithms further improve visualization of both normal and pathological structures.[12,13] However, the high-resolution technique comes at the expense of increased image noise, particularly in the paravertebral regions and across the shoulders (Figure 4-3). However, this does not interfere with diagnosis in the majority of patients. For obese patients, thicker collimations of 2.5 to 3 mm should be considered when thinner images are nondiagnostic because of severe image noise.

Two widely used supplementary HRCT techniques are prone imaging and scans performed at end-expiration. Prone images aid the assessment of early pulmonary fibrosis and differentiate subpleural changes from dependent atelectasis.[14]

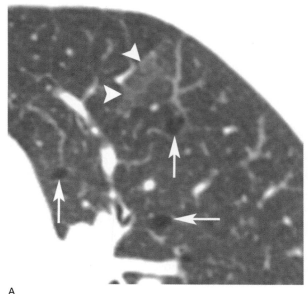

A

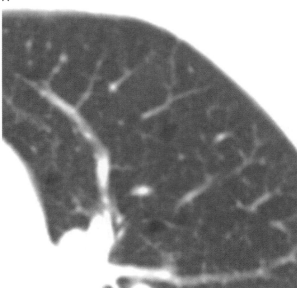

B

Fig. 4-2 Volumetric HRCT at varying slice reconstructions. Ground-glass opacity *(arrowheads)* seen on the 1.25-mm slice thickness image (**A**) is not visible on the 2.5-mm slice thickness image (**B**), and centrilobular emphysema *(arrows)* becomes less conspicuous.

Dependent subpleural lines can be seen in up to 35% of normal subjects and are thought to be more common with increasing age.[14] This can be misinterpreted as either early interstitial lung disease in normal lungs, or dependent opacity in patients who really have early interstitial lung disease. Expiratory

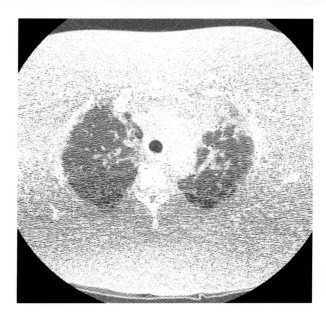

Fig. 4-3 Axial HRCT using 1-mm collimation in a large patient with image quality severely degraded by increased image noise.

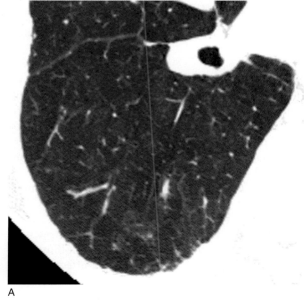

A

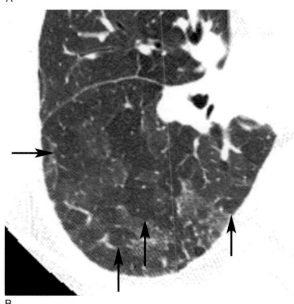

B

Fig. 4-4 Air trapping caused by early bronchiolitis obliterans in a lung transplant recipient without bronchiectasis. **A,** Minimal inhomogeneity of the lung parenchyma at inspiration. **B,** Several secondary pulmonary lobules fail to increase normally in attenuation on expiration *(arrows)*, resulting in more obvious inhomogeneity. Normal lung parenchyma should increase in attenuation on expiration.

images are useful for detecting air trapping of small airway disease. Normally, images at expiration demonstrate smaller lung size and increased lung attenuation compared with the inspiratory images. Air trapping is identified as areas of lung parenchyma that fail to increase in attenuation with expiration. Air trapping may aid in differentiating small airway disease from vascular causes of mosaic attenuation. The degree of air trapping has been shown to correlate with the degree of obstructive impairment in lung function in small airway disease.[15] Isolated air trapping in the absence of abnormalities on inspiratory HRCT images may be the only radiological evidence of small airway diseases, such as asthma or bronchiolitis obliterans, and may be found before the development of anatomic abnormalities such as bronchiectasis or bronchial wall thickening (Figure 4-4).[16]

The accuracy of HRCT has been well established. In the diagnosis of usual interstitial pneumonia, typical findings of basilar subpleural honeycombing are pathognomonic and obviate the need for surgical lung biopsy in cases with appropriate clinical findings.[17-19] HRCT accurately identifies the presence of emphysema and differentiates forms of cystic lung diseases, such as eosinophilic granuloma, and lymphangioleiomyomatosis.[20] In early asbestosis, HRCT abnormalities may precede clinical evidence of deterioration in pulmonary function, and typical findings have again made biopsy unnecessary.[21,22] In the assessment of bronchiectasis, the high diagnostic accuracy of HRCT has made bronchography obsolete.[23]

MULTISLICE HRCT TECHNIQUES

Multislice HRCT may be used in a variety of modes to acquire high-resolution images of the lung parenchyma. Scanning simultaneously using multiple detectors allows multiple true axial images to be acquired simultaneously. Technical parameters and image quality do not differ significantly from standard single-slice HRCT.[24]

Both phantom and clinical studies have demonstrated that the image quality of helical HRCT is diagnostically equivalent to axial HRCT techniques. Sixteen-row MSCT using a beam pitch of 1.375 (detector pitch 6) and detector collimations of 0.625 mm and 1.25 mm has an effective slice thickness of 0.8 mm and 1.25 mm, respectively (GE LightSpeed QXi technical specifications; GE Medical Systems, Milwaukee, Wisconsin). Novel reconstruction algorithms minimize the increase in effective slice thickness associated with helical imaging. When using a 35-cm SFOV and a 512×512 image matrix, the pixel size is 0.68 mm in the x and y axes. Honda et al. (2001)[24] evaluated the image quality of 4-row multislice helical HRCT on cadaveric lungs with a range of interstitial lung diseases and phantoms, by varying the scanning parameters. With visual assessment, the image quality using a 4×1.25-mm detector configuration and pitch 3 was inferior to standard incremental HRCT. At a pitch of 6, there was further slight deterioration in image quality, with slight blurring of intralobular reticular opacities. Image noise was increased, and artifacts radiating from objects of much greater attenuation than their surroundings were encountered. However, these findings minimally affected diagnostic quality. Using the 4×1.25-mm MSCT and pitch 6 led to a loss of diagnostic efficacy in only one examination (5%). Dense centrilobular nodules, ground-glass opacities, emphysema, honeycombing, and architectural distortion were all accurately depicted.

Two subsequent clinical studies have demonstrated no significant difference in overall image quality between 4×1-mm MSCT using a pitch of 6, and standard axial HRCT techniques.[25,26] Schoepf et al. (2001)[25] randomly allocated 67 patients with known or suspected interstitial lung disease to multislice HRCT and standard axial HRCT. Observers, blinded to the technique, scored the examinations for overall image quality, spatial and contrast resolution, artifacts, and diagnostic quality. No significant difference was found in the two techniques. Mehnert et al. (2000)[26] examined 20 patients with interstitial lung disease using both multislice HRCT and standard axial HRCT. There was significantly better spatial resolution on axial HRCT, with better depiction of small vessels and bronchi, whereas multislice HRCT better depicted intralobular septa and was less prone to cardiac and respiratory motion artifact. Overall, the differences were not considered diagnostically relevant.

The acquisition of isotropic data volume allows images to be reconstructed in any plane and at varying collimation (Figure 4-5). Initial studies, using normal cadaveric lung phantoms, compared coronal reconstructions of MSCT data with direct coronal MSCT. Using 4×0.5-mm MSCT and a pitch of 6, there was no significant difference in image quality between coronal reconstructions of axially acquired data and the direct coronal studies.[27] In clinical practice, Remy-Jardin et al. (2003)[28] compared the diagnostic accuracy of 1.25-mm axial images and 1.0-mm coronal images both interspaced by 10-mm intervals, which were reconstructed from volumetric 4×1-mm MSCT in 50 patients with known or suspected interstitial lung disease. The coronal reconstructions resulted in significantly fewer images for interpretation compared to the axial reconstructions (mean 19 versus 28 images). Discrepancies in final diagnoses between the two groups occurred in four patients (8%). In two cases this was thought to be the result of interpretive inexperience (using the coronal images rather than the technical failings of MSCT). In one case small linear opacities were visualized only on the axial images and not on either the axial or coronal interspaced techniques, and in one patient, evidence of sarcoidosis was visualized only on the coronal images, but not the axial images. The quality of both image sets was considered compatible with the search for interstitial lung disease.

Volumetric imaging allows novel reconstruction methods to be used, such as maximum intensity projections (MIP), sliding thin-slab maximum intensity projections (STS-MIP), and minimum intensity projections (Min-IP).[29] MIP images are two-dimensional views generated from projections of the greatest attenuation encountered within a stack of images or volume of data. Projections can be generated along any axis or plane from the data volume, as is commonly done in CT angiography. STS-MIP images are targeted reconstructions of

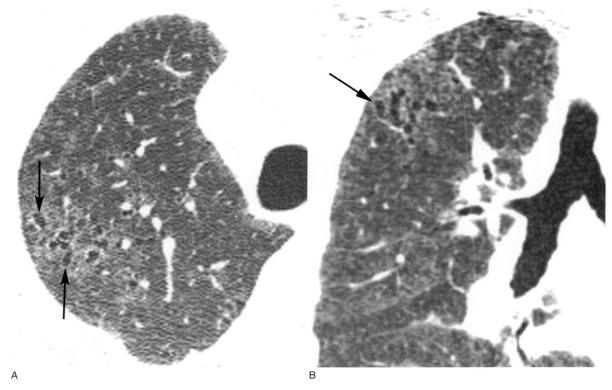

A   B

Fig. 4-5 Bronchiectasis versus honeycombing on incremental versus volumetric HRCT. **A,** Axial interspaced HRCT suggests honeycomb fibrosis at the apex of the right lung. **B,** Volumetric HRCT reconstructed in the coronal plane demonstrates that the round low attenuation structures seen in cross-section actually connect in a tubular branching shape, representing bronchiectasis.

limited data volumes of varying thickness along any axis or plane. They select a region of interest and remove the overlying structures that may mask pathology. Unlike conventional thick reconstructions, STS-MIP images preserve spatial resolution and emphasize structures of increased attenuation (Figure 4-6); however, the details of low-attenuation areas are suppressed.

Both experimental and clinical studies have demonstrated the effectiveness of STS-MIP images for differentiating vascular structures from small pulmonary nodules.[30-32] One clinical study compared 5-mm–thick MIP images with conventional 8-mm CT images and 1-mm HRCT images for the evaluation of suspected nodular disease in 81 patients. The diseases included were coal worker's pneumoconiosis, sarcoidosis, various causes of bronchiolitis, and extrinsic allergic alveolitis. STS-MIP images at 5-mm slice thickness were found to be superior for identifying small pulmonary nodules less than or equal to 3 mm, including both solid soft-tissue attenuation nodules and non-solid or ground-glass nodules. In 17 patients (21%), both 8-mm conventional CT or 1-mm HRCT examinations were inconclusive; in these cases the MIP images demonstrated nodules and accurately depicted their distribution (Figure 4-7).[30]

Min-IP images demonstrate the lowest attenuation in a data volume and are effective in demonstrating emphysema, regions of air trapping, and lung cysts; however, details in areas of increased attenuation are suppressed, such as vessels. For the identification of emphysema, Min-IP images are more sensitive and equally specific as standard HRCT.[31-33] In a series of 27 patients who underwent resection for lung cancer, 21 of whom had emphysema histologically, the presence and severity of emphysema were correctly identified in 13 patients on HRCT, and 17 in patients on Min-IP images; neither method resulted in a false positive. The 82% sensitivity of Min-IP images was greater than HRCT images; both techniques were 100% specific.[33] Both MIP and Min-IP have limitations, as each enhance or suppress areas of low and high attenuation,

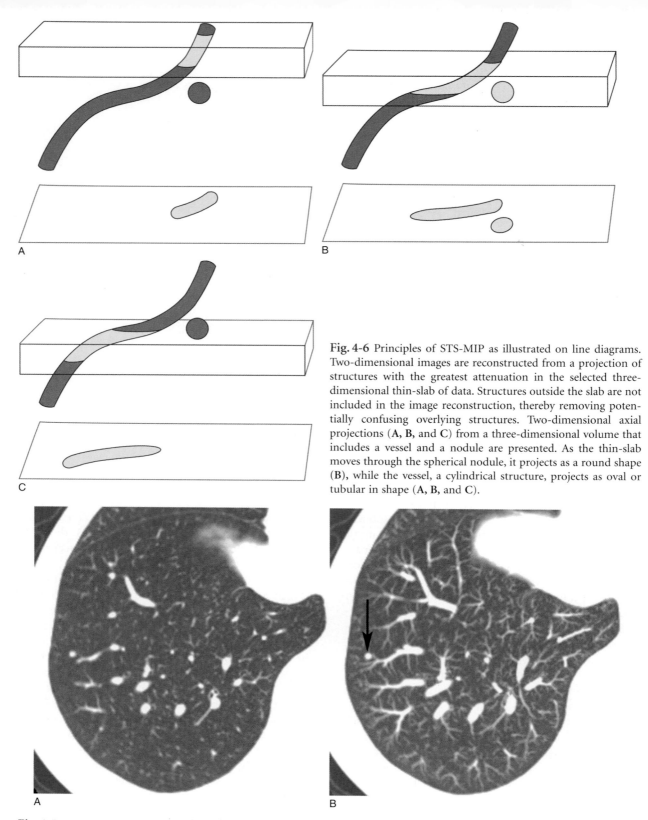

Fig. 4-6 Principles of STS-MIP as illustrated on line diagrams. Two-dimensional images are reconstructed from a projection of structures with the greatest attenuation in the selected three-dimensional thin-slab of data. Structures outside the slab are not included in the image reconstruction, thereby removing potentially confusing overlying structures. Two-dimensional axial projections (**A, B,** and **C**) from a three-dimensional volume that includes a vessel and a nodule are presented. As the thin-slab moves through the spherical nodule, it projects as a round shape (**B**), while the vessel, a cylindrical structure, projects as oval or tubular in shape (**A, B,** and **C**).

Fig. 4-7 Impact of volumetric image reconstruction on a small pulmonary nodule. **A,** A small pulmonary nodule is difficult to identify on a single thin-slice image volumetric HRCT axial image. **B,** On 5-mm thick STS-MIP, the vessels appear cylindrical and not nodular, while nodules maintain their round shape *(arrow)*, facilitating detection of nodules.

respectively. In addition, both have the potential to mask pathology. For example, endobronchial lesions may be obscured if a mass is surrounded by air on a Min-IP slab.

STS-MIP increases the detection of small nodules, and Min-IP aids in the identification of abnormal areas of low attenuation. Both techniques have limitations, which may mask the presence of pathology. There are currently no sufficient studies for determining whether these techniques can replace traditional axial thin slice reformats. Therefore, they should not be used as a primary review method but as a complement to conventional thin collimation image reconstructions.

ARTIFACTS

Volumetric imaging may produce artifacts uniquely associated with helical imaging. Helical artifacts include black and white linear opacities that radiate out from objects with an attenuation that varies greatly from the surrounding structures, such as the pulmonary vasculature surrounded by aerated lung parenchyma. This has been called the "hurricane artifact" and may obscure fine abnormalities, such as intralobular reticular opacities, centrilobular emphysema, and ground-glass opacity.[34] The "hurricane artifact" results from the cone geometry of the x-ray beam and partial volume effects; this artifact increases with increasing pitch. With intravenous contrast-enhanced MSCT, a series of black and white bands may project from vessels containing highly concentrated contrast media. This may be related to the helical artifact just described, together with motion artifact from rapidly moving contrast media.[34] For this reason, parenchymal abnormalities should only be evaluated on nonenhanced helical HRCT images (Figure 4-8).

Incremental axial scanning is usually acquired with a series of breath holds, whereas volumetric images are obtained in a single breath hold, a potential problem for dyspneic patients. There is conflicting evidence from 4-row and 8-row MSCT clinical studies regarding the frequency of respiratory motion artifact. Kelly et al.[34a] compared 40 studies of 4-row and 7 cases of 8-row volumetric HRCT, with prone axial HRCT images obtained during the same examination. With the use of a scoring system of findings indicating respiratory motion artifacts, including double-imaged structures and blurring of pulmonary vessels, the volumetric

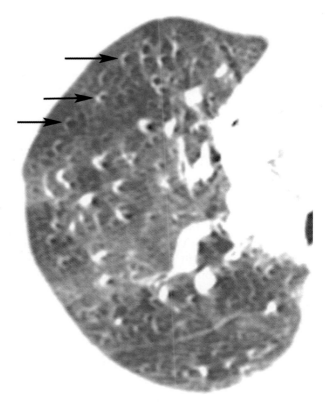

Fig. 4-8 Helical artifact with intravenous contrast enhancement, with linear opacities radiating from high attenuation structures (arrows), such as contrast-enhanced vessels, can make accurate assessment of the lung parenchyma difficult.

HRCT studies demonstrated significantly greater respiratory motion artifacts. Other authors have reported no increase in respiratory motion artifacts. In an evaluation of the image quality of volumetric HRCT, 70 patients were randomly allocated to 4 × 1 mm volumetric HRCT with scan durations of between 22 to 32 seconds, or axial HRCT with multiple breath holds of 1.5 seconds. With the use of a scoring system that assessed spatial resolution, depiction of bronchial walls, and presence of motion and streak artifacts, there was no significant difference in image quality between the two sets of studies.[25] In 20 patients who underwent examinations that included both 4 × 1 mm volumetric HRCT obtained in a single breath hold and axial HRCT with multiple 1-second breath holds, respiratory motion was identified in 11% of axial HRCT and 4% of volumetric HRCT images. In addition, with volumetric HRCT there were fewer images with cardiac motion artifacts (8% volumetric versus 24% axial HRCT).[26]

As the number of detectors increases and gantry rotation time decreases, scan times will continue to fall and respiratory motion artifacts will be further reduced. Compared with 4-row MSCT, current 16-row MSCT reduces scan times by a factor of 4 and can perform a volumetric inspiratory HRCT of the entire lungs in 6 to 11 seconds. This is up to four times faster with 64-row MSCT scanners.

RADIATION DOSE

One concern regarding the use of volumetric HRCT is the potentially increased radiation dose to the patient. Radiation dose has a linear relationship to the tube current (mA), and low-dose volumetric HRCT techniques can use low mA to reduce patient dose. Phantom studies using cadaveric lungs indicate that with 120 kVp, mA can be reduced to 40 mA before image noise obscures faint structures such as centrilobular nodules.[35] A small study of 12 patients with an average weight of 70 kg (154 lb) and suspected bronchiectasis or lung cancer found that low-dose volumetric HRCT resulted in increased image noise; however, subjective image quality was not significantly impaired by reducing the tube current from 150 mA to 40 mA.[36] The same authors applied these findings in a subsequent clinical study of 52 patients with known or suspected small airway disease who underwent both standard incremental HRCT (120 kVp, 170 mA, 1-mm collimation at 10-mm intervals) and volumetric HRCT (120 kVp; 40 mA; 3-mm collimation, pitch 2; 24-second breath hold). The volumetric technique identified a greater number of bronchiectatic segments and small pulmonary nodules. Interobserver agreement was high with both techniques, and both techniques were comparable in identifying pulmonary abnormalities other than bronchiectasis, including bronchiolitis, active pulmonary tuberculosis, lymphangitic spread of tumor, and emphysema.[36] Another investigation of volumetric HRCT evaluated 4-row MSCT with varying mA (10, 20, 40, 70, 100, and 170; 120 kVp; 2.5-mm collimation; pitch 1.5; 2.5-mm image reconstruction thickness; bone reconstruction algorithm) in a small group of patients with suspected bronchiectasis (mean weight of 61 kg [134 lb]). Image quality was subjectively reduced when tube current fell below 70 mA, as judged by two radiologists blinded to the tube current used.[37]

The protocol listed in Table 4-1 suggests using 80 mA with 120 kVp for patients weighing less than

Table 4-1	Volumetric HRCT Protocol
Indications	Focal abnormalities associated with diffuse parenchymal lung disease
Protocol designed for	LightSpeed 16-row
Patient preparation	None
First series	Supine inspiration
Oral contrast	None
IV contrast	None
Tube settings	
kVp	120
mA	80 if the patient weighs less than 54.4 kg (120 lb) 160 if the patient weighs more than 54.4 kg (120 lb)
Gantry speed (sec)	0.7
Table speed (mm/rotation)	27.5
Table speed (mm/s)	39
Slice collimation (mm)	1.25
Anatomical coverage	Lung apices to bases
Reconstruction kernel	High spatial resolution (bone)
Breath hold	Inspiration
Window setting HU	Width 1000 Level −600
Postprocessing	As required

54.4 kg (120 lb), and increasing the mA to 160 for heavier patients. The estimated effective dose of this technique at 80 mA is 2.9 mSv for a supine study of the lungs (mean length of 27 cm in full inspiration) compared with 6.5 mSv at 180 mA. In identical patients, the effective dose of standard-dose HRCT using 1.25-mm thick slices at 10-mm intervals in full inspiration is calculated to be 4.3 mSv. By comparison, the effective dose of a PA radiograph is between 0.01 and 0.05 mSv.

USES OF MULTISLICE HRCT

Axial incremental HRCT typically involves 1-mm slices at 10-mm intervals. This technique obtains representative images of the lung parenchyma. From these, the overall distribution of disease and pattern of abnormality are used to render a diagnosis, which has proved to be highly accurate in the evaluation of diffuse diseases. Indeed, the diagnostic accuracy of HRCT may be maintained even if single images are obtained from only three levels of the parenchyma in usual interstitial pneumonitis, reducing image number and radiation dose.[38,39] However, for the detection of focal pulmonary abnormalities, such as small nodules, incremental axial HRCT is inferior to conventional CT.[10] Unlike helical CT, incremental HRCT suffers from the lack of anatomical contiguity between images. The interspaced technique may miss focal abnormalities, and the narrow collimation hampers nodule detection by making tubular structures (e.g., vessels) appear round and therefore difficult to distinguish from true nodules. Small, dilated airways can appear as cysts on incremental axial HRCT. The ability to scroll through a stack of contiguous images generated by helical CT and recognize the cylindrical nature of these small, low-attenuation structures helps avoid this confusion.

Volumetric HRCT images the entire lung parenchyma. Images from the data volume can be reconstructed both at narrow-slice thickness to detect subtle interstitial abnormalities and again at thicker collimation to avoid missing focal abnormalities, such as small nodules. Therefore, volumetric HRCT has the ability to evaluate both the diffuse and focal manifestations of interstitial lung disease, emphysema, and small airway disease. Potential indications for volumetric HRCT are discussed next.

Evaluation of Emphysema

Emphysema is characterized by abnormal permanent enlargement of the airspaces distal to the terminal bronchiole, accompanied by destruction of the alveolar walls. The predominant form, centrilobular emphysema, is strongly associated with cigarette smoking. Early HRCT abnormalities include areas of low attenuation located near the center of the secondary pulmonary lobule interspersed with normal lung parenchyma (Figure 4-9).

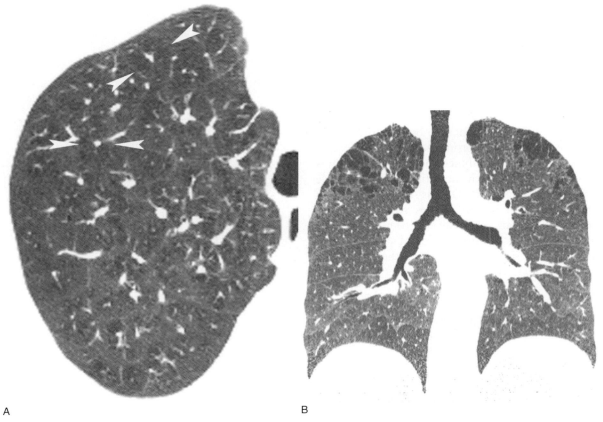

A

B

Fig. 4-9 **Emphysema on volumetric HRCT. A,** Axial image demonstrates areas of low attenuation, with intervening normal lung parenchyma *(arrowheads)*. Note the central opacity indicating the central arteriole within the destroyed secondary pulmonary lobule. **B,** Coronal reconstructions in a different patient demonstrate the upper lobe predominant distribution of disease in a single image; the patient has both centrilobular and paraseptal emphysema.

The changes usually predominate in the upper lobes.[40,41] Panacinar emphysema is usually associated with alpha-1-antitrypsin deficiency and is exacerbated by smoking. It is characterized by uniform destruction of the entire acinus with a predilection for the lower lobes. The imaging characteristics are confluent areas of low attenuation involving the entire lobules with minimal normal intervening lung parenchyma (Figure 4-10).

Patients with severe forms of both types of emphysema are often considered for either lung volume reduction surgery (LVRS) or lung transplantation.[42,43] The success of LVRS is greatest in patients with disease localized to the upper lobes; in transplantation candidates, asymmetric disease may alter the choice of which lung to transplant.[42] CT of the lung parenchyma is commonly performed to evaluate the symmetry and severity of underlying lung disease and to look for occult lung cancers, which are found in up to 5% of patients.[44-46] The presence of a neoplasm may preclude or alter the choice of surgery.

While incremental axial HRCT techniques accurately identify the presence of both emphysema and bronchiectasis and can subjectively evaluate their severity, helical CT techniques are used with the density mask technique to quantify the severity of emphysema based on lung attenuation and to look for lung nodules that may represent lung cancer.[41,47-50] In the past, both an incremental HRCT and a helical CT had to be performed in the same patient, increasing radiation exposure. Volumetric HRCT combines the two and obtains the necessary clinical information from a single inspiratory acquisition. This is reconstructed at both narrow collimation images to evaluate the parenchymal detail, and thicker contiguous slice reconstructions to identify incidental cancers, while also permitting quantification using the volumetric whole lung data set.

Evaluation of Pulmonary Fibrosis

Axial incremental HRCT is widely used for the diagnosis and management of interstitial lung disease, such as pulmonary fibrosis (i.e., usual interstitial pneumonitis). There is a greater risk of lung cancer in patients with pulmonary fibrosis.[51] The incidence of lung cancer is estimated at between 4.4% and 9.8% in patients with usual interstitial pneumonia[52-54] and is thought to be an independent risk factor to smoking, with a relative risk of

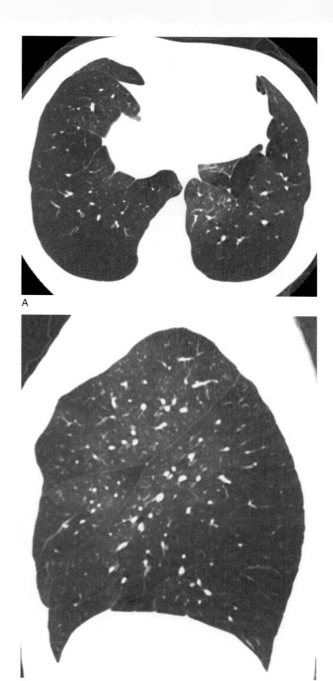

A

B

Fig. 4-10 Severe panacinar emphysema due to alpha-1-antitrypsin deficiency on volumetric HRCT. Axial (A) and sagittal (B) reconstructions demonstrate confluent regions of low attenuation, with no intervening normal lung. The sagittal images readily demonstrate the lower lobe predominance on a single image.

approximately 7.3.[53,54] Squamous cell carcinomas predominate and often occur within areas of fibrosis; as many as 50% are found incidentally (Figure 4-11).[55,56] As with emphysema imaging, volumetric HRCT allows evaluation of detailed lung architecture on narrow image reconstructions; therefore, septal lines, fibrosis, and ground-glass opacity can be readily identified, as well as thicker image reconstructions to look for lung nodules that may represent cancer. Small dilated bronchi may appear as round cysts on axial images and may be incorrectly interpreted as lung cysts or honeycombing; the multiplanar reconstructions made possible from the volumetric data set allow these to be differentiated.

Because of its relatively recent development, the evidence supporting the use of volumetric HRCT in the evaluation of other diffuse interstitial lung diseases (e.g., idiopathic pneumonias) is currently limited. The potential advantages of this technique in the evaluation of diffuse interstitial lung diseases include the improved depiction of the craniocaudal distribution of disease, the identification of associated small nodules, and the accurate differentiation of honeycombing from peripheral bronchiectasis. Volumetric HRCT lends itself to potential quantitative analysis of interstitial lung disease, using computer-assisted diagnostic tools. These may provide a functional analysis of parenchymal abnormalities and an objective comparison of sequential studies.[57]

Evaluation of Hemoptysis

Hemoptysis has many causes, including neoplasia, bronchiectasis, pneumonia, and bronchitis.[58] Helical tracheobronchial CT and direct visualiza-

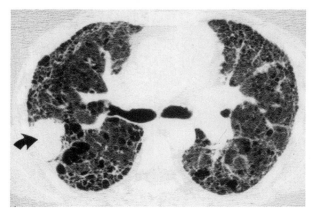

Fig. 4-11 Axial HRCT showing the development of a lung carcinoma *(arrow)* in a patient with usual interstitial pneumonitis.

tion of the lumen of the tracheobronchial lumen with fiberoptic bronchoscopy (FOB) have complementary roles in the investigation of hemoptysis. Whereas FOB is used in older patients with a smoking history and a focally abnormal chest radiograph (mass, atelectasis, or cavity) for histological diagnosis, helical CT is used to evaluate the extent of extraluminal disease and the airway distal to stenoses that a bronchoscope cannot pass through.[59] When the chest radiograph is normal or does not localize a finding, the diagnostic yield of FOB is lower and identifies malignancy in approximately 6% of smokers more than 40 years of age.[60] FOB is also less useful for identifying tumors in the lung periphery[60,61] and is not as accurate as CT for identifying peripheral airway disease.[62] For example, in a study of 40 patients with hemoptysis and a normal chest radiograph, normal FOB, and normal sputum examinations, helical CT identified a potential cause in half the patients; the pathologies identified included bronchiectasis, infective airspace disease (including active tuberculosis), primary and secondary lung neoplasms, arteriovenous vascular malformations, and one case of eosinophilic granuloma.[63] Traditionally, a helical CT was performed to evaluate the central tracheobronchial tree, and HRCT was performed to evaluate the lung parenchyma and small airways. Now, volumetric HRCT can do both with a single inspiratory acquisition reconstructed to evaluate both and can allow CT virtual bronchoscopy.

CT with virtual bronchoscopic reconstruction is moderately sensitive for the detection of central airway neoplasia in patients with hemoptysis. In one series of 136 consecutive patients with symptoms or radiographic findings suspicious for neoplasia, single-slice helical CT using 3-mm collimation was 68% sensitive and 90% specific for the detection of endobronchial tumors; 32% of lobar and segmental stenoses and all lesions limited to the mucosa were not identified.[64] The largest MSCT study to date reported 83% sensitivity and 100% specificity for identifying endobronchial lesions in 44 patients with known malignancy, using 4 × 1.25-mm MSCT with virtual bronchoscopy. As in SDCT studies, limitations of MSCT include the identification of peripheral stenoses and mucosal abnormalities.[65] Two small studies using 4 × 1-mm MSCT have reported sensitivities of 90% and specificities of 95% for bronchial strictures, with equal accuracy in the evaluation of central and peripheral airways.[66,67] MSCT accurately evaluates peripheral bronchial strictures beyond the range of a bronchoscope but is limited by its inability to identify the subtle mucosal changes of early malignancies recognized by direct visualization with bronchoscopy.

The diagnostic accuracy of axial HRCT in the evaluation of bronchiectasis is well established[23,68,69] and is greater than bronchoscopy.[62] Standard axial HRCT identifies 87% of pulmonary segments affected with bronchiectasis before pulmonary resection.[68] Volumetric contiguous HRCT increases the diagnostic accuracy of CT by 15% for bronchiectasis in comparison to standard interspaced axial HRCT.[70] Contiguous images help to differentiate mucous-filled bronchi from vessels and nodules and help miss focal areas of bronchiectasis, particularly of small peripheral bronchi (Figure 4-12). Coronal multiplanar reconstructions are particularly useful for identifying dilated airways oriented in the craniocaudal direction.[71]

Mild cylindrical bronchiectasis can be difficult to identify and usually manifests as dilated airways that extend to within 1 cm of the pleural surface.[68] A luminal diameter greater than the adjacent artery, or a total diameter of the airway greater than 1.5 times the adjacent vessel, is considered abnormally dilated.[68,72] However, normal subjects have apparent bronchial dilation using these criteria.[73] The most specific sign is a lack of normal tapering of the airway,[68,73] a finding that can be difficult to evaluate on axial incremental HRCT. This is due to the lack of anatomical continuity between images, particularly for bronchi seen in cross-section and not with their long axis in the axial scan plane. Volumetric HRCT allows the small airways to be visualized in any scan plane, regardless of their anatomical orientation with anatomical continuity (Figure 4-13). A small study using low-dose volumetric MSCT for detection of bronchiectasis confirms increased detection of abnormal lung segments using volumetric evaluation compared with axial incremental HRCT.[36]

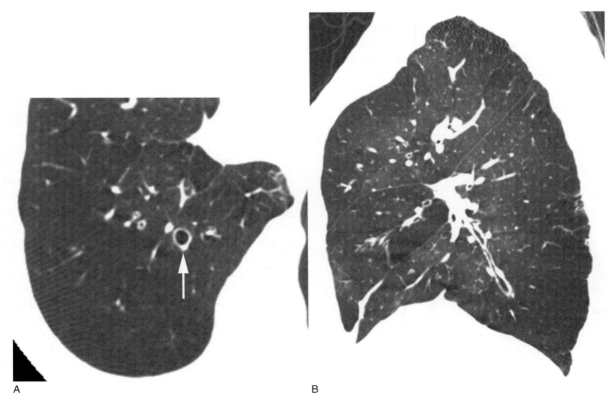

A   B

Fig. 4-12 Severe emphysema and airway dilation on volumetric HRCT. A, Axial image demonstrates airway dilation *(arrow).* **B,** Sagittal image reconstructions reveal the extent of disease.

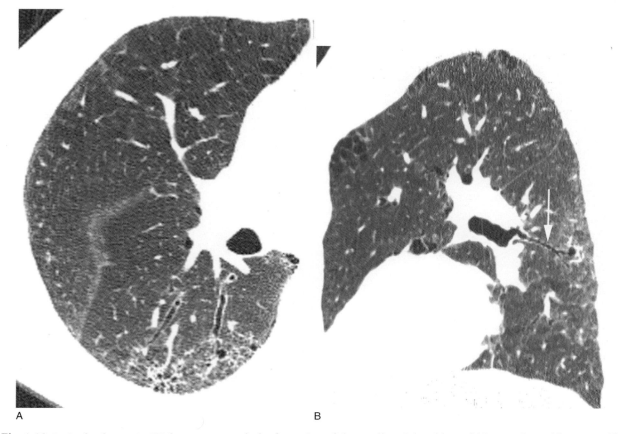

A   B

Fig. 4-13 **Sagittal volumetric CT demonstrates a lack of tapering of the small peripheral bronchi in a patient with nonspecific interstitial pneumonia. A,** Apparent lung cysts of honeycombing on axial incremental HRCT. **B,** Sagittal image reconstructions show these to be areas of traction bronchiectasis *(arrow)*.

Evaluation of Oncology Patients with Respiratory Complaints

Respiratory symptoms are common among oncology patients, with dyspnea being the fourth most common symptom of cancer patients presenting to the emergency department of one large oncology center.[74] Dyspnea is an ominous sign with a poor outcome, particularly in lung cancer patients. Symptoms can indicate either disease progression with direct involvement of the respiratory system by malignancy, such as lymphangitic spread of tumor and hematogenously disseminated lung metastases, or indirect respiratory complications, such as post-obstructive atelectasis or pleural effusions. Alternatively, symptoms may indicate the development of radiation lung injury or drug-induced lung toxicity after treatment. Oncology patients often have underlying co-morbid conditions (e.g., chronic obstructive pulmonary disease, heart failure) and are predisposed to numerous pulmonary patholo-

gies, such as venous thromboembolic disease and infection.[75,76]

HRCT is well known to be superior to both plain radiography and conventional CT in the evaluation of parenchymal abnormalities, including the lymphangitic spread of tumor.[77,78] HRCT findings include irregular thickening of the bronchovascular structures and exaggerated the centrilobular structures and result from foci of tumor and associated edema within the lymphatics of the pulmonary interstitium. Involvement of the interlobular septa leads to smooth or irregular interlobular septal thickening. Multiple polygonal shapes may form as the septal lines unite around the periphery of the secondary pulmonary lobule (Figure 4-14).[77,78]

CT is superior to chest radiographs for detecting radiation-related lung injury (Figure 4-15).[79] The radiological findings are characteristically confined to the treatment field and have a varied but clear temporal progression.[79-81] Acute radiation

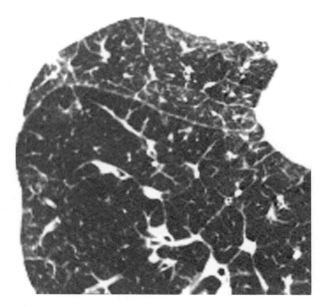

Fig. 4-14 Axial HRCT of lymphangitic spread of tumor caused by breast cancer demonstrates increased septal lines forming polygonal shapes. Multiple small nodules are within the parenchyma and against the oblique fissure.

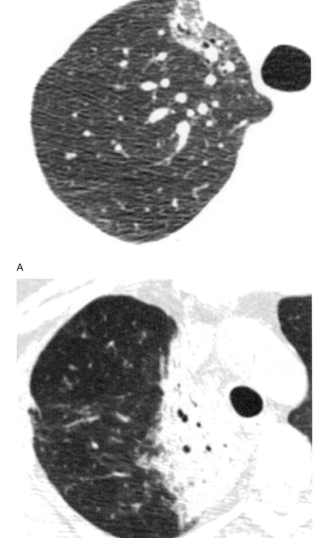

A

B

Fig. 4-15 Volumetric HRCT of early and late stage radiation-induced fibrosis. A, In a patient treated for Hodgkin's lymphoma, early radiation lung injury appears as ground-glass opacity within the radiation field that is distinguished from other causes of consolidation by its non-anatomical contour. Three-dimensional radiotherapy planning increasingly leads to curved, rather than the traditional straight, borders of the radiotherapy field. B, In a patient treated for thyroid carcinoma, late radiation fibrosis appears as progressive loss of volume in the lung included in the radiation field and traction bronchiectasis.

pneumonitis is frequent and usually clinically silent[82]; the CT findings include diffuse ground-glass opacities, which develop into patchy airspace disease in the treatment field. The onset of CT findings has a varied time course and can develop within 1 week of therapy, usually peaking 3 to 4 months after therapy.[79-81] Later radiation fibrosis can be associated with a dyspnea, a dry cough, and the development of cor pulmonale.[82] The CT findings are airspace disease progressing to a well-defined parenchymal opacity outlining the radiation therapy field, associated with architectural distortion such as traction bronchiectasis, which indicates underlying fibrosis. These findings may develop within 3 months of treatment, or many years later, but are typically stable after 1 to 2 years.[80,81] Radiotherapy changes can be difficult to distinguish from tumor recurrence or infection but are distinct in their temporal relationship with therapy and findings that conform to the radiotherapy field rather than anatomical boundaries. With CT, the straight boundaries of the treatment field are clearly seen, although they may be more difficult to recognize when multidirectional three-dimensional therapy fields are used.[83]

In half of oncology patients, pulmonary symptoms result from multiple etiologies. Therefore, an incremental axial HRCT scanning protocol tailored to evaluate for lymphangitic tumor spread, or thick-collimation helical CT to evaluate lung nodules and lymph node enlargement, will miss other disease processes.[74] Volumetric HRCT allows the evaluation of the many causes of pulmonary symptoms from one volumetric scanning acquisition reconstructed at greater slice thickness to evaluate for the progression of masses and lymph node disease, and at thinner collimation for more detailed parenchymal abnormalities related to therapy or lymphangitic tumor spread; although intravenous contrast can create some artifacts, as described earlier, it can also permit the evaluation of pulmonary embolism. Volumetric CT therefore allows a combined and detailed assessment of the many focal and parenchymal abnormalities that may contribute to the pulmonary symptoms of oncology patients.

CONCLUSION

Volumetric HRCT allows complete evaluation of diffuse interstitial lung disease, focal lung pathologies, and the large and small airways. Until the development of faster MSCT scanners, this had not been technically possible. Low-dose techniques can be used to reduce the radiation dose. In patients in whom volumetric HRCT is being considered, the advantages of accurate diagnosis may outweigh the increased radiation dose.

Acknowledgments

We are very grateful for the invaluable assistance of Medical Physicist Manos Christodoulou and Media Coordinator Sarah Abate.

REFERENCES

1. Itoh H, Tokunaga S, Asamoto H, et al: Radiologic-pathologic correlations of small lung nodules with special reference to peribronchiolar nodules, *Am J Roentgenol* 130:223-231, 1978.
2. Littleton JT, Shaffer KA, Callahan WP, et al: Temporal bone: comparison of pluridirectional tomography and high resolution computed tomography, *Am J Roentgenol* 137:835-845, 1981.
3. Shaffer KA, Haughton VM, Wilson CR: High resolution computed tomography of the temporal bone, *Radiology* 134:409-414, 1980.
4. Todo G, Ito H, Nakano Y, et al: High resolution CT (HRCT) for the evaluation of pulmonary peripheral disorders, *Rinsho Hoshasen* 27:1319-1326, 1982.
5. Nakata H, Kimoto T, Nakayama T, et al: Diffuse peripheral lung disease: evaluation by high-resolution computed tomography, *Radiology* 157:181-185, 1985.
6. Webb WR, Stein MG, Finkbeiner WE, et al: Normal and diseased isolated lungs: high-resolution CT, *Radiology* 166:81-87, 1988.
7. Weibel ER: Fleischner Lecture. Looking into the lung: what can it tell us? *Am J Roentgenol* 133:1021-1031, 1979.
8. Murata K, Itoh H, Todo G, et al: Centrilobular lesions of the lung: demonstration by high-resolution CT and pathologic correlation, *Radiology* 161:641-645, 1986.
9. Schurawitzki H, Stiglbauer R, Graninger W, et al: Interstitial lung disease in progressive systemic sclerosis: high-resolution CT versus radiography, *Radiology* 176:755-759, 1990.
10. Remy-Jardin M, Remy J, Deffontaines C, et al: Assessment of diffuse infiltrative lung disease: comparison of conventional CT and high-resolution CT, *Radiology* 181:157-162, 1991.
11. Mathieson JR, Mayo JR, Staples CA, et al: Chronic diffuse infiltrative lung disease: comparison of diagnostic accuracy of CT and chest radiography, *Radiology* 171:111-116, 1989.
12. Murata K, Khan A, Rojas KA, et al: Optimization of computed tomography technique to demonstrate the fine structure of the lung, *Invest Radiol* 23:170-175, 1988.
13. Mayo JR, Webb WR, Gould R, et al: High-resolution CT of the lungs: an optimal approach, *Radiology* 163:507-510, 1987.
14. Aberle DR, Gamsu G, Ray CS, et al: Asbestos-related pleural and parenchymal fibrosis: detection with high-resolution CT, *Radiology* 166:729-734, 1988.
15. Arakawa H, Webb WR, McCowin M, et al: Inhomogeneous lung attenuation at thin-section CT: diagnostic value of expiratory scans, *Radiology* 206:89-94, 1998.
16. Arakawa H, Webb WR: Air trapping on expiratory high-resolution CT scans in the absence of inspiratory scan abnormalities: correlation with pulmonary function tests and differential diagnosis, *Am J Roentgenol* 170:1349-1353, 1998.
17. Raghu G, Mageto YN, Lockhart D, et al: The accuracy of the clinical diagnosis of new-onset idiopathic pulmonary fibrosis and other interstitial lung disease: a prospective study, *Chest* 116:1168-1174, 1999.
18. Nishimura K, Kitaichi M, Izumi T, et al: Usual interstitial pneumonia: histologic correlation with high-resolution CT, *Radiology* 182:337-342, 1992.
19. Tung KT, Wells AU, Rubens MB, et al: Accuracy of the typical computed tomographic appearances of fibrosing alveolitis, *Thorax* 48:334-338, 1993.
20. Bonelli FS, Hartman TE, Swensen SJ, et al: Accuracy of high-resolution CT in diagnosing lung diseases, *Am J Roentgenol* 170:1507-1512, 1998.
21. Akira M, Yokoyama K, Yamamoto S, et al: Early asbestosis: evaluation with high-resolution CT, *Radiology* 178:409-416, 1991.
22. Staples CA, Gamsu G, Ray CS, et al: High resolution computed tomography and lung function in asbestos-exposed workers with normal chest radiographs, *Am Rev Respir Dis* 139:1502-1508, 1989.

23. Young K, Aspestrand F, Kolbenstvedt A: High resolution CT and bronchography in the assessment of bronchiectasis, *Acta Radiol* 32:439-441, 1991.
24. Honda O, Johkoh T, Tomiyama N, et al: High-resolution CT using multislice CT equipment: evaluation of image quality in 11 cadaveric lungs and a phantom, *Am J Roentgenol* 177:875-879, 2001.
25. Schoepf UJ, Bruening RD, Hong C, et al: Multislice helical CT of focal and diffuse lung disease: comprehensive diagnosis with reconstruction of contiguous and high-resolution CT sections from a single thin-collimation scan, *Am J Roentgenol* 177:179-184, 2001.
26. Mehnert F, Pereira PL, Dammann F, et al: High resolution multislice CT of the lung: comparison with sequential HRCT slices, *Rofo Fortschr Geb Rontgenstr Neuen Bildgeb Verfahr* 172:972-977, 2000.
27. Honda O, Johkoh T, Yamamoto S, et al: Comparison of quality of multiplanar reconstructions and direct coronal multislice CT scans of the lung, *Am J Roentgenol* 179:875-879, 2002.
28. Remy-Jardin M, Campistron P, Amara A, et al: Usefulness of coronal reformations in the diagnostic evaluation of infiltrative lung disease, *J Comput Assist Tomogr* 27:266-273, 2003.
29. Napel S, Rubin GD, Jeffrey RB, Jr: STS-MIP: a new reconstruction technique for CT of the chest, *J Comput Assist Tomogr* 17:832-838, 1993.
30. Remy-Jardin M, Remy J, Artaud D, et al: Diffuse infiltrative lung disease: clinical value of sliding-thin-slab maximum intensity projection CT scans in the detection of mild micronodular patterns, *Radiology* 200:333-339, 1996.
31. Bhalla M, Naidich DP, McGuinness G, et al: Diffuse lung disease: assessment with helical CT-preliminary observations of the role of maximum and minimum intensity projection images, *Radiology* 200:341-347, 1996.
32. Coakley FV, Cohen MD, Johnson MS, et al: Maximum intensity projection images in the detection of simulated pulmonary nodules by spiral CT, *Br J Radiol* 71:135-140, 1998.
33. Remy-Jardin M, Remy J, Gosselin B, et al: Sliding thin slab, minimum intensity projection technique in the diagnosis of emphysema: histopathologic-CT correlation, *Radiology* 200:665-671, 1996.
34. Johkoh T, Honda O, Mihara N, et al: Pitfalls in the interpretation of multislice-row helical CT images at window width and level setting for lung parenchyma, *Radiat Med* 19:181-184, 2001.
34a. Kelly DM, Hasegawa I, Borders R, et al: High-resolution CT using MSCT: Comparison of degree of motion artifact between volumetric and axial methods. *Am J Roentgenol* 182:757-759, 2004.
35. Johkoh T, Honda O, Yamamoto S, et al: Evaluation of image quality and spatial resolution of low-dose high-pitch multislice-row helical high-resolution CT in 11 autopsy lungs and a wire phantom, *Radiat Med* 19:279-284, 2001.
36. Jung KJ, Lee KS, Kim SY, et al: Low-dose, volumetric helical CT: image quality, radiation dose, and usefulness for evaluation of bronchiectasis, *Invest Radiol* 35:557-563, 2000.
37. Yi CA, Lee KS, Kim TS, et al: Multidetector CT of bronchiectasis: effect of radiation dose on image quality, *Am J Roentgenol* 181:501-505, 2003.
38. Leung AN, Staples CA, Muller NL: Chronic diffuse infiltrative lung disease: comparison of diagnostic accuracy of high-resolution and conventional CT, *Am J Roentgenol* 157:693-696, 1991.
39. Kazerooni EA, Martinez FJ, Flint A, et al: Thin-section CT obtained at 10-mm increments versus limited three-level thin-section CT for idiopathic pulmonary fibrosis: correlation with pathologic scoring, *Am J Roentgenol* 169:977-983, 1997.
40. Thurlbeck WM, Muller NL: Emphysema: definition, imaging, and quantification: *Am J Roentgenol* 163:1017-1025, 1994.
41. Murata K, Khan A, Herman PG: Pulmonary parenchymal disease: evaluation with high-resolution CT, *Radiology* 170:629-635, 1989.
42. Fishman A, Martinez F, Naunheim K, et al: A randomized trial comparing lung-volume-reduction surgery with medical therapy for severe emphysema, *N Engl J Med* 348:2059-2073, 2003.
43. Trulock EP, III: Lung Transplantation for COPD, *Chest* 113:269S-276S, 1998.
44. Kazerooni EA, Chow LC, et al: Preoperative examination of lung transplant candidates: value of chest CT compared with chest radiography, *Am J Roentgenol* 165:1343-1348, 1995.
45. Rozenshtein A, White CS, Austin JH, et al: Incidental lung carcinoma detected at CT in patients selected for lung volume reduction surgery to treat severe pulmonary emphysema, *Radiology* 207:487-490, 1998.
46. Ojo TC, Martinez F, Paine R, III, et al: Lung volume reduction surgery alters management of pulmonary nodules in patients with severe COPD, *Chest* 112:1494-1500, 1997.
47. Spouge D, Mayo JR, Cardoso W, et al: Panacinar emphysema: CT and pathologic findings, *J Comput Assist Tomogr* 17:710-713, 1993.
48. Cederlund K, Bergstrand L, Hogberg S, et al: Visual grading of emphysema severity in candidates for lung volume reduction surgery. Comparison between HRCT, spiral CT and "density-masked" images, *Acta Radiol* 43:48-53, 2002.
49. Muller NL, Staples CA, Miller RR, et al: "Density mask." An objective method to quantitate emphysema using computed tomography, *Chest* 94:782-787, 1988.
50. Sashidhar K, Gulati M, Gupta D, et al: Emphysema in heavy smokers with normal chest radiography. Detection and quantification by HCRT, *Acta Radiol* 43:60-65, 2002.
51. Bouros D, Hatzakis K, Labrakis H, et al: Association of malignancy with diseases causing interstitial pulmonary changes, *Chest* 121:1278-1289, 2002.
52. Kusajima K, Murata Y, Ohshi F, et al: Characteristics of chronic interstitial pneumonia seen in the lung operated for lung cancer, *Nihon Kyobu Shikkan Gakkai Zasshi* 30:1673-1681, 1992.
53. Hubbard R, Venn A, Lewis S, et al: Lung cancer and cryptogenic fibrosing alveolitis. A population-based cohort study, *Am J Respir Crit Care Med* 161:5-8, 2000.
54. Turner-Warwick M, Lebowitz M, Burrows B, et al: Cryptogenic fibrosing alveolitis and lung cancer, *Thorax* 35:496-499, 1980.
55. Kawasaki H, Nagai K, Yokose T, et al: Clinicopathological characteristics of surgically resected lung cancer associated with idiopathic pulmonary fibrosis, *J Surg Oncol* 76:53-57, 2001.
56. Aubry MC, Myers JL, Douglas WW, et al: Primary pulmonary carcinoma in patients with idiopathic pulmonary fibrosis, *Mayo Clin Proc* 77:763-770, 2002.

57. Hoffman EA, Reinhardt JM, Sonka M, et al: Characterization of the interstitial lung diseases via density-based and texture-based analysis of computed tomography images of lung structure and function, *Acad Radiol* 10:1104-1118, 2003.

58. Hirshberg B, Biran I, Glazer M, et al: Hemoptysis: etiology, evaluation, and outcome in a tertiary referral hospital, *Chest* 112:440-444, 1997.

59. Weaver LJ, Solliday N, Cugell DW: Selection of patients with hemoptysis for fiberoptic bronchoscopy, *Chest* 76:7-10, 1979.

60. Lederle FA, Nichol KL, Parenti CM: Bronchoscopy to evaluate hemoptysis in older men with nonsuspicious chest roentgenograms, *Chest* 95:1043-1047, 1989.

61. Set PA, Flower CD, Smith IE, et al: Hemoptysis: comparative study of the role of CT and fiberoptic bronchoscopy, *Radiology* 189:677-680, 1993.

62. McGuinness G, Beacher JR, Harkin TJ, et al: Hemoptysis: prospective high-resolution CT/bronchoscopic correlation, *Chest* 105:1155-1162, 1994.

63. Millar AB, Boothroyd AE, Edwards D, et al: The role of computed tomography (CT) in the investigation of unexplained haemoptysis, *Respir Med* 86:39-44, 1992.

64. Lacasse Y, Martel S, Hebert A, et al: Accuracy of virtual bronchoscopy to detect endobronchial lesions, *Ann Thorac Surg* 77:1774-1780, 2004.

65. Finkelstein SE, Schrump DS, Nguyen DM, et al: Comparative evaluation of super high-resolution CT scan and virtual bronchoscopy for the detection of tracheobronchial malignancies, *Chest* 124:1834-1840, 2003.

66. Hoppe H, Dinkel HP, Walder B, et al: Grading airway stenosis down to the segmental level using virtual bronchoscopy, *Chest* 125:704-711, 2004.

67. Hoppe H, Walder B, Sonnenschein M, et al: Multidetector CT virtual bronchoscopy to grade tracheobronchial stenosis, *Am J Roentgenol* 178:1195-1200, 2002.

68. Kang EY, Miller RR, Muller NL: Bronchiectasis: comparison of preoperative thin-section CT and pathologic findings in resected specimens, *Radiology* 195:649-654, 1995.

69. Grenier P, Maurice F, Musset D, et al: Bronchiectasis: assessment by thin-section CT, *Radiology* 161:95-99, 1986.

70. Engeler CE, Tashjian JH, Engeler CM, et al: Volumetric high-resolution CT in the diagnosis of interstitial lung disease and bronchiectasis: diagnostic accuracy and radiation dose, *Am J Roentgenol* 163:31-35, 1994.

71. Sung YM, Lee KS, Yi CA, et al: Additional coronal images using low-milliamperage multislice-row computed tomography: effectiveness in the diagnosis of bronchiectasis, *J Comput Assist Tomogr* 27:490-495, 2003.

72. Kim SJ, Im JG, Kim IO, et al: Normal bronchial and pulmonary arterial diameters measured by thin section CT, *J Comput Assist Tomogr* 19:365-369, 1995.

73. Lynch DA, Newell JD, Tschomper BA, et al: Uncomplicated asthma in adults: comparison of CT appearance of the lungs in asthmatic and healthy subjects, *Radiology* 188:829-833, 1993.

74. Escalante CP, Martin CG, Elting LS, et al: Dyspnea in cancer patients. Etiology, resource utilization, and survival-implications in a managed care world, *Cancer* 78:1314-1319, 1996.

75. Reuben DB, Mor V: Dyspnea in terminally ill cancer patients, *Chest* 89:234-236, 1986.

76. Kvale PA, Simoff M, Prakash UB: Lung cancer. Palliative care, *Chest* 123:284S-311S, 2003.

77. Stein MG, Mayo J, Muller N, et al: Pulmonary lymphangitic spread of carcinoma: appearance on CT scans, *Radiology* 162:371-375, 1987.

78. Munk PL, Muller NL, Miller RR, et al: Pulmonary lymphangitic carcinomatosis: CT and pathologic findings, *Radiology* 166:705-709, 1988.

79. Ikezoe J, Takashima S, Morimoto S, et al: CT appearance of acute radiation-induced injury in the lung, *Am J Roentgenol* 150:765-770, 1988.

80. Libshitz HI: Radiation changes in the lung, *Semin Roentgenol* 28:303-320, 1993.

81. Libshitz HI, Shuman LS: Radiation-induced pulmonary change: CT findings, *J Comput Assist Tomogr* 8:15-19, 1984.

82. Davis SD, Yankelevitz DF, Henschke CI: Radiation effects on the lung: clinical features, pathology, and imaging findings, *Am J Roentgenol* 159:1157-1164, 1992.

83. Koenig TR, Munden RF, Erasmus JJ, et al: Radiation injury of the lung after three-dimensional conformal radiation therapy, *Am J Roentgenol* 178:1383-1388, 2002.

5

Multislice Computed Tomography in the Investigation of Pulmonary Thromboembolic Disease

Bobby Bhartia
Smita Patel
Ella A. Kazerooni

ACUTE THROMBOEMBOLIC DISEASE

The brilliant nineteenth century pathologist, Rudolf Virchow, was the first to recognize that pulmonary emboli (PE) originate from distant sites of venous thrombosis, and that both PE and deep vein thrombosis (DVT) are facets of the same disease process.[1] In the United States, venous thromboembolic disease is the third most common cause of cardiovascular death following myocardial infarction and stroke, and it is the most common unsuspected postmortem diagnosis.[2,3] These findings highlight both the low sensitivity of clinical assessment and the lack of a single accurate test for the diagnosis of thromboembolic disease.

With the development of helical computed tomography (CT), the first prospective case study by Remy-Jardin et al. (1992)[4] reported the potential value of CT, with 100% sensitivity for the diagnosis of central PE in 42 patients using single-slice CT (SSCT). Advances in multislice CT (MSCT) have further improved the ability of CT to visualize the smaller pulmonary arteries consistently, bringing CT to the forefront in the diagnostic algorithm of this elusive condition.

Natural History of Pulmonary Thromboembolic Disease

The majority of DVT arises in the veins of the lower limbs. The incidence of DVT is strongly related to increasing age, underlying malignancy, recent surgery, and immobilization.[2] Most DVT begins as asymptomatic thrombi caudal to the popliteal veins. Symptoms usually develop with extension of thrombus into and proximal to the popliteal veins and are associated with an increased risk of PE. The incidence of clinically important PE with infrapopliteal DVT is approximately 1%; therefore, anticoagulation in asymptomatic ambulatory patients with infrapopliteal DVT is not recommended.[3] In patients with symptomatic DVT in or proximal to the popliteal veins, 35% to 51% have a high probability ventilation-perfusion (VQ) scintigraphy result, which is associated with PE in 96% of cases.[5-7] However, because of the low sensitivity of using a high-probability VQ scintigraphy to diagnose (sensitivity 41%), the incidence of silent PE in proximal DVT is probably higher still.[8]

Untreated mortality from PE is 26%, and untreated isolated DVT is 16%.[3] Even with therapy, mortality from PE is 12% to 15% and 6% from DVT. This is partly due to the association of thromboembolic disease with co-morbid conditions, such as malignancy. However, 45% of deaths from venous thromboembolic disease are primarily attributed to PE.[9] Therapy is not without risks. Morbidity from anticoagulation is approximately 6.5% per year, which increases with age and the presence of co-morbid conditions.[10,11] Furthermore, there is a 1.9% to 3% risk of intracranial hemorrhage with thrombolytic therapy.[9] Accurate diagnosis is therefore critical.

Diagnosis of Pulmonary Embolism

Clinical Diagnosis and D-Dimer

History and physical examination are known to be inaccurate for the diagnostic evaluation of suspected venous thromboembolic disease. Several attempts have been made to increase the accuracy of clinical diagnosis with formalized assessments.[12,13] A prospective study using the Wells clinical score stratified 1239 inpatients and outpatients into low, moderate, and high-risk groups. There was a 3.4%, 27.8%, and 78.4% prevalence of PE in each group, respectively. Although clinical assessment can determine the likelihood of disease, it is unable to diagnose or exclude the presence of PE in an individual patient.

D-Dimer assays improve the clinician's ability to exclude thromboembolic disease. D-Dimer is a fibrin degradation product and is therefore elevated in the presence of thrombus. A normal D-dimer assay has a very high negative predictive value to exclude thromboembolic disease. However, an elevated assay is very nonspecific and may be seen with many inflammatory processes. There are two broad groups of D-dimer assays.[14] The first group includes the enzyme-linked immunosorbent assays (ELISA) and "rapid" ELISA, which are highly sensitive for thrombus. A normal assay has a 99.3% negative predictive value and therefore virtually excludes thromboembolic disease.[15] However, only 31% of patients evaluated for suspected venous thromboembolic disease have a normal assay. In the remaining 69%, the specificity of a positive D-dimer ELISA for thromboembolism is low. The second group includes whole blood D-dimer assays. These are simpler to perform, but they have a lower sensitivity of 85% and cannot exclude the presence of venous thromboembolism alone.[16] When combined with a low Wells clinical score, there is a 2% prevalence of thromboembolic disease with a normal whole blood assay, decreasing the suspicion of PE in a large proportion of patients, which virtually eliminates the need for further tests.[17]

Chest Radiography

In patients with cardiopulmonary disorders, the chest radiograph is often the first radiological investigation. It has both a low sensitivity and specificity for PE and is used primarily to exclude other diagnoses that mimic PE and for the interpretation of VQ scintigraphy. From retrospective analysis of the Prospective Investigation of Pulmonary Embolism Diagnosis (PIOPED) study data by Worsley et al. (1993),[18] 88% of patients with PE have abnormal radiographs, but so do 82% of patients without PE. Of the specific radiological signs attributed to PE, only oligemia (Westermark's sign) is found significantly more often in patients with PE than those without PE (8% versus 4%). Enlargement of the central pulmonary arteries (Fleischner's sign) and pleural-based opacities (Hampton's hump) are identified with similar frequency in patients with and without PE.[18] In 117 patients with PE but no prior history of cardiopulmonary disease, 64% had abnormal radiographs, and no signs were specific for PE.[19]

COMPUTED TOMOGRAPHY

Advances in MSCT

MSCT has several advantages over SSCT, which are particularly useful for the detection of PE. These include improved z-axis resolution and shorter scanning times, which reduce motion artifacts. In addition, the volume of contrast required to obtain optimal pulmonary artery opacification can be reduced.

Z-Axis Resolution

MSCT has overcome a major limitation of SSCT in thoracic imaging by increasing the scan range in a reasonable breath hold at optimal slice thickness. Increased width of the detector array and advances in gantry rotation speed and tube performance permit more rapid acquisition of volumetric data. Segmentation of the detector array results in simultaneous reduction in slice thickness and increased z-axis resolution. This addresses a persistent concern regarding the poor depiction of the peripheral pulmonary arteries with SSCT. Initial reports of high sensitivity and specificity for SSCT did not include analysis of subsegmental arteries and demonstrated poor sensitivity for PE in the subsegmental pulmonary arteries.[4,20] For example, Goodman et al.[21] demonstrated a sensitivity of SSCT using 5-mm collimation of 86% for the central pulmonary arteries, but only 63% when the subsegmental arteries were included in the analysis. A series of subsequent studies confirm the reduced sensitivity of SSCT for evaluating the subsegmental pulmonary arteries.[22-24]

At conventional angiography, 6% to 30% of patients have isolated subsegmental or smaller emboli, and an estimated 20% of all emboli occur in the horizontally oriented middle lobe or lingula

segmental arteries.[25-27] Arteries in or oblique to the CT scan plane are particularly prone to volume-averaging artifacts and rely on high z-axis resolution for accurate depiction.[20] Reducing the reconstruction slice thickness improves z-axis resolution and improves visualization of the small arteries (Figure 5-1). Reducing collimation from 3 mm to 2 mm on SSCT increases visualization of subsegmental arteries from 37% to 61% in optimal studies.[28] However, reducing the slice thickness on SSCT comes at the expense of an extended breath hold, which is a problem for dyspneic patients, and a common symptom of PE.

MSCT partially overcomes these problems. Narrow slice reconstruction has led to progressive improvement in visualization of subsegmental arteries. Using 4-row MSCT at 1.25-mm slice thickness in an optimal group of patients without prior pulmonary disease and an optimal contrast bolus, 94% of fourth order (subsegmental) and 74% of fifth order arteries are well visualized.[29] In patients with a high burden of respiratory disease, using MSCT at 1.25-mm slice thickness visualizes 78% of subsegmental arteries.[30] Reducing reconstruction thickness from 3 mm to 1 mm, with 4-row MSCT, leads to a 40% improvement in the detection of subsegmental PE (see Figure 5-1). Additional benefits of narrower slice thickness include improved interobserver agreement for the diagnosis of PE and a decreased number of indeterminate CT results.[31]

Reduced Scan Times

Respiratory motion artifact, a common cause of suboptimal studies, exacerbates partial volume artifacts of arteries in or near the scan plane and leads to loss of continuity of arteries in the z-axis, resulting in interpretative difficulty. The reduced scan time of MSCT reduces motion artifacts, particularly in patients with underlying respiratory disease.[32] A scan range of 15 to 20 cm from the mid-dome of the diaphragm to above the aortic arch takes 32 to 43 seconds with SSCT at 3-mm collimation and pitch of 1.6. Studies in patients who were unable to maintain a breath hold for this period of time involves compromising slice thickness, pitch, or range. MSCT not only allows imaging of the same range, but also permits evaluation of the entire lung using 1.25-mm collimation in 15 to 28 seconds on 4-row MSCT, and 7 to 13 seconds using 16-row CT (Table 5-1). The

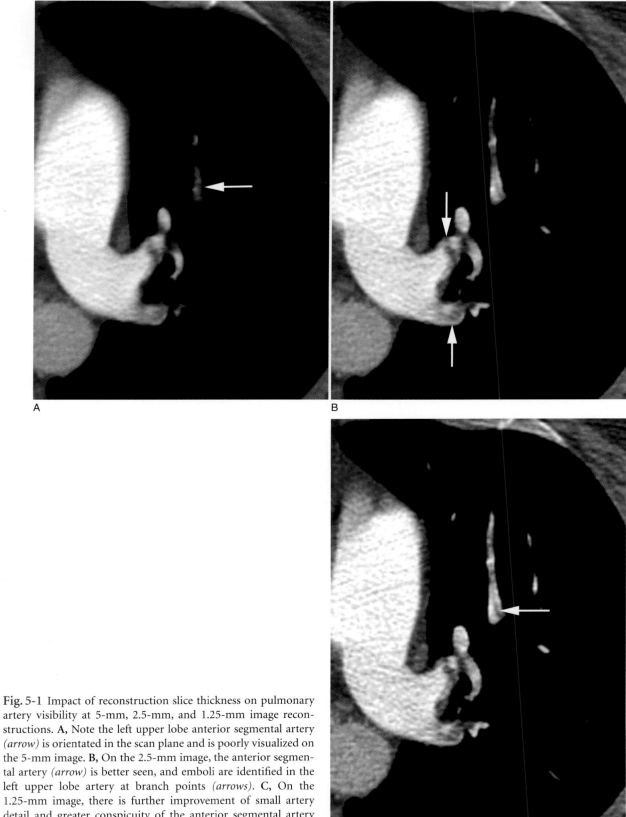

Fig. 5-1 Impact of reconstruction slice thickness on pulmonary artery visibility at 5-mm, 2.5-mm, and 1.25-mm image reconstructions. **A,** Note the left upper lobe anterior segmental artery *(arrow)* is orientated in the scan plane and is poorly visualized on the 5-mm image. **B,** On the 2.5-mm image, the anterior segmental artery *(arrow)* is better seen, and emboli are identified in the left upper lobe artery at branch points *(arrows)*. **C,** On the 1.25-mm image, there is further improvement of small artery detail and greater conspicuity of the anterior segmental artery embolism *(arrow)*.

Table 5-1 Suggested Imaging Protocols for CT Pulmonary Angiography

Indications			Suspected thromboembolic disease	
			Thin collimation	Ultrathin collimation
Protocol designed for	LightSpeed QXi 4-row	LightSpeed Ultra 8-row	LightSpeed 16 16-row*	LightSpeed 16 16-row*
Patient preparation	NPO for 6 hours if possible			
First series	CT pulmonary angiography			
Oral contrast	None			
IV contrast	Yes	Yes	Yes	Yes
Concentration	300 mg/ml			
Volume: (ml)/rate(ml/s)/delay	130-150/4/calculated to end 5 sec after the contrast bolus			
Saline chaser	50/4/0			
Tube settings kVp	140	140	140	140
mA	380	380	400	400
Gantry speed (sec)	0.8	0.7	0.7	0.7
Table speed (mm/rotation)	7.5	13.5	27.5*	13.75*
Table speed (mm/sec)	9.4	19.3	39.3	19.6
Slice collimation (mm)	1.25	1.25	1.25*	0.625*
Breath hold	Inspiration			
Anatomical coverage	Mid-diaphragm to lung apices (25 cm)			
Acquisition time(s)	27.6	13.8	7.0*	13.5*
Reconstruction kernel	Standard			
Reconstruction thickness (mm)	1.25	1.25	1.25	0.625
Effective slice thickness (mm)	2.5	1.6	1.6	0.8
Reconstruction interval (mm)	0.625	0.625	0.625	0.625
Window settings	Typically WW 500, WL 50			
Postprocessing	None			

*The 16-row scanner allows a choice of rapid acquisition using a 1.25 mm collimation, which is particularly useful in dyspneic patients, or thinner collimation for greater spatial resolution.

development of 64-row MSCT will further reduce this by another factor of four.

The lung bases, a common site of emboli, demonstrate the greatest movement from diaphragmatic motion during the respiratory cycle. Scanning in the caudal to cranial direction reduces motion artifacts by imaging the lung bases at the beginning of the breath hold. In addition, imaging the superior mediastinum later in the study reduces beam-hardening artifact from concentrated iodinated contrast in the superior vena cava (SVC) (Figure 5-2).

Contrast Volume Reduction

A shorter acquisition time permits a reduction in the volume of intravenous contrast material needed to optimally opacify the pulmonary arteries. The use of a saline chasing bolus following the contrast with a dual-chamber power injector further reduces the volume of contrast required. Although this has not been formally investigated in the diagnosis of PE, replacing 30% of a contrast bolus with an equivalent volume of saline during coronary CT

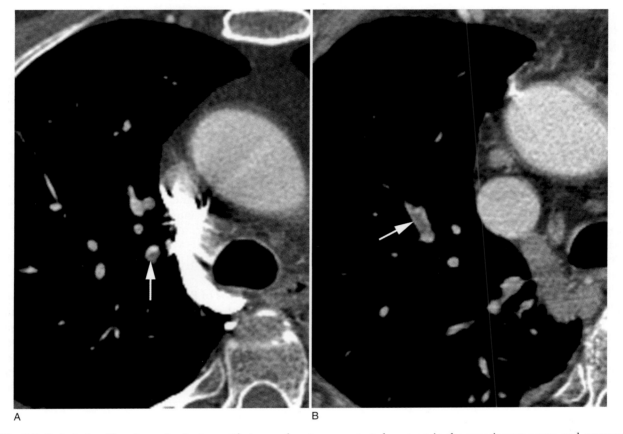

A   B

Fig. 5-2 Technical artifact: beam-hardening artifact secondary to concentrated contrast in the superior vena cava and azygous vein. **A,** This produces a "pseudo" filling defect *(arrow)* in the right upper lobe apical segmental artery, mimicking pulmonary embolism that was not present or changed shape on images above and below the one presented here. **B,** In another patient, scanning the superior mediastinum later in the study reduces this artifact and reveals a right upper lobe apical subsegmental artery embolism *(arrow).*

angiography demonstrated no significant difference in the level of peak arterial enhancement within the coronary arteries.[33] Furthermore, beam-hardening artifacts caused by concentrated contrast in the SVC are also reduced.

In patients who are allergic to iodinated contrast, gadolinium-based contrast agents may be used for MSCT pulmonary angiography. The current evidence for use of this technique is limited to research models and sporadic case reports.[34,35]

CTPA Technique

Table 5-1 suggests parameters for CTPA using 4-, 8-, and 16-row MSCT. The aim is to perform the study at the thinnest slice thickness achievable in a single inspiratory breath hold, minimizing respiratory motion artifact to optimize visualization of

subsegmental arteries. If even a short breath hold is not possible, quiet respiration can be substituted. Given the short acquisition time of MSCT, respiration can usually be suspended in intubated patients.

The intravenous cannula for contrast injection should not be distal to the antecubital fossa. The arms should be placed above the patient's head, outside the scan field, without flexing the elbow. Leaving the arm used for injection by the patient's side avoids an inadvertent delay in the bolus that is the result of either extrinsic venous compression at the flexed antecubital fossa or compression of the subclavian vein at the level of the first rib, which unfortunately increases image noise. Power injectors are required for rapid contrast delivery in order to obtain adequate pulmonary artery enhancement. Increasing the rate of contrast injection leads to earlier and greater arterial enhancement, independent of the iodine concentration of the contrast agent.[36]

Incorrect timing of image acquisition relative to the contrast bolus is a common cause of suboptimal studies. The time to peak pulmonary artery enhancement following injection of contrast into the antecubital fossa at 4 m/sec is approximately 20 seconds, and this may be used empirically as the scan delay time in patients with normal cardiac function. Individually timed studies, using either a test bolus or a bolus tracking method, are available, but currently there is limited evidence regarding their use in CTPA. When comparing empirical timing to the test bolus timing methods in 85 patients, significantly greater objective pulmonary artery enhancement was demonstrated using the test bolus, but this did not translate into observable differences in image quality. In addition, 16% of the test bolus studies had to be excluded from the analysis because of uninterpretable time-density curves resulting from technical difficulties.[37] A saline bolus may be used to follow the iodinated contrast, effectively chasing the contrast from the antecubital vein into the pulmonary artery circulation and reducing total contrast volume. Further evaluation of this method is required because accurate bolus timing becomes even more critical with shorter study times. We time the study to end 5 seconds after the end of the contrast bolus and use a saline chaser bolus. In cases with poor cardiac reserve, we use a timing bolus.

Electrocardiographic (ECG)-gated MSCT is increasingly being used in cardiac imaging. The addition of ECG-gating to CT pulmonary angiography reduces the presence of cardiac motion artifacts within the middle, lingular, and medial basilar lower lobe pulmonary arteries but has not been shown to improve diagnostic accuracy or confidence.[38] In addition, ECG-gating increases radiation dose and increases acquisition time twofold to fourfold, increasing the likelihood of respiratory motion artifact in patients who are already dyspneic.

Image Interpretation

The near isotropic data set generated from MSCT pulmonary angiography comes at the expense of a large number of images. Images may be reconstructed with overlapping reconstructions using a standard soft tissue kernel. Soft-copy computer workstation interpretation is particularly beneficial in the diagnosis of PE, because the ability to easily follow arteries to their origin avoids the potential for mistaking pulmonary veins or mucous-filled bronchi for pulmonary arteries. Soft-copy interpretation also reduces interpretation time and increases diagnostic accuracy.[39] The ability to reformat images in other planes may be useful to differentiate small mural thrombi from peribronchial lymph nodes.[40] Depending on the attenuation of contrast within the pulmonary arteries, the window level and width is altered to be slightly wider than standard soft tissue windows to avoid obscuring small emboli within intensely enhancing pulmonary arteries.[41]

Direct and Indirect Signs of PE

The diagnosis of PE on CT hinges on the direct visualization of emboli. CT signs can be divided into direct findings of PE and ancillary findings that suggest PE (Table 5-2). Specific findings are filling defects, which completely occlude a well-enhanced pulmonary artery with or without (vessel cutoff sign) visualization of the distal non-opacified artery (Figure 5-3), or a partially occluded artery with a surrounding rim of contrast identified as the "rim" sign when seen in short axis, or the "railway track" sign in long axis (Figure 5-4).[4]

Ancillary signs may suggest the need for further diagnostic testing for PE when CT is inconclusive. The significant ancillary findings on CT differ from those reported on plain radiography. In a large chest radiographic study by Worsley et al. (1993),[18] oligemia was the only finding identified significantly more frequently in the presence of PE. On CT, two small studies indicate that pleural-based, wedge-shaped opacities (incidence 62% with PE versus 27% without PE) (Figure 5-5), linear parenchymal

Table 5-2 Signs of acute pulmonary embolism	
Specific signs	**Ancillary signs**
Rim sign	Pleural-based parenchymal opacities +/− enhancement
Railway track sign	Linear parenchymal bands
Vessel cutoff sign	

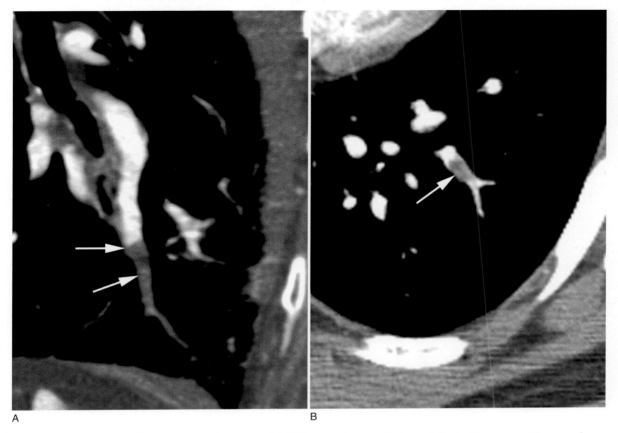

Fig. 5-3 Vessel cutoff sign of pulmonary embolism. **A,** Multiplanar reformat of a lower lobe basilar segmental artery shows an embolism as an abrupt lack of enhancement of the distal artery *(arrows)*. **B,** In a different patient, an embolism partially occludes the artery *(arrow),* with enhancement of the distal artery.

bands (incidence 46% with PE versus 21% without PE), and central pulmonary arterial enlargement occur significantly more frequently in patients with PE than in patients without PE.[42,43] The triangular, pleural-based parenchymal opacities may contain air bronchograms and presumably represent pulmonary infarcts or the CT equivalent of a chest radiographic Hampton's hump. Pleural-based parenchymal opacities that enhance are thought to be complicated by hemorrhage.[42] Linear parenchymal bands are of uncertain etiology and may represent sequela of prior infarction. Nonpleural-based opacities, isolated atelectasis, and pleural effusions are common but do not occur significantly more frequently in the presence of PE.[43]

Pitfalls in the Diagnosis of PE

Pitfalls in the diagnosis of PE can be divided into technical pitfalls and interpretative pitfalls.

Technical Pitfalls

These include poor arterial opacification caused by incorrect bolus timing (Figure 5-6) and beam-hardening artifact, particularly from dense contrast in the SVC, which creates bands of low attenuation in the adjacent arteries of the right upper lobe. Partial volume artifacts are increased by respiratory and cardiac motion. The latter are most common in the lingula and left lower lobe. Advances in MSCT and attention to bolus delivery technique reduce these artifacts. A recently described artifact, known as a "transient interruption of contrast," may be more common with the rapid scanning capability of MSCT (Figure 5-7).[44] During deep inspiration at the beginning of the scan, the negative intrathoracic pressure draws non-opacified blood from the inferior vena cava into the right atrium, creating a column of non-opacified blood that flows through the pulmonary vasculature that may be mistaken

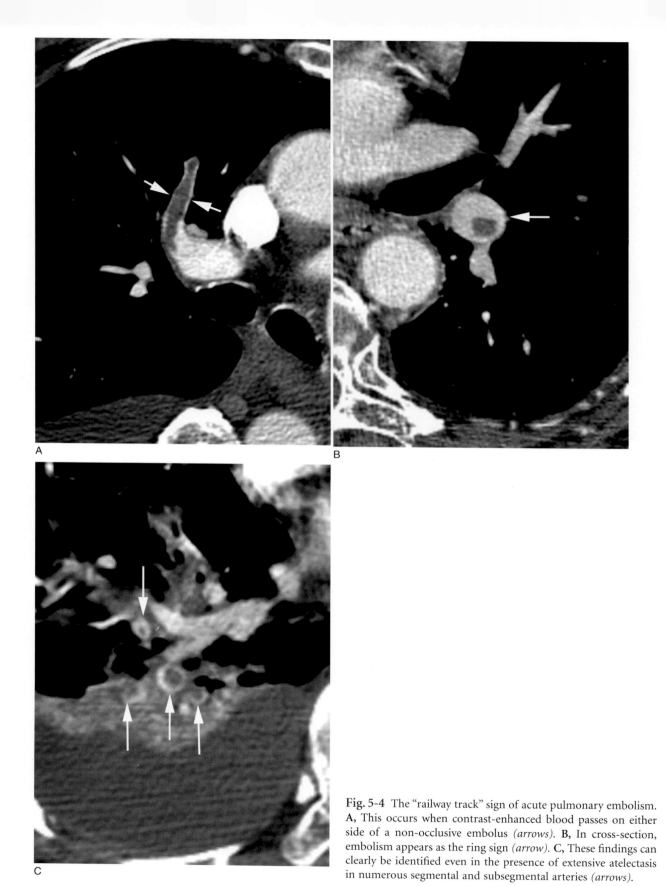

Fig. 5-4 The "railway track" sign of acute pulmonary embolism. **A,** This occurs when contrast-enhanced blood passes on either side of a non-occlusive embolus *(arrows)*. **B,** In cross-section, embolism appears as the ring sign *(arrow)*. **C,** These findings can clearly be identified even in the presence of extensive atelectasis in numerous segmental and subsegmental arteries *(arrows)*.

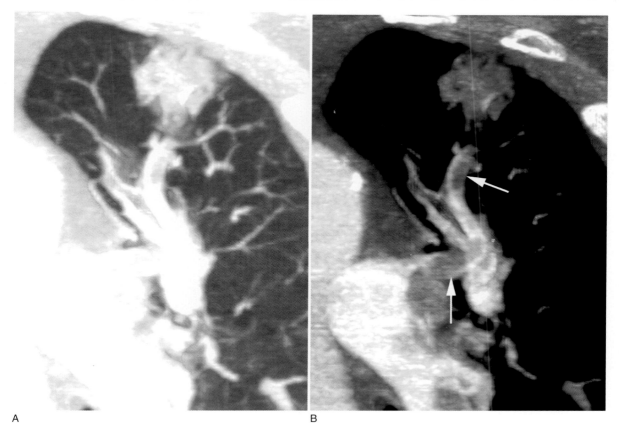

A   B

Fig. 5-5 Pleural-based parenchymal opacity: an indirect sign of pulmonary embolism. In this patient with multiple pulmonary emboli, coronal reformatted images demonstrate a pleural-based opacity in the left upper lobe apical segment on lung windows (**A**). **B**, Image at soft-tissue windows demonstrates emboli *(arrows)* in the lobar and segmental artery supplying this segment, indicating that the pleural-based opacity represents a pulmonary infarct.

for emboli. This artifact can be reduced by hyperventilating the patient before the study.

Interpretative Pitfalls

Non-opacified pulmonary veins and mucous-filled bronchi can be confused with non-opacified pulmonary arteries (Figure 5-8). Soft-copy interpretation and a systematic approach for analyzing pulmonary arteries are recommended to ensure that non-opacified structures are within the arterial tree. Peribronchial lymph nodes can occasionally be confused with mural thrombi but are less of a problem with reduced slice thicknesses of fast MSCT scanners and soft-copy reporting (Figure 5-9). Multiplanar reformats (MPR) may further reduce this pitfall. In rare cases, beam hardening from venous and pulmonary artery catheters

causes a streak artifact that either mimics or obscures PE.

MSCT and Ventilation/Perfusion Scintigraphy

VQ scintigraphy has long been the primary imaging modality for the diagnosis of PE. Unlike both CT and catheter pulmonary angiography, VQ scans provide only indirect evidence of PE and are of limited value in patients with underlying pulmonary disease. The PIOPED study determined the accuracy of VQ scans in a prospective comparison with catheter pulmonary angiography in patients with suspected acute PE.[8] High-probability VQ scintigraphy has a positive predictive value of 88% for PE, increasing to 96% when combined with a high

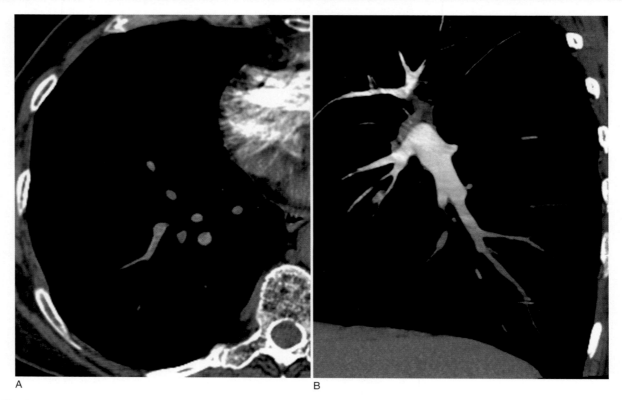

A   B

Fig. 5-6 Technical pitfall: poor contrast enhancement of the pulmonary arteries. **A,** Axial image through the right lower lobe. **B,** Sagittally reconstructed image of the right lung demonstrates poor enhancement of the pulmonary arteries caused by scanning too early. Note the gradient of improved enhancement as the scan proceeded from the caudal to the cranial direction. This can be differentiated from the vessel cutoff sign by gradual and not abrupt margin of poor enhancement and the uniform involvement of the arteries at any given craniocaudal level.

clinical suspicion for PE. A normal or near-normal examination has a high negative predictive value, with only 4% of patients having PE. Unfortunately, in the PIOPED study, only 27% of studies fall into these two diagnostic categories, and only 41% of patients with a PE have a high probability study. Furthermore, 90% of patients without PE have an abnormal isotope study, which is an indicator of low specificity.

Most studies comparing CT to VQ scintigraphy have used SSCT technology. In a prospective study of 139 patients, Mayo et al. (1997)[45] demonstrated that SSCT is more likely to be correctly interpreted than scintigraphy (92% versus 74%) and has greater interobserver agreement. A negative CT excludes the diagnosis of PE as effectively as a normal VQ study or a normal catheter pulmonary angiogram. A study comparing the clinical outcome of 198 patients with negative CTPA using 3-mm SSCT to patients with low probability or normal

VQ scans found that the frequency of subsequent clinically apparent PE is 1% with negative CTPA. This rate was not significantly different when compared to patients with low probability or normal VQ scintigraphy.[46]

Comparing 4 × 1-mm MSCT with VQ scintigraphy in 94 patients, Coche et al.[47] demonstrated both higher sensitivity (96% versus 86%) and specificity (98% versus 88%) for the diagnosis of PE with MSCT. In patients with discordant MSCT and VQ results, MSCT correlated with the findings at catheter angiography in 91% of cases (*n* = 10). Furthermore, CT provided an alternative diagnosis in 29% of patients in whom PE was excluded.

When used as the initial imaging modality, CT leads to a higher number of confident diagnoses and is better at demonstrating alternative pathology that may be responsible for patient symptoms.[48] The increased diagnostic accuracy of MSCT has led to

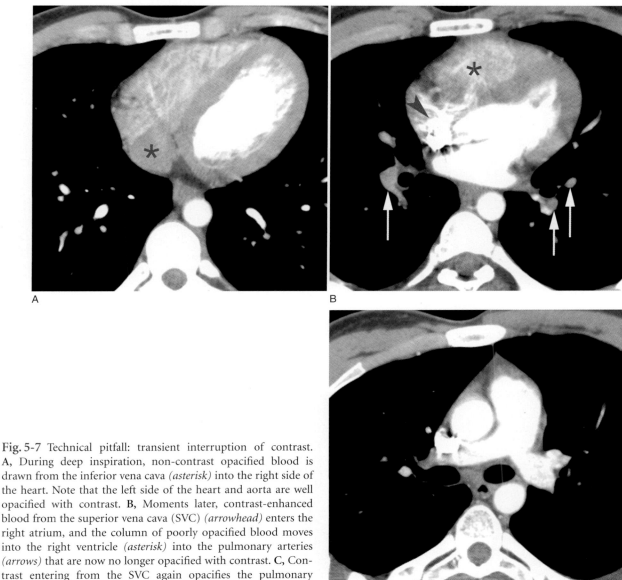

Fig. 5-7 Technical pitfall: transient interruption of contrast. **A,** During deep inspiration, non-contrast opacified blood is drawn from the inferior vena cava *(asterisk)* into the right side of the heart. Note that the left side of the heart and aorta are well opacified with contrast. **B,** Moments later, contrast-enhanced blood from the superior vena cava (SVC) *(arrowhead)* enters the right atrium, and the column of poorly opacified blood moves into the right ventricle *(asterisk)* into the pulmonary arteries *(arrows)* that are now no longer opacified with contrast. **C,** Contrast entering from the SVC again opacifies the pulmonary arteries. (Images courtesy of Dr. M. Gosselin, Oregon Health and Science University.)

CT challenging VQ as the primary modality of choice in the investigation of thromboembolic disease, particularly in patients with underlying respiratory disorders.

MSCT and Catheter Pulmonary Angiography

Like CTPA, catheter angiography directly visualizes acute PE as filling defects and has long been held as the gold standard for diagnosing PE. Several studies have demonstrated a deterioration in angiographic interobserver agreement as the branch order of arteries being visualized increases, with poor agreement particularly in subsegmental arteries.[49-51] This suggests that emboli within subsegmental arteries are at the limit of angiography resolution. Baile et al. (2000)[52] compared 1-mm helical CT and catheter angiography following the injection of artificial emboli of equivalent size to subsegmental emboli into the pulmonary arteries of pigs, using

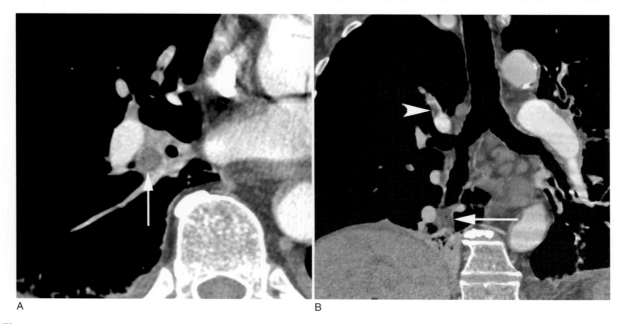

Fig. 5-8 Interpretive pitfall: mucus plugging mimicking pulmonary embolism. **A,** Low-attenuation filling defect in the right lower lobe bronchus *(arrow)* on an axial image may be mistaken for an embolism. **B,** Multiplanar reformat shows the mucous-filled bronchus *(arrow)* and a real embolism originating in the right upper lobe pulmonary artery *(arrowhead).*

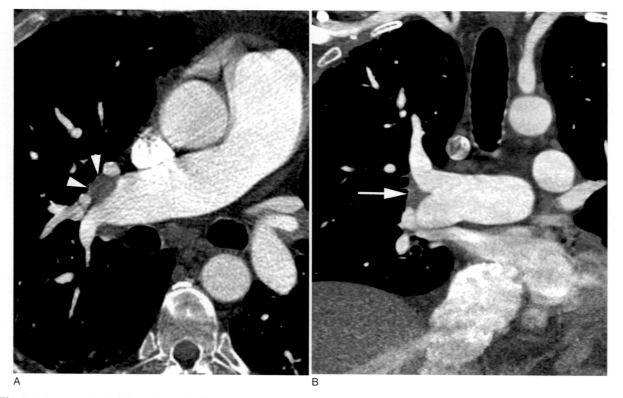

Fig. 5-9 Interpretive pitfall: peribronchial lymphoid tissue mimicking pulmonary embolism. **A,** Low-attenuation round "pseudo" filling defect in the right pulmonary artery *(arrowheads)* represents a hilar lymph node *(arrow)* on a multiplanar coronal reformatted image (**B**).

autopsy as an independent reference test. There was a significant difference in the sensitivity between catheter angiography and CTPA.[52] The authors suggested that with the advent of multiple detectors, CT may surpass the accuracy of angiography.

Improved visualization of subsegmental pulmonary arteries and greater intraobserver agreement call into question whether pulmonary angiography should continue to be considered the standard by which MSCT is judged, or whether MSCT has already exceeded the accuracy of catheter pulmonary angiography. Not only is catheter angiography less readily available than CT, it does not demonstrate alternative pathology and has a morbidity, although small, that is greater than CT. Similar to CT, following a negative catheter angiogram, there is a 1.6% to 1.7% incidence of PE.[53,54]

The Evidence for MSCT in the Diagnosis of Acute Pulmonary Embolism

Improved visualization of the subsegmental arteries[28-30] with thinner slice reconstruction translates into an improved diagnostic accuracy of MSCT for the detection of subsegmental pulmonary emboli, when compared with SSCT.[31] Currently there is limited research on the diagnostic accuracy of MSCT compared with the current reference test of catheter angiography. In 157 patients with suspected acute PE, imaged with a dual-detector CT with an effective slice thickness of 2.7-mm and using catheter angiography as the reference test, CT demonstrated a 90% sensitivity and a 94% specificity. CTPA depicted more subsegmental emboli than selective angiography, which raises the question of which test is correct. It also raises the question about the role of pulmonary angiography, which may be an imperfect gold standard against which to judge CT.[55] A second study using 4-row

MSCT with 2.5-mm collimation in 93 patients with catheter angiography as the reference test (Winer-Muram HT et al., Society of Thoracic Radiology Annual Meeting, 2004), reported a sensitivity of 100% and specificity of 89% for MSCT in the detection of PE.

If we accept that CTPA using SSCT may miss isolated subsegmental PE, the low risk of fatal PE after a negative SSCT pulmonary angiogram calls into question the benefit of treating isolated subsegmental emboli. The largest outcome study followed 993 patients for 3 months following a negative SSCT pulmonary angiogram. The study found a 0.5% recurrence of thromboembolic disease and a 0.3% incidence of fatal pulmonary emboli.[56] Multiple subsequent outcome studies following negative CTPA performed with SSCT report an average recurrence rate of 1.3% and a rate of fatal PE of 0.3%. A small number of outcome studies following negative MSCT for PE demonstrate comparable low rates of recurrent thromboembolism (Table 5-3). Mortality rates in these studies are complicated by deaths related to co-morbid conditions. When 91 patients were followed-up for 3 months after a negative CTPA using 4×1-mm MSCT, there was a single recognized fatal PE in a patient who was not anticoagulated despite known deep vein thrombus.[32] In 85 patients reviewed clinically over 9 months following a negative 4×1.25 MSCT for PE, there was one nonfatal PE, producing a negative predictive value of 98%. This study is limited by a lack of autopsy data in 17 patients who were thought to have died from unrelated causes.[57] The benefit of treating isolated subsegmental emboli in healthy people is therefore uncertain. Treatment may be beneficial for the prevention of chronic pulmonary hypertension in patients with multiple small emboli and in patients with limited cardiopulmonary reserve. However, a 1-year follow-up of 344 patients with no evidence of PE following 2-mm SSCT found no significant

Table 5-3   Clinical outcome after negative MSCT for pulmonary embolism

First author	Year	Study design	N	Follow-up duration (months)	Overall patient deaths (N)	Recurrent DVT (%)	Recurrent PE (%)
Remy-Jardin[32]	2002	Prospective	91	3	1	–	1
Donato[109]	2003	Retrospective	239	3	33	1.7	0.4
Coche[47]	2003	Prospective	65	3-6	Not stated	0	0
Kavanagh[57]	2004	Prospective	85	9	17	–	0

difference in the incidence of clinically apparent PE between patients with or without underlying pulmonary disease.[58] The current PIOPED II study is designed to determine the diagnostic accuracy of state-of-the-art MSCT compared with a reference test of negative VQ studies, pulmonary angiography, lower extremity ultrasound, and clinical outcome.

CT Venography

Case reports of incidental iliofemoral thrombi date back to the early days of CT. Initial studies of direct CT venography following cannulation of the dorsal veins of the foot indicate an accuracy comparable to conventional fluoroscopic venography.[59,60] The development of indirect CT venography (CTV) allows the option of a rapid combined assessment for both PE and DVT in a single examination. Loud et al. (1998)[61] first demonstrated the potential use of indirect CTV following CTPA, avoiding the need for pedal cannulation.

The lower limb veins can be imaged once the lower limb venous system is adequately opacified following the contrast administration for CTPA. A variety of techniques have been investigated, ranging from spaced incremental CT to helical MSCT, with the scan range extending from the upper calf to the iliac crests or the diaphragm; all demonstrate similar accuracy rates for detecting DVT (see Table 5-6).[62-67] The recommended technique is helical CT, which will minimize the

possibility of missing small thrombi between incremental images. This technique does not require the use of additional iodinated contrast. Published studies of combined CTPA and CTV use doses varying from 100 ml of 300 mg/ml to 140 ml of 370 mg/ml of iodinated contrast. The minimal venous enhancement required to consider a study technically adequate is 80 HU. A retrospective study of 429 patients administered 150 ml of 240 mg/ml iodinated contrast and imaged at 180 seconds demonstrated a mean enhancement of 97 (SD ± 20) HU. Enhancement of less than 61 HU was seen in less than 5% of patients.[68]

Maximum enhancement timing of the peripheral venous system varies because of poor cardiac output or the presence of peripheral vascular disease. Published studies have used delays of between 145 and 210 seconds from the end of the contrast injection. The optimal delay for veins above the knee is thought to be 180 seconds from the end of contrast injection, because 85% of subjects are within 10% of their peak venous enhancement at this time.[69,70]

In our protocol (Table 5-4) following a 180-second delay, a spiral study of the lower limb veins is performed from the iliac crests to 2 cm below the tibial plateaus to minimize the risk of missing small thrombi. Imaging the abdomen has a low yield of isolated proximal inferior vena cava thrombus in the absence of more distal thrombus or PE.[65] Viewing images with a narrow window width helps differentiate enhanced veins from thrombus and

Table 5-4 Suggested Imaging Protocols for Indirect CT Venography		
Second series		**CT venography**
Oral contrast	None	
IV contrast	No additional intravenous contrast	
	4-row MSCT	16-row MSCT
Tube settings		
kVp	120	120
mA	190	190
Gantry speed (sec)	1.1	1.0
Table speed (mm/sec)	7.5	27.5
Slice collimation (mm)	7.5	7.5
Anatomical coverage	Iliac crests to 2 cm below the tibial plateaus	
Reconstruction kernel	Standard	Standard
Reconstruction thickness (mm)	7.5	7.5
Reconstruction interval (mm)	7.5	7.5
Window settings	Width 500, level 50	Width 500, level 50
Postprocessing	None	

adjacent soft tissue, caused by the less marked enhancement of the lower limb veins.

Signs and Pitfalls of Indirect CTV

Thrombi are visualized as low-attenuation intraluminal filling defects that completely or partially occlude a vein (Table 5-5). Partially occluding thrombi may be free-floating or adherent to the wall. Ancillary signs include venous dilation compared with the contralateral limb, mural enhancement of the vasa vasorum, infiltration of the perivenous fat, and the presence of collateral vessels (Figure 5-10).[71]

Table 5-5	Signs of acute deep vein thrombosis on indirect CT venography
Specific signs	**Ancillary signs**
Central or eccentric filling defect	Venous dilation Mural enhancement Perivenous infiltration Collateral vessels

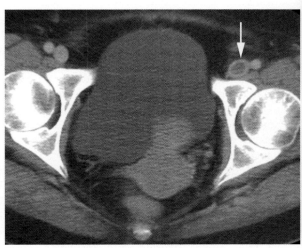

A

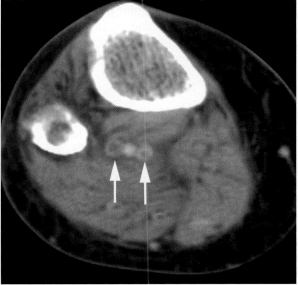

B

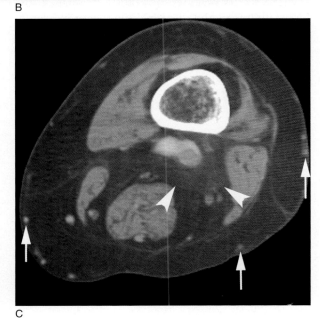

C

Fig. 5-10 Indirect CT venography with deep venous thrombosis. Note the low-attenuation filling defects that completely occlude the left femoral vein (**A**) *(arrow)* and infrapopliteal right calf veins (**B**) *(arrows)*. **C**, Perivenous stranding *(arrowheads)* and dilation of collateral veins *(arrows)* are ancillary findings of deep venous thrombosis.

Technical pitfalls include beam-hardening artifacts from metallic prostheses and cortical bone and inadequate venous enhancement. Interpretative errors include venous valves, which may appear as low-attenuation filling defects that dilate the vein but are not visualized on consecutive images. Contiguous acquisition may help to avoid this error. Variations in vascular anatomy, particularly venous duplication, can lead to missed diagnosis.[72] Chronic venous thrombosis may lead to eccentric mural thrombi in small-caliber veins without mural enhancement or perivenous stranding. In the absence of ancillary signs, it is not possible to accurately differentiate acute from chronic thrombi.[73] In subacute and chronic thrombi, the vein may subsequently partially calcify and recanalize, leading to intraluminal webs, or fibrose and appear as a nonenhancing tract in the expected location of the vein.

The Evidence for CT Venography

Several studies have evaluated whether the addition of CTV to CTPA alters clinical practice. In a study of 800 patients with suspected acute PE in an emergency department setting, 5% had a positive CTPA venous alone, 4% had positive CTPA and CTV, and 2% had isolated positive CTV and a negative CTPA.[74] The authors noted the logistical advantage of a combined examination and concluded that it significantly increased the detection rate of venous thromboembolic disease. Subsequent studies confirm a 2% to 5% detection rate of isolated DVT.[65,66,75,76] Coche et al. (2001)[66] imaged the whole abdomen and identified significant incidental abdominal pathology in 6% of patients.

Studies investigating the accuracy of CTV have used ultrasonography as the reference test (Table 5-6). At least six additional studies have been published since 1998, all demonstrating good correlation with ultrasonography. The largest study by Loud et al. (2000)[64] was a retrospective review of 308 patients who underwent combined CTPA and CTV using incremental CT (5- to 10-mm collimation; 50-mm intervals) with bilateral lower limb ultrasonography as a reference test. Only two false-negative and no false-positive studies were reported, yielding a sensitivity of 97% and a specificity of 100%. Among other prospective studies, sensitivities ranged from 93% to 100%; specificities ranged from 97% to 100%. Interobserver agreement is good to excellent, with kappa values ranging from 0.59 to 0.88.[66,77] A single study by Peterson et al. (2001)[78] reported a reduced sensitivity of 71%. This lower sensitivity was thought to be related to selection bias, because this was a retrospective study of patients who had both CTPA/CTV and ultrasonography, not consecutive patients evaluated with both tests; therefore, patients with obviously normal CTV or ultrasonography may have not undergone both tests, and the population was skewed toward patients with nondiagnostic or inconclusive CTV examinations.

Rademaker et al. (2001)[79] evaluated the additional radiation dose of adding indirect CTV to CTPA. The effective dose of CTV using a single SSCT technique (8-mm collimation, pitch 3, 120 kVp, and 170 mA) was 2.3 to 2.7 mSv. Compared with CTPA alone, ovarian and testicular doses are increased by a factor of 500 and 2000, respectively.[79] This dose is less than that from dual-phase hepatic

Table 5-6 Results of CT venography trials

Author	Year	Patients	Scanning method slice/reconstruction (mm)	Sensitivity	Specificity	PPV	NPV
Garg[62]	2000	68	Incremental 10/20	100	97	71	100
Duwe[63]*	2000	74	SD helical 10/pitch 1	89	94	67	98
Loud[64]	2000	71†	Incremental 5-10/50	100	100	100	100
Loud[65]*	2001	308†	Incremental 5-10/50	97	100	100	99
Coche[66]	2001	65	MD helical 2 × 6.5/pitch 1.5	93	97	93	97
Peterson[78]*	2001	136	MD helical 1 × 7.5/pitch 3	53	93	53	97
Begemann[67]	2003	41	MD helical 4 × 2.5/pitch 1.25	100	96.6	91.7	100

*Retrospective design.
†Overlap of patients.

CT and translates into a risk of hereditary genetic defects of 1 : 15,000 to 20,000. Although careful consideration should be given to the use of CTV, especially in younger patients, this should be weighed against the considerable morbidity and mortality of undiagnosed and untreated thromboembolic disease.

The addition of CTV to CTPA creates a single radiological evaluation for the presence of venous thromboembolic disease. Current treatments with oral anticoagulants in venous thromboembolism reflect the concept that both PE and DVT are facets of the same disease. Duration of treatment is determined by the presence of underlying risk factors and not by the site of thrombus.[80-82] Patients with first-time idiopathic proximal DVT or PE and underlying long-term risk factors, such as thrombophilia or factor V Leiden deficiency, have an increased risk of recurrent thromboembolism. They should receive a longer course of anticoagulation compared with patients with temporary risk factors such as surgery or trauma, regardless of the site of thrombus.

Vena cava filters are an effective form of venous thromboembolic disease therapy for patients with contraindications to anticoagulants, in those who develop complications related to anticoagulation, and in patients for whom adequate anticoagulation fails to prevent recurrent PE.[83] A further indication is the identification of a free-floating iliofemoral thrombus in the absence of PE. Prophylactic filter placement is increasingly used in the prevention of pulmonary embolism in trauma and high-risk orthopedic patients. Prophylactic filter placement should be considered in patients too hemodynamically unstable to tolerate further PE or following massive or recurrent PE. Filter placement is indicated in patients with cor pulmonale secondary to PE and may be considered in patients with cor pulmonale of other etiologies.

Chronic Thromboembolic Disease and Pulmonary Hypertension

Pulmonary hypertension is hemodynamically defined as the resting mean pulmonary arterial pressure of greater than 25 mm Hg.[84,85] The etiologies of pulmonary hypertension can be broadly divided into three categories: precapillary, postcapillary, and pulmonary disorders (Table 5-7). In a small study of 62 patients, Remy-Jardin et al. (1997)[86] performed a follow-up CT with a mean of 11 months following the initial diagnosis of acute PE and found that 52% of patients had either incomplete resolution of PE or developed chronic PE despite therapy. A proportion of these patients will progress to chronic pulmonary hypertension with remodeling of the pulmonary vasculature. The true incidence of chronic pulmonary hypertension is uncertain, but it is thought to be 0.5% to 5% of patients who survive an acute PE. It may also occur in patients without a previous clinical diagnosis of thromboembolism that may have been silent.[84,87,88] A prospective study following 223 patients with adequately treated acute PE identified recurrent thromboembolic disease in 14% of patients, with 62% occurring after cessation of anticoagulation.[89] Symptomatic and angiographic evidence of chronic thromboembolic pulmonary hypertension (CTEPH) developed in 4% of the 223 patients after 2 years, with two patients having recognized recurrent PE. Risk factors for the development of CTEPH included younger age, idiopathic etiology of PE, large initial PE, and a prior episode of PE.

Chronic thromboembolic disease with vascular remodeling is a unique form of pulmonary hypertension and is potentially curable with pulmonary

Table 5-7 Etiology of pulmonary hypertension

Precapillary (arterial)		Pulmonary disorders	Postcapillary (venous)
Cardiac: left to right shunts		COPD	Left atrial, valvular or ventricular disorders
Emboli	Thrombi	Interstitial lung disease	
	Tumor	Chronic hypoxia	Stenosis/compression of
	Parasites		pulmonary veins
	Foreign bodies		Primary venoocclusive disease
Collagen vascular disease			
Primary pulmonary hypertension			
Drugs			

endarterectomy. Assessment of patients for this procedure involves recognizing pulmonary hypertension and differentiating CTEPH from other causes of pulmonary hypertension. Signs of chronic pulmonary thromboembolism include pulmonary hypertension, incomplete resolution of thrombus, remodeling of the pulmonary arteries, and lung parenchymal changes (Table 5-8).

Pulmonary hypertension leads to thickening or dilation of the right atrium and ventricle with straightening or leftward bowing of the intraventricular septum (Figure 5-11). Long-standing pulmonary hypertension leads to dilation of the central pulmonary arteries. Estimates of the normal upper limit for the MPA diameter vary. A simple rule is that the diameter is normally smaller than the diameter of the aorta in patients less than 50 years of age.[90-92] Bronchial artery dilation (>1.5 mm) indicates the presence of an abnormal systemic to pulmonary arterial shunt and is a feature of chronic thromboembolic hypertension, which correlates with a favorable outcome after thromboembolectomy.[93,94]

Pulmonary vascular changes include the visualization of chronic thrombus, with webs and bands, or eccentric thrombus adherent to the vessel walls. The thrombus may become calcified (Figure 5-12).[95-98] Well-defined filling defects within the pulmonary arteries are rarely seen. Central thrombi occasionally occur in primary pulmonary hypertension.[99] Vascular remodeling leads to abrupt narrowing and focal dilation or outpouching of the arteries.

Parenchymal changes include mosaic attenuation and air trapping. A mosaic pattern of attenuation is an uncommon finding in acute PE.[42,43,100] Animal models suggest that it is unlikely to develop for up to 12 weeks following an acute thromboembolic event.[101,102] Mosaic attenuation is common in CTEPH and is a specific finding that may differentiate CTEPH from primary and other secondary causes of pulmonary hypertension.[103,104] The mosaic attenuation of CTEPH represents both air trapping caused by secondary changes in the small airways supplied, and not just vascular occlusion.[105]

Favorable surgical candidates are those with proximal vessel involvement with sparing of the peripheral vasculature. The imaging diagnosis of CTEPH has relied on isotope perfusion lung scanning with confirmation and assessment of surgical operability using catheter angiography and angioscopy.[106,107] CT has traditionally been used to exclude other secondary causes of pulmonary hypertension and is not currently used to confirm the diagnosis or to stage the patient. In part, this is due to poor depiction of the changes of segmental arteries with SSCT.[95,108] The role of MSCT in diagnosing and staging CTEPH has not been fully evaluated.

CONCLUSION

Advances in MSCT technology have overcome several limitations of SSCT in the evaluation of venous thromboembolic disease, particularly in the evaluation of segmental and subsegmental PE. This should translate into an increased diagnostic accuracy, but data to support this are currently limited. The advantage of MSCT pulmonary angiography compared with other imaging modalities, and the potential for the combined evaluation of lower limb veins and pulmonary arteries, may eventually lead to MSCT becoming the test of choice for imaging suspected venous thromboembolic disease with one diagnostic examination.

Table 5-8 CT findings of chronic thromboembolic pulmonary hypertension

Pulmonary hypertension	Pulmonary vascular	Parenchymal
Right atrial and ventricular enlargement	Vascular webs and bands	Mosaic attenuation
Enlargement of central arteries	Eccentric thrombus	Air trapping
Bronchial artery shunts	Calcified thrombus	
	Vascular remodeling	

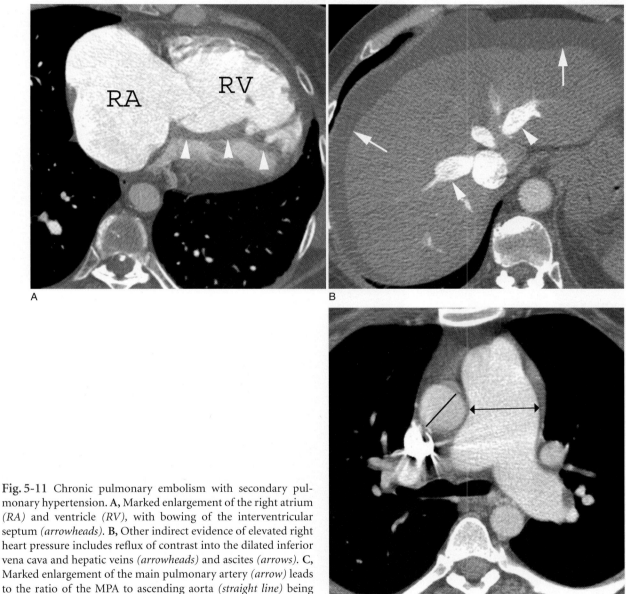

Fig. 5-11 Chronic pulmonary embolism with secondary pulmonary hypertension. **A,** Marked enlargement of the right atrium *(RA)* and ventricle *(RV)*, with bowing of the interventricular septum *(arrowheads)*. **B,** Other indirect evidence of elevated right heart pressure includes reflux of contrast into the dilated inferior vena cava and hepatic veins *(arrowheads)* and ascites *(arrows)*. **C,** Marked enlargement of the main pulmonary artery *(arrow)* leads to the ratio of the MPA to ascending aorta *(straight line)* being greater than 1.

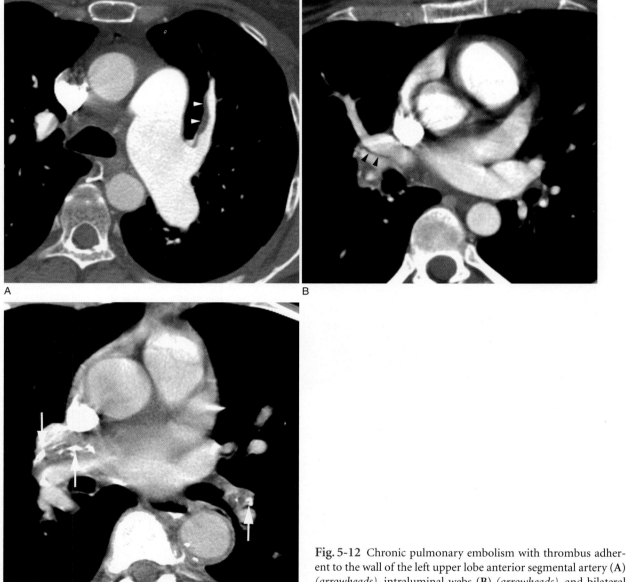

Fig. 5-12 Chronic pulmonary embolism with thrombus adherent to the wall of the left upper lobe anterior segmental artery (**A**) *(arrowheads)*, intraluminal webs (**B**) *(arrowheads)*, and bilateral calcified thrombus (**C**) *(arrows)*.

Acknowledgment

We are very grateful for the invaluable assistance of CT technologists Ian Case and Karen Barber.

REFERENCES

1. Virchow RLK: Die Cellularpathologie in ihrer Begrundung auf physiologische und pathologische Gewebelehre, Berlin: Verlag von August Hirschwald, 1862.

2. White RH: The epidemiology of venous thromboembolism, *Circulation* 107:I4-I8, 2003.

3. Kelly J, Hunt BJ: Do anticoagulants improve survival in patients presenting with venous thromboembolism? *J Intern Med* 254:527-539, 2003.

4. Remy-Jardin M, Remy J, Wattinne L, et al: Central pulmonary thromboembolism: diagnosis with spiral volumetric CT with the single-breath-hold technique–comparison with pulmonary angiography, *Radiology* 185:381-387, 1992.

5. Huisman MV, Buller HR, Ten Cate JW, et al: Unexpected high prevalence of silent pulmonary embolism in patients with deep venous thrombosis, *Chest* 95:498-502, 1989.

6. Dorfman GS, Cronan JJ, Tupper TB, et al: Occult pulmonary embolism: a common occurrence in deep venous thrombosis, *Am J Roentgenol* 148:263-266, 1987.

7. Moser KM, Fedullo PF, LitteJohn JK, et al: Frequent asymptomatic pulmonary embolism in patients with deep venous thrombosis, *JAMA* 271:223-225, 1994.

8. Value of the ventilation/perfusion scan in acute pulmonary embolism. Results of the Prospective Investigation of Pulmonary Embolism Diagnosis (PIOPED). The PIOPED Investigators, *JAMA* 263:2753-2759, 1990.

9. Goldhaber SZ, Visani L, De Rosa M: Acute pulmonary embolism: clinical outcomes in the International Cooperative Pulmonary Embolism Registry (ICOPER), *Lancet* 353:1386-1389, 1999.

10. Levine MN, Raskob G, Landefeld S, et al: Hemorrhagic complications of anticoagulant treatment, *Chest* 114:511S-523S, 1998.

11. Beyth RJ, Quinn LM, Landefeld CS: Prospective evaluation of an index for predicting the risk of major bleeding in outpatients treated with warfarin, *Am J Med* 105:91-99, 1998.

12. Wells PS, Ginsberg JS, Anderson DR, et al: Use of a clinical model for safe management of patients with suspected pulmonary embolism, *Ann Intern Med* 129:997-1005, 1998.

13. Wicki J, Perneger TV, Junod AF, et al: Assessing clinical probability of pulmonary embolism in the emergency ward: a simple score, *Arch Intern Med* 161:92-97, 2001.

14. Kearon C: Diagnosis of pulmonary embolism, *CMAJ* 168:183-194, 2003.

15. Perrier A, Desmarais S, Miron MJ, et al: Non-invasive diagnosis of venous thromboembolism in outpatients, *Lancet* 353:190-195, 1999.

16. Ginsberg JS, Wells PS, Kearon C, et al: Sensitivity and specificity of a rapid whole-blood assay for D-dimer in the diagnosis of pulmonary embolism, *Ann Intern Med* 129:1006-1011, 1998.

17. Wells PS, Anderson DR, Rodger M, et al: Derivation of a simple clinical model to categorize patients probability of pulmonary embolism: increasing the models utility with the SimpliRED D-dimer, *Thromb Haemost* 83:416-420, 2000.

18. Worsley DF, Alavi A, Aronchick JM, et al: Chest radiographic findings in patients with acute pulmonary embolism: observations from the PIOPED Study, *Radiology* 189:133-136, 1993.

19. Stein PD, Terrin ML, Hales CA, et al: Clinical, laboratory, roentgenographic, and electrocardiographic findings in patients with acute pulmonary embolism and no pre-existing cardiac or pulmonary disease, *Chest* 100:598-603, 1991.

20. Remy-Jardin M, Remy J, Deschildre F, et al: Diagnosis of pulmonary embolism with spiral CT: comparison with pulmonary angiography and scintigraphy, *Radiology* 200:699-706, 1996.

21. Goodman LR, Curtin JJ, Mewissen MW, et al: Detection of pulmonary embolism in patients with unresolved clinical and scintigraphic diagnosis: helical CT versus angiography, *Am J Roentgenol* 164:1369-1374, 1995.

22. Drucker EA, Rivitz SM, Shepard JA, et al: Acute pulmonary embolism: assessment of helical CT for diagnosis. *Radiology* 209:235-241, 1998.

23. Ruiz Y, Caballero P, Caniego JL, et al: Prospective comparison of helical CT with angiography in pulmonary embolism: global and selective vascular territory analysis. Interobserver agreement, *Eur Radiol* 13:823-829, 2003.

24. Stone E, Roach P, Bernard E, et al: Use of computed tomography pulmonary angiography in the diagnosis of pulmonary embolism in patients with an intermediate probability ventilation/perfusion scan, *Intern Med J* 33:74-78, 2003.

25. Stein PD, Henry JW: Prevalence of acute pulmonary embolism in central and subsegmental pulmonary arteries and relation to probability interpretation of ventilation/perfusion lung scans, *Chest* 111:1246-1248, 1997.

26. Oser RF, Zuckerman DA, Gutierrez FR, et al: Anatomic distribution of pulmonary emboli at pulmonary angiography: implications for cross-sectional imaging, *Radiology* 199:31-35, 1996.

27. de Monye W, van Strijen MJ, Huisman MV, et al: Suspected pulmonary embolism: prevalence and anatomic distribution in 487 consecutive patients. Advances in New Technologies Evaluating the Localisation of Pulmonary Embolism (ANTELOPE) Group, *Radiology* 215:184-188, 2000.

28. Remy-Jardin M, Remy J, Artaud D, et al: Peripheral pulmonary arteries: optimization of the spiral CT acquisition protocol, *Radiology* 204:157-163, 1997.

29. Ghaye B, Szapiro D, Mastora I, et al: Peripheral pulmonary arteries: how far in the lung does multi-detector row spiral CT allow analysis? *Radiology* 219:629-636, 2001.

30. Patel S, Kazerooni EA, Cascade PN: Pulmonary embolism: optimization of small pulmonary artery visualization at multi-detector row CT. *Radiology* 227:455-460, 2003.

31. Schoepf UJ, Holzknecht N, Helmberger TK, et al: Subsegmental pulmonary emboli: improved detection with thin-collimation multi-detector row spiral CT, *Radiology* 222:483-490, 2002.

32. Remy-Jardin M, Tillie-Leblond I, Szapiro D, et al: CT angiography of pulmonary embolism in patients with underlying respiratory disease: impact of multislice CT on image quality and negative predictive value, *Eur Radiol* 12:1971-1978, 2002.

33. Cademartiri F, Mollet N, van der Lugt A, et al: Non-invasive 16-row multislice CT coronary angiography: usefulness of saline chaser, *Eur Radiol* 14:178-183, 2004.

34. Bae KT, McDermott R, Gierada DS, et al: Gadolinium-enhanced computed tomography angiography in multi-detector row computed tomography: initial observations, *Acad Radiol* 11:61-68, 2004.

35. Coche EE, Hammer FD, Goffette PP: Demonstration of pulmonary embolism with gadolinium-enhanced spiral CT, *Eur Radiol* 11:2306-2309, 2001.

36. Cademartiri F, van der Lugt A, Luccichenti G, et al: Parameters affecting bolus geometry in CTA: a review, *J Comput Assist Tomogr* 26:598-607, 2002.

37. Hartmann IJ, Lo RT, Bakker J, et al: Optimal scan delay in spiral CT for the diagnosis of acute pulmonary embolism, *J Comput Assist Tomogr* 26:21-25, 2002.

38. Marten K, Engelke C, Funke M, et al: ECG-gated multi-slice spiral CT for diagnosis of acute pulmonary embolism, *Clin Radiol* 58:862-868, 2003.

39. Reiner BI, Siegel EL, Hooper FJ: Accuracy of interpretation of CT scans: comparing PACS monitor displays and hardcopy images, *Am J Roentgenol* 179:1407-1410, 2002.

40. Simon M, Boiselle PM, Choi JR, et al: Paddle-wheel CT display of pulmonary arteries and other lung structures: a new imaging approach, *Am J Roentgenol* 177:195-198, 2001.

41. Brink JA, Woodard PK, Horesh L, et al: Depiction of pulmonary emboli with spiral CT: optimization of display window settings in a porcine model, *Radiology* 204:703-708, 1997.

42. Coche EE, Muller NL, Kim KI, et al: Acute pulmonary embolism: ancillary findings at spiral CT, *Radiology* 207:753-758, 1998.

43. Shah AA, Davis SD, Gamsu G, et al: Parenchymal and pleural findings in patients with and patients without acute pulmonary embolism detected at spiral CT, *Radiology* 211:147-153, 1999.

44. Gosselin MV, Rassner UA, Thieszen SL, et al: Contrast dynamics during CT pulmonary angiogram: analysis of an inspiration associated artifact, *J Thorac Imaging* 19:1-7, 2004.

45. Mayo JR, Remy-Jardin M, Muller NL, et al: Pulmonary embolism: prospective comparison of spiral CT with ventilation-perfusion scintigraphy, *Radiology* 205:447-452, 1997.

46. Goodman LR, Lipchik RJ, Kuzo RS, et al: Subsequent pulmonary embolism: risk after a negative helical CT pulmonary angiogram–prospective comparison with scintigraphy, *Radiology* 215:535-542, 2000.

47. Coche E, Verschuren F, Keyeux A, et al: Diagnosis of acute pulmonary embolism in outpatients: comparison of thin-collimation multi-detector row spiral CT and planar ventilation-perfusion scintigraphy, *Radiology* 229:757-765, 2003.

48. Cross JJ, Kemp PM, Walsh CG, et al: A randomized trial of spiral CT and ventilation perfusion scintigraphy for the diagnosis of pulmonary embolism, *Clin Radiol* 53:177-182, 1998.

49. Quinn MF, Lundell CJ, Klotz TA, et al: Reliability of selective pulmonary arteriography in the diagnosis of pulmonary embolism, *Am J Roentgenol* 149:469-471, 1987.

50. Diffin DC, Leyendecker JR, Johnson SP, et al: Effect of anatomic distribution of pulmonary emboli on interobserver agreement in the interpretation of pulmonary angiography, *Am J Roentgenol* 171:1085-1089, 1998.

51. Stein PD, Henry JW, Gottschalk A: Reassessment of pulmonary angiography for the diagnosis of pulmonary embolism: relation of interpreter agreement to the order of the involved pulmonary arterial branch, *Radiology* 210:689-691, 1999.

52. Baile EM, King GG, Muller NL, et al: Spiral computed tomography is comparable to angiography for the diagnosis of pulmonary embolism, *Am J Respir Crit Care Med* 161:1010-1015, 2000.

53. Henry JW, Relyea B, Stein PD: Continuing risk of thromboemboli among patients with normal pulmonary angiograms, *Chest* 107:1375-1378, 1995.

54. Novelline RA, Baltarowich OH, Athanasoulis CA, et al: The clinical course of patients with suspected pulmonary embolism and a negative pulmonary arteriogram, *Radiology* 126:561-567, 1978.

55. Qanadli SD, Hajjam ME, Mesurolle B, et al: Pulmonary embolism detection: prospective evaluation of dual-section helical CT versus selective pulmonary arteriography in 157 patients, *Radiology* 217:447-455, 2000.

56. Swensen SJ, Sheedy PF, II, Ryu JH, et al: Outcomes after withholding anticoagulation from patients with suspected acute pulmonary embolism and negative computed tomographic findings: a cohort study, *Mayo Clin Proc* 77:130-138, 2002.

57. Kavanagh EC, O'Hare A, Hargaden G, et al: Risk of pulmonary embolism after negative MSCT pulmonary angiography findings, *Am J Roentgenol* 182:499-504, 2004.

58. Tillie-Leblond I, Mastora I, Radenne F, et al: Risk of pulmonary embolism after a negative spiral CT angiogram in patients with pulmonary disease: 1-year clinical follow-up study, *Radiology* 223:461-467, 2002.

59. Zerhouni EA, Barth KH, Siegelman SS: Demonstration of venous thrombosis by computed tomography, *Am J Roentgenol* 134:753-758, 1980.

60. Baldt MM, Zontsich T, Stumpflen A, et al: Deep venous thrombosis of the lower extremity: efficacy of spiral CT venography compared with conventional venography in diagnosis, *Radiology* 200:423-428, 1996.

61. Loud PA, Grossman ZD, Klippenstein DL, et al: Combined CT venography and pulmonary angiography: a new diagnostic technique for suspected thromboembolic disease, *Am J Roentgenol* 170:951-954, 1998.

62. Garg K, Kemp JL, Wojcik D, et al: Thromboembolic disease: comparison of combined CT pulmonary angiography and venography with bilateral leg sonography in 70 patients, *Am J Roentgenol* 175:997-1001, 2000.

63. Duwe KM, Shiau M, Budorick NE, et al: Evaluation of the lower extremity veins in patients with suspected pulmonary embolism: a retrospective comparison of helical CT venography and sonography. 2000 ARRS Executive Council Award I. American Roentgen Ray Society, *Am J Roentgenol* 175:1525-1531, 2000.

64. Loud PA, Katz DS, Klippenstein DL, et al: Combined CT venography and pulmonary angiography in suspected thromboembolic disease: diagnostic accuracy for deep venous evaluation, *Am J Roentgenol* 174:61-65, 2000.

65. Loud PA, Katz DS, Bruce DA, et al: Deep venous thrombosis with suspected pulmonary embolism: detection with combined CT venography and pulmonary angiography, *Radiology* 219:498-502, 2001.

66. Coche EE, Hamoir XL, Hammer FD, et al: Using dual-detector helical CT angiography to detect deep venous thrombosis in patients with suspicion of pulmonary embolism: diagnostic value and additional findings, *Am J Roentgenol* 176:1035-1039, 2001.

67. Begemann PG, Bonacker M, Kemper J, et al: Evaluation of the deep venous system in patients with suspected pulmonary embolism with multi-detector CT: a prospective study in comparison to Doppler sonography, *J Comput Assist Tomogr* 27:399-409, 2003.

68. Bruce D, Loud PA, Klippenstein DL, et al: Combined CT venography and pulmonary angiography: how much venous enhancement is routinely obtained? *Am J Roentgenol* 176:1281-1285, 2001.

69. Yankelevitz DF, Gamsu G, Shah A, et al: Optimization of combined CT pulmonary angiography with lower extremity CT venography, *Am J Roentgenol* 174:67-69, 2000.

70. Szapiro D, Ghaye B, Willems V, et al: Evaluation of CT time-density curves of lower-limb veins, *Invest Radiol* 36:164-169, 2001.

71. Katz DS, Loud PA, Klippenstein DL, et al: Extra-thoracic findings on the venous phase of combined computed tomographic venography and pulmonary angiography, *Clin Radiol* 55:177-181, 2000.

72. Ghaye B, Szapiro D, Willems V, et al: Pitfalls in CT venography of lower limbs and abdominal veins, *Am J Roentgenol* 178:1465-1471, 2002.

73. Katz DS, Loud PA, Bruce D, et al: Combined CT venography and pulmonary angiography: a comprehensive review, *Radiographics* 22 Spec No:S3-19; discussion S20-14, 2002.

74. Richman PB, Wood J, Kasper DM, et al: Contribution of indirect computed tomography venography to computed tomography angiography of the chest for the diagnosis of thromboembolic disease in two United States emergency departments, *J Thromb Haemost* 1:652-657, 2003.

75. Cham MD, Yankelevitz DF, Shaham D, et al: Deep venous thrombosis: detection by using indirect CT venography. The Pulmonary Angiography-Indirect CT Venography Cooperative Group, *Radiology* 216:744-751, 2000.

76. Walsh G, Redmond S: Does addition of CT pelvic venography to CT pulmonary angiography protocols contribute to the diagnosis of thromboembolic disease? *Clin Radiol* 57:462-465, 2002.

77. Garg K, Kemp JL, Russ PD, et al: Thromboembolic disease: variability of interobserver agreement in the interpretation of CT venography with CT pulmonary angiography, *Am J Roentgenol* 176:1043-1047, 2001.

78. Peterson DA, Kazerooni EA, Wakefield TW, et al: Computed tomographic venography is specific but not sensitive for diagnosis of acute lower-extremity deep venous thrombosis in patients with suspected pulmonary embolus, *J Vasc Surg* 34:798-804, 2001.

79. Rademaker J, Griesshaber V, Hidajat N, et al: Combined CT pulmonary angiography and venography for diagnosis of pulmonary embolism and deep vein thrombosis: radiation dose, *J Thorac Imaging* 16:297-299, 2001.

80. British Thoracic Society guidelines for the management of suspected acute pulmonary embolism, *Thorax* 58:470-483, 2003.

81. Kearon C: Duration of therapy for acute venous thromboembolism, *Clin Chest Med* 24:63-72, 2003.

82. Schulman S: Unresolved issues in anticoagulant therapy, *J Thromb Haemost* 1:1464-1470, 2003.

83. Streiff MB: Vena caval filters: a comprehensive review, *Blood* 95:3669-3677, 2000.

84. Frazier AA, Galvin JR, Franks TJ, et al: From the archives of the AFIP: pulmonary vasculature: hypertension and infarction, *Radiographics* 20:491-524; quiz 530-531, 532, 2000.

85. Chemla D, Castelain V, Herve P, et al: Haemodynamic evaluation of pulmonary hypertension, *Eur Respir J* 20:1314-1331, 2002.

86. Remy-Jardin M, Louvegny S, Remy J, et al: Acute central thromboembolic disease: posttherapeutic follow-up with spiral CT angiography, *Radiology* 203:173-180. 1997.

87. Moser KM, Auger WR, Fedullo PF: Chronic major-vessel thromboembolic pulmonary hypertension, *Circulation* 81:1735-1743, 1990.

88. Fedullo PF, Auger WR, Kerr KM, et al: Chronic thromboembolic pulmonary hypertension, *N Engl J Med* 345: 1465-1472, 2001.

89. Pengo V, Lensing AW, Prins MH, et al: Incidence of chronic thromboembolic pulmonary hypertension after pulmonary embolism, *N Engl J Med* 350:2257-2264, 2004.

90. Edwards PD, Bull RK, Coulden R: CT measurement of main pulmonary artery diameter, *Br J Radiol* 71:1018-1020, 1998.

91. Kuriyama K, Gamsu G, Stern RG, et al: CT-determined pulmonary artery diameters in predicting pulmonary hypertension, *Invest Radiol* 19:16-22, 1984.

92. Ng CS, Wells AU, Padley SP: A CT sign of chronic pulmonary arterial hypertension: the ratio of main pulmonary artery to aortic diameter, *J Thorac Imaging* 14:270-278, 1999.

93. Kauczor HU, Schwickert HC, Mayer E, et al: Spiral CT of bronchial arteries in chronic thromboembolism, *J Comput Assist Tomogr* 18:855-861, 1994.

94. Ley S, Kreitner KF, Morgenstern I, et al: Bronchopulmonary shunts in patients with chronic thromboembolic pulmonary hypertension: evaluation with helical CT and MR imaging, *Am J Roentgenol* 179:1209-1215, 2002.

95. Schwickert HC, Schweden F, Schild HH, et al: Pulmonary arteries and lung parenchyma in chronic pulmonary embolism: preoperative and postoperative CT findings, *Radiology* 191:351-357, 1994.

96. Auger WR, Fedullo PF, Moser KM, et al: Chronic major-vessel thromboembolic pulmonary artery obstruction: appearance at angiography, *Radiology* 182:393-398, 1992.

97. King MA, Ysrael M, Bergin CJ: Chronic thromboembolic pulmonary hypertension: CT findings, *Am J Roentgenol* 170:955-960, 1998.

98. Remy-Jardin M, Remy J, Louvegny S, et al: Airway changes in chronic pulmonary embolism: CT findings in 33 patients, *Radiology* 203:355-360, 1997.

99. Moser KM, Fedullo PF, Finkbeiner WE, et al: Do patients with primary pulmonary hypertension develop extensive central thrombi? *Circulation* 91:741-745, 1995.

100. Johnson PT, Wechsler RJ, Salazar AM, et al: Spiral CT of acute pulmonary thromboembolism: evaluation of pleuroparenchymal abnormalities, *J Comput Assist Tomogr* 23:369-373, 1999.

101. Im JG, Choi YW, Kim HD, et al: Thin-section CT findings of the lungs: experimentally induced bronchial and pulmonary artery obstruction in pigs, *Am J Roentgenol* 167:631-636, 1996.

102. Kim TK, Im JG, Kim SH, et al: Experimentally induced pulmonary arterial occlusion with detachable balloon in pigs: thin-section CT findings, *Acad Radiol* 5:822-831, 1998.

103. Bergin CJ, Rios G, King MA, et al: Accuracy of high-resolution CT in identifying chronic pulmonary thromboembolic disease, *Am J Roentgenol* 166:1371-1377, 1996.

104. Sherrick AD, Swensen SJ, Hartman TE: Mosaic pattern of lung attenuation on CT scans: frequency among patients with pulmonary artery hypertension of different causes, *Am J Roentgenol* 169:79-82, 1997.

105. Arakawa H, Stern EJ, Nakamoto T, et al: Chronic pulmonary thromboembolism. Air trapping on computed tomography and correlation with pulmonary function tests, *J Comput Assist Tomogr* 27:735-742, 2003.

106. Auger WR, Channick RN, Kerr KM, et al: Evaluation of patients with suspected chronic thromboembolic pulmonary hypertension, *Semin Thorac Cardiovasc Surg* 11:179-190, 1999.

107. Williamson TL, Kim NH, Rubin LJ: Chronic thromboembolic pulmonary hypertension, *Prog Cardiovasc Dis* 45:203-212, 2002.

108. Bergin CJ, Sirlin CB, Hauschildt JP, et al: Chronic thromboembolism: diagnosis with helical CT and MR imaging with angiographic and surgical correlation, *Radiology* 204:695-702, 1997.

109. Donato AA, Scheirer JJ, Atwell MS, et al: Clinical outcomes in patients with suspected acute pulmonary embolism and negative helical computed tomographic results in whom anticoagulation was withheld, *Arch Intern Med* 163:2033-2038, 2003.

6

Cardiac Multislice Computed Tomography

Friedrich Knollmann

EVOLUTION OF CORONARY CT

Cardiac CT has gained tremendous interest since the introduction of 4-row detector multislice CT (MSCT) in 1998. Cardiac applications have been cited as a major benefit of MSCT since its inception, and the main interest was in noninvasive coronary angiography. Coronary calcium scoring was another area of research interest early on, and some manufacturers have argued for the replacement of electron beam CT by 4-row MSCT units.

Indications for Coronary MSCT

With an evidence-based medicine approach, it becomes important to review current guidelines that offer recommendations for the test. Evidence-based medicine is intended as an alternative approach to opinion-based medicine and relies on a formalized approach of reviewing medical intelligence. One approach to identify guidelines is the online resource "National Guideline Clearinghouse" (http://www.guideline.gov). A search in this database for "coronary artery computed tomography" has revealed 11 citations, only two of which were relevant to our subject. Interestingly, the guideline "ACR Appropriateness Criteria™ for acute chest pain—no ECG evidence of myocardial ischemia/ infarction" has a different focus than the guideline "ACC/AHA guidelines for coronary angiography. A report of the American College of Cardiology/ American Heart Association Task Force on Practice Guidelines (Committee on Coronary Angiography)." Both guidelines were issued in 1998 and 1999, respectively, at a time when the published data on coronary CTA were very limited; thus neither reflects today's state of knowledge on coronary CT. One therefore needs to review the more current literature directly to derive conclusions on this subject.

More detailed consensus documents are available for the case of coronary artery calcium quantification with electron beam CT, which has been in clinical use since 1990. One important guideline titled "Coronary artery calcification: pathophysiology, epidemiology, imaging methods, and clinical implications" has been published by a working group of the American Heart Association as a Medical/Scientific Statement[1] in 1996. This statement concludes that at that time, data were insufficient to replace stress testing in patients with typical symptoms by electron beam CT (EBCT) calcium scoring, although the role for asymptomatic patients with conventional risk factors was still unclear. In 2000, a document issued by the AHA and the American College of Cardiology[2] found that the test is not recommendable for diagnosing obstructive coronary disease because of its low specificity, although the available data did still not suffice to determine if EBCT calcium scoring would add predictive intelligence in asymptomatic individuals over that of conventional risk factors. Thus, the conclusion was that further prospective study results from studies such as the MESA trial were needed. The conclusions from an AHA prevention conference were similar, in that CT calcium scoring was not routinely recommended for asymptomatic individuals based on the lack of supportive data, although by conventional wisdom, it was deemed possibly acceptable in patients with intermediate risk.[3] Conversely, coronary calcium quantification is accepted as an important risk marker by a more recent European guideline.[4] Based on these divergent assessments, one could doubt that evidence-based medicine principles have replaced opinion-based medicine in current guidelines.

Critics of coronary calcium scoring have argued that the value of the technique as an independent predictor of coronary risk remained unclear. One prospective study demonstrated that calcium scores do differentiate low-risk from high-risk subjects independently in a subgroup of patients with intermediate risk as in the Framingham score, although the method allowed little additional insight in patients with low or very high conventional risk factors.[5]

More than 5 years after the introduction of 4-row MSCT, only a handful of solid, citable reports on coronary CT can be found in the medical literature (Table 6-1). Other publications largely confirm the accuracies reported in these publications but may not give sufficient detail for the assessment of the evalauble case rate.[6,7] The evaluable case rate is a real world measure of the percentage of patients in whom all coronary artery segments of interest could be evaluated (i.e., in how many patients of the study population a definite diagnosis of high-grade coronary stenosis was possible). This measure is important because the percentage of evaluable coronary segments alone may mask the fact that a single segment with motion artifacts in an individual patient may render the test useless, although the number of evaluable segments in a larger cohort may look impressively high. For example, the middle third of the right coronary artery and the circumflex branch of the left

Table 6-1   Diagnostic performance of CT in the detection of severe coronary artery stenosis

Method	Reference	Sensitivity	Specificity	Beta blocker	Evaluable case rate
EBCT	8	92%	94%	—	78/125 (63%)
4-row MSCT	9	91%	84%	—	19/64 (30%)
12-row MSCT	10	92%	93%	+	57/77 (74%)

coronary artery are notoriously susceptible to motion artifacts. It is self-explanatory that the clinical usefulness of the test is determined by the percentage of patients in whom the expected diagnosis can be made.

Based on published guidelines, no established indication for using coronary MSCT angiography has been approved. Similarly, coronary artery calcium quantification by CT has not yet been established, although its acceptance is increasing. One limitation of the mentioned investigations is that only vessels with a diameter more than 1.5 mm were included, and only the proximal main arteries in the case of EBCT and 4-row MSCT. Thus, smaller vessel segments and collateral circulation could not be assessed. Also, it may be difficult on CT to determine if a vessel is occluded or smaller than 1.5 mm as an anatomical variant based on this standard.

Thus, coronary MSCT angiography stands ready to enter clinical routine but remains a matter of clinical research at the moment. Clinical experience indicates that many patients seek a noninvasive coronary MSCT angiogram as a replacement of cardiac catheterization, often at a time when catheterization has been recommended by the patient's cardiologist. To elucidate potentially acceptable indications for the coronary CTA, a review of the established indications for cardiac catheterization is needed. According to the current guidelines of the American College of Cardiology and the American Heart Association (ACC/AHA),[8] the indications for performing cardiac catheterization follow criteria of evidence-based medicine. In their guidelines, patients with stable angina (CCS class III and IV, which is defined by angina after climbing one flight of stairs or less); those with high-risk, noninvasive testing for myocardial ischemia; and individuals who have been resuscitated from sudden cardiac death constitute a recommendable indication for catheterization. Patients within this group have a high likelihood of severe coronary stenosis, and many of them need either percutaneous treatment or bypass surgery. For both treatments, even a highly accurate noninvasive test such as coronary MSCT angiography would increase the costs of treatment, potentially delay therapy, but only very seldom reveal a normal coronary artery tree. Thus, such patients are poor candidates for coronary MSCT. According to the ACC/AHA guidelines, the usefulness of cardiac catheterization is less well established in patients with stable CCS class III or IV angina who improve to class I or II

with medical treatment, patients who cannot be risk-stratified by other methods, and patients with non–high-risk abnormalities in noninvasive tests. Coronary calcification is not deemed an indication for coronary angiography. The noninvasive risk assessment in these guidelines is based on stress testing criteria, which may involve thallium scintigraphy or stress echocardiography. It is in patients with these less well-established indications for performing coronary angiography that MSCT may replace the invasive test, although this role has not yet been accepted by the guidelines. For some of these indications, the presence of nonrandomized studies has been deemed sufficient to establish the indication for angiography within the guidelines. Because such studies are available for MSCT angiography today, one could argue that coronary MSCT should be included in such guidelines in future editions, either as a noninvasive test whose outcome defines the progression to invasive tests, or as an alternative to catheterization in the less well-established indications. However, it is imperative for all coronary CT procedures discussed here that the patient's history be carefully reviewed with respect to the well-established indications for performing catheterization.

From another perspective, coronary MSCT angiography would be ineffective in a patient population in whom 50% or more had signifcant stenotic disease and would thus proceed to catheterization anyway. It is also implausible that the test be performed in patients with a very low likelihood of stenotic disease, namely in asymptomatic patients. Thus, the target group for effective coronary MSCT angiography is clearly limited. It should be noted that the published data on the diagnostic accuracy of coronary CTA pertain to patient groups with an established indication for coronary catheterization, which is not the ideal target group for CTA.

Heart Rate Management

Heart rate is a major determinant of image quality in coronary CT. Several studies have found that with 4-row MSCT and a gantry speed of 0.5 seconds, heart rates of more than 60 bpm lead to an unacceptable number of nondiagnostic coronary CTA studies. Thus, heart rate is the primary determinant of the evaluable case rate for coronary CTA. Despite the introduction of faster gantry speeds with 16-row MSCT units, heart rates over 70 bpm

Table 6-2 Recommended beta blocker drugs for preconditioning cardiac MSCT patients

Drug	Route of administration	Dose
Metoprolol	IV	5 mg (max 20 mg)
Metoprolol	Orally	95 mg
Esmolol	IV	1 mg/kg body weight

still limit image quality to an extent that patients who are expected to exceed a heart rate of 60 bpm in a pre-study breath hold maneuver should undergo pharmaceutical treatment. Most commonly, beta blockers are used to reduce the heart rate. Since the patient's heart rate is most often unknown before the patient is present at the CT suite, IV beta blockers have the advantage of immediate action and are thus favored. Patients should be routinely advised to take their normal medications on the day of the examination. Also, patients should be advised to abstain from coffee and nicotine on the day of the examination to help achieve an acceptable heart rate. The general precautions for IV contrast administration including the contraindication for patients on metformin remain unaffected.

In a small series of cardiac CT exams, however, in which beta blockers were administered when patients' heart rates exceeded 70 bpm, the maximum heart rate during the actual CT scan was still beyond the desired range. One reason for this effect is that the rapid IV administration of a monomeric, nonionic contrast agent bolus causes tachycardia just at the moment of the scan. It remains to be seen if use of a much more expensive dimeric contrast agent (iodixanol) can improve this effect. Table 6-2 lists recommended beta blocker drugs for preconditioning cardiac MSCT patients.

Protocol Choices for the Calcium Scoring Series

Rationale

The cardiac MSCT protocol defined in Table 6-3 warrants explanation. In its first series, coronary artery calcifications are quantified. Unfortunately, calcium quantification of coronary artery calcium has evolved into a highly controversial topic since its inception as an electron-beam CT test. To date,

at least 20 different CT systems are marketed for the purpose of coronary artery scoring, and it is growing increasingly difficult to keep track of all candidates. In an attempt to consolidate the multitude of technical approaches, a so-called calcium mass determination has been devised,[9] which is based on a static phantom with defined calcium content. This method does not improve the risk classification, nor the reproducibility of the resultant score index.[10]

Clinical data bases for this scoring method are largely unavailable at this time, and one has to fear that the variety of scoring methods may further discredit the test. The purpose of the calcium scoring series in the "exclude coronary heart disease" protocol is twofold: (1) with very high calcification, the contrast-assisted coronary CTA can safely be skipped, because severe calcifications may render an angiographic run nondiagnostic. This is typically the case with an Agatston Score Equivalent of above 800 when a submillimeter slice thickness is used, and with lower score values with thicker slices; (2) coronary calcium load is increasingly accepted as a valuable indicator of coronary risk and offers additional intelligence about an angiographic series.

Scan Parameters

The exact parameters of the calcium scoring series are based on electron-beam CT protocols. Thus, the 2.5-mm slices simulate the 3-mm EBCT slices, and the EKG-synchronization by prospective triggering at 40% of the RR-interval is also derived from EBCT-protocols. Although the 80 mA tube current results in relatively noisy images (mAs less than 40), no data have been made public that would indicate a clinical benefit of a low-noise protocol. The relatively noisy images shall suffice for the purpose of cardiac risk assessment, as evidenced by the large clinical experience with EBCT calcium scoring. One major advantage of this protocol is its low radiation dose. Several authors have argued for helical

Table 6-3   Cardiac CT Protocol

Indication	Patient with atypical chest symptoms, referred to rule out coronary artery disease
Protocol designed for (scanner type)	LightSpeed VCT
Patient preparation	No coffee or smoking before the exam, patient fills out cardiac questionnaire before exam
	Breath hold trained before scan. If heart rate exceeds 70 bpm, give IV beta blocker if possible (contraindications!)
First Series	Coronary calcium scoring
Oral contrast	—
IV contrast administration	—
Tube settings	kV 120
	mA 80
Gantry speed (sec)	0.35
Table speed (mm/sec)	Sequential mode (Cine segment axial)
Slice thickness (mm)	2.5
Anatomical coverage	Carina—2 cm below diaphragm
Reconstruction kernel	Standard
Breath hold	Inspiration
Window settings	
Postprocessing	Calculation of calcium score on workstation
Other	Prospectively ECG-triggered at 70% of the RR-interval
Typical dose	CTDI 1.52 mGy, DLP: 18 mGycm at 120 mm scan length
Second Series	Coronary CT angiogram
Oral contrast	—
IV contrast administration	Iopromide, 300 mg I/cc
Volume/injection rate/delay	1. 90 ml / 5 ml/s / bolus tracking
	2. Saline chaser 40 ml / 5 ml/s / starts upon completion of contrast injection
Tube settings	kV 120
	mA 500 EKG-based dose modulation, maximum 500 mA (50-90% of RR-interval), min 120 mA
Detector configuration	64 *0.625 mm
Gantry speed (sec)	0.35
Table speed (mm/sec)	8 mm/rotation, retrospective EKG-gating
Reconstructed slice thickness	0.63 mm
Anatomical coverage	Carina—2 cm below diaphragm
Reconstruction kernel	Standard
Breath hold	Inspiration
Window settings	800/90
Postprocessing	Image reconstruction with segmented algorithm ("snapshot segment") at 50%, 70%, and 80% of the cardiac cycle length
	Review of axials
	Focused vessel tracking of suspicious segments
	Volume rendering (VRT) for documentation
Other	Additional image reconstruction series using other cardiac phases and multisegmented reconstruction algorithms according to the discretion of the attending radiologist
Typical dose	CTDI = 43.6 mGy, DLP = 743 mGycm at 14 cm scan length

calcium scoring protocols by claiming a better reproducibility of the resultant score. Notably, the comparison of reproducibility as the mean repeatability of calcium scores is statistically erroneous,[11] which makes such arguments invalid. Even if an improved reproducibility of a helical technique could be demonstrated, it would be of questionable use for risk-stratification or to rule out heavy calcification. The benefit would be reserved for follow-up studies in controlled clincal trials. At this time, the effects of increasing calcium load for an individual are largely unknown.

With the present protocol, the total calcium score is primarily calculated with the Agatston-Janowitz algorithm, because extensive results with this method are readily available in the literature. Other scoring methods such as the calculation of calcified plaque volume (volume score) or mass (mass score) have theoretical advantages but lack clinical evidence of superior diagnostic capabilities.

Protocol Choices for the CTA Series

The parameter selection for the CTA series is highly dependent on the exact CT unit used. Generally, the smallest slice thickness that is feasible is used to achieve the best spatial resolution. With the C-150 EBCT unit, 3-mm slices were the smallest practical choice, since the prospective trigger mode with one image position per cardiac cycle and a resultant breath hold time of 20 to 35 seconds limit the feasiblity of smaller slice thicknesses. With this approach, the evaluation of distal coronary artery segments with a typical vessel diameter of 2 mm or less is not routinely feasible. With the newer eSpeed EBT-unit, 1.5-mm slices can be acquired within the same time. The 4-row MSCT units typically use 1.25-mm slices, which can be reconstructed with a 50% slice overlap to improve the evaluation of small vessel segments. In 8-row MSCT, the 1.25-mm slice thickness is still the smallest practical choice, although the scan duration is significantly improved. With 16-row MSCT, the smallest slice thickness is typically 0.5 mm (Toshiba Aquillion 16), 0.63 mm (GE LightSpeed 16 and LightSpeed 16 pro) or 0.75 mm (Siemens Sensation 16, Sensation Cardiac, Philipps Mx8000 IDT). With 64-row MSCT, the z-axis resolution has been further improved, although the detector element size of the LightSpeed VCT unit has remained unchanged at 0.625 mm. This smaller slice thickness is particularly important if the analysis is focused on coronary artery stent patency, distal coronary artery segments, and small branches (such as septal branches of the left coronary artery),[12] coronary bypass anastomoses, or coronary plaque morphology. The effect of slice thickness on image detail is illustrated in Figure 6-1, which shows an isolated porcine heart. The coronary arteries have been filled with a barium sulfate contrast agent to mimic the contrast encountered in human coronary CTA using IV iodinated contrast agents. All images are volume-rendering reconstruction with the same rendering parameters. The benefit of a smaller slice thickness is a more detailed reproduction of the smaller vessel segments. Some branches only become visible with a smaller slice thickness.

Slice thickness also determines table feed, since it is generally necessary to use a table pitch of no more than 0.3 for most heart rates in EKG-gated image reconstruction. The table speed and its relation to heart rate also determines which reconstruction options will be available.

Generally, for heart rates of 40 to 65 bpm, the snaphot segment algorithm has been recommended; for heart rates between 66 and 92 bpm, a two-segment "snapshot burst" algorithm is recommended. The availability of segmented reconstruction algorithms depends on the following combinations of gantry speed, heart rate, and table pitch:

No. of Segments	Heart Rate (bpm)	Pitch	Gantry Speed (s)
1	40-	0.22	0.4
1	45-	0.24	0.4
1	50-	0.26	0.4
1	55-	0.28	0.4
2		0.26	0.4
4	65-	0.3	0.5
4	76-	0.26	0.4
4	93-	0.26	0.5
4	106	0.275	0.4

With the most widely used cardiac CT systems (Siemens Somatom Sensation or GE LightSpeed series), reconstruction algorithms are available that select the suitable number of segments for reconstruction based on the available image and EKG data. Although no direct comparison on the benefit of a multisegment algorithm in patients has been published, in vitro data demonstrate that the two-sector reconstruction method reduces motion artifacts at critical time points.[13] In our clinical experience, however, the benefit of the two-segment reconstruction technique is not evident, and since its applicability depends on a reduced pitch factor,

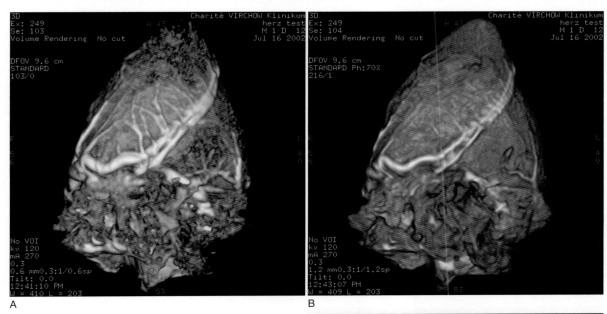

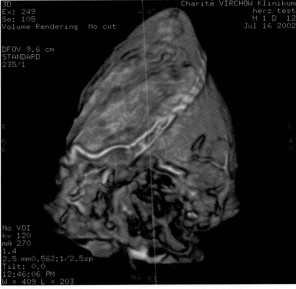

Fig. 6-1 A, Role of slice thickness for image detail in coronary CT angiography: Slice thickness 0.63 mm, reconstruction increment 0.63 mm. B, Slice thickness 1.25 mm, reconstruction increment 1.25 mm. C, Slice thickness 2.5 mm, reconstruction increment 2.5 mm.

we doubt that the concomitant radiation exposure can be justified.

POSTPROCESSING AND IMAGE INTERPRETATION

Calcium Scoring

Interpretation of coronary artery calcium load is facilitated by a consensus document from the EBCT working group of the German Cardiac Society. According to this document, the first step is classi-fying coronary calcium load as minimal (TCS < 10), moderate (TCS < 101), significant (TCS < 400), extensive (TCS < 1001), and severe (> 1000), followed by a comparison with age- and gender-adjusted reference groups.[14] A score that exceeds the 75th percentile of this reference group indicates a high cardiac risk profile.

Coronary CTA

Review of axial images remains the most important step in image analysis (Figure 6-2). Volume-rendering reconstruction has proved useful for the

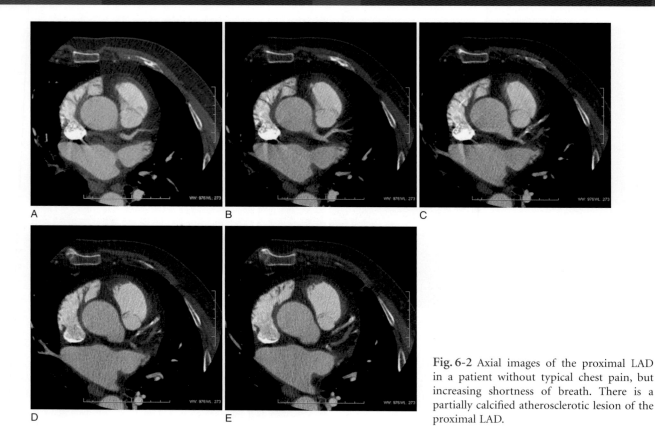

Fig. 6-2 Axial images of the proximal LAD in a patient without typical chest pain, but increasing shortness of breath. There is a partially calcified atherosclerotic lesion of the proximal LAD.

documentation and communication of findings, both with patients and referring physicians. A direct comparison of different reconstruction methods has confirmed that the review of axial images yields the best diagnostic result of all isolated approaches.[15] Volume-rendering reconstructions are also extremely helpful for determining the presence of certain image artifacts, since they provide a good overview of a vessel's course. However, the same vessel segment can be reconstructed with very different results depending on the volume-rendering parameters.

For a better understanding of the lesion geometry, a sliding thin slab maximum intensity projection (STS-MIP) of this vessel segment was reconstructed with two different window settings (Figure 6-3). It is immediately obvious that the MIP reconstruction on Figure 6-3, *B* suggests a more severe degree of stenosis than that on Figure 6-3, *A*. This case illustrates how display settings suggest different diagnoses and thus can be used to dramatically change the interpretation of a coronary CTA study.

Volume-rendering reconstruction faces a similar dilemma (Figure 6-4). Our index case illustrates that with the volume-rendering parameters in Figure 6-4, *A*, no luminal stenosis can be discerned, although a widening of the more distal part of the lesion is apparent. Such an effect is plausible, since the buildup of atherosclerotic material is known to grow "outward" initially, an effect also known as remodeling of the coronary artery wall. In contrast, the volume-rendering parameters in Figure 6-4, *B* suggest high-grade stenosis. Again, both findings can be supported, depending on the selection of volume-rendering technique (VRT) parameters, which makes this method a less reliable candidate for the diagnosis or exclusion of high-grade coronary artery stenosis.

One promising method to overcome the uncertainties associated with MIP and VRT reconstruction is the use of reformatation techniques, which preserve the inherent spatial resolution of the axial images. To include curved vessel segments, an automatic vessel tracking technique is helpful to document the vessel course in a single view.

Such algorithms identify the course of the target vessel after a starting point and some optional landmarks and the end point have been identified

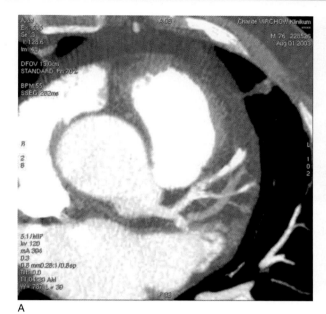

A

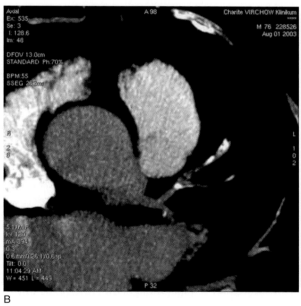

B

Fig. 6-3 Axial maximum intensity projections (MIPs) of the proximal LAD at different window settings illustrate the susceptibility to window settings of MIPs.

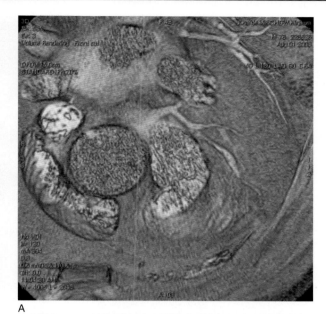

A

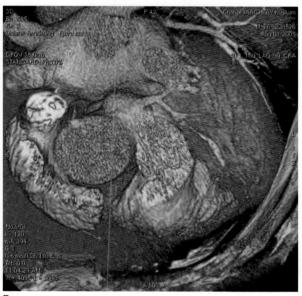

B

Fig. 6-4 Volume-rendering technique (VRT) reconstructions of a coronary CTA data set illustrate how different rendering parameters can change the visual diagnosis of coronary artery stenosis.

manually in the axial images, usually a matter of less than a minute (Figures 6-5 and 6-6).*

In the curved reformat, the entire course of the LAD is depicted (Figure 6-7). This view can be rotated along the long axis of the artery to further

*Advanced Vessel Analysis software, Advantage Windows Workstation V4.1, GE Medical Systems, Milwaukee, Wisconsin.

enhance the confidence in the diagnosis. In this case, despite severe calcification, a diagnosis of severe LAD stenosis was depicted. The patient underwent coronary catheterization, a greater than 70% stenosis of the proximal LAD was confirmed and treated by angioplasty, and a stent was implanted. The lower part of both figures reproduce an automatic measurement of coronary artery diameter, which

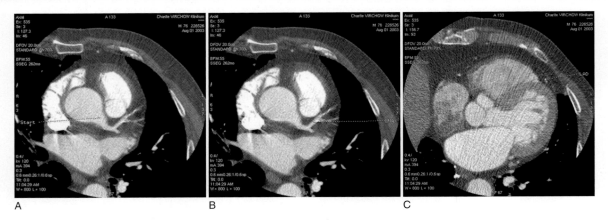

Fig. 6-5 A-C, Marking of start and end points for the left main stem and LAD for automatic vessel tracking.

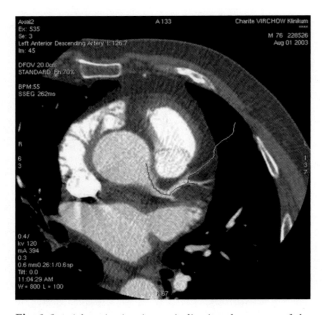

Fig. 6-6 Axial projection image indicating the course of the LAD as detected by the vessel-tracking algorithm.

still needs manual confirmation. This method is a CT counterpart to quantitative coronary angiography.

Another valuable software feature allows the reconstruction of images perpendicular to the vessel axis, which supports the identification of high-grade stenosis and the assessment of plaque morphology.

One important application is the exclusion of high-grade coronary stenosis, which can be conveniently and convincingly documented in a few image reconstructions, if the diagnosis is based on the interactive cine review of the thin axial images (Figure 6-8).

The volume-rendering reconstruction in Figure 6-9 is an illustration of excluded coronary stenosis that documents the patency of the major branches and curved reformats of the LAD, circumflex branch, and right coronary artery.

In clinical practice, there is a definite risk of overestimating coronary stenosis as compared with coronary angiography. In a prospective comparison of patients who were scheduled for cardiac surgery, all instances of significant coronary stenosis were detected.

For an analysis of false-positive CT results, the first step is a review of the diagnostic accuracy of the gold standard, coronary angiography. Unfortunately, this present gold standard has substantial inaccuracies when compared with a pathological standard: in an early investigation of postmortem coronary angiography, only 61% of all nonfocally stenosed coronary segments were correctly identified by direct-injection coronary angiography, and only 11% of all focally diseased segments were correctly classified.[16] The tendency of coronary angiography to underestimate histologically significant coronary disease has been noted early after the introduction of selective coronary angiography.[17] In another comparison of left main coronary artery diameters upon in vivo coronary angiography with subsequent histological correlation, the degree of stenosis differed significantly between the two in 71% of cases,[18] and coronary angiography more commonly underestimated the degree of stenosis. Two factors predispose lesions to be underestimated by coronary angiography: diffuse disease and eccentric atherosclerotic disease.[18] Both factors are revealed upon cross-sectional examinations such as histopathology and, of course, MSCT.

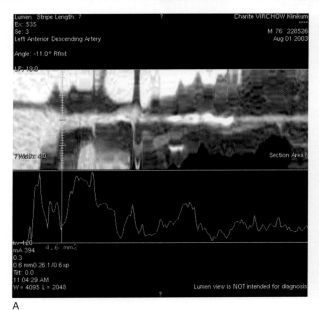

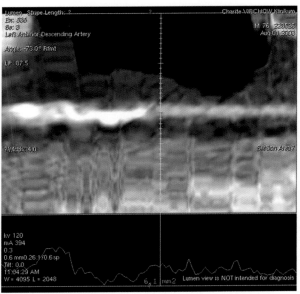

Fig. 6-7 A-B, The curved reformat of the proximal LAD provides a convenient overview of the vessel lumen along its course.

For the interpretation of coronary CT findings, it is important to note that a 50% reduction in coronary artery diameter corresponds to a luminal area reduction of 75%, and that a diameter reduction of 70% corresponds to a luminal area reduction of 91% (Figure 6-10).

While CT displays the luminal area, the projection technique displays a diameter scale of luminal

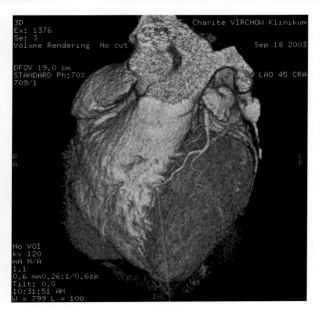

Fig. 6-8 VRT reconstruction of a patient in whom significant coronary stenosis was ruled out by CTA *(arrow).*

patency, and this difference alone may cause divergent assessments.

Special Case: Patients with a Coronary Stent Implant

In patients with a coronary stent implant, obstructive coronary disease has already been established. Calcium scoring protocols have no role in such patients, since the metal stent implants cannot be differentiated from calcification, and the coronary risk is already known to be very high.

Although the most recent developments in stent design have improved outcome, stent thrombosis and restenosis remain important concerns.[19] According to the AHA guidelines, the sole fact that a stent has been implanted is not an indication for coronary angiography. However, asymptomatic patients undergo routine coronary angiography after stent implantation at many institutions, and a noninvasive alternative would be highly desirable. The rationale for examining asymptomatic patients in this case is that the rate of stent thrombosis or restenosis is still considerable (Figure 6-11), and more than half of these individuals remain asymptomatic.[20] Although early reports have demonstrated an impressive diagnostic accuracy of an EBCT dynamic scan technique,[21,22] our experience

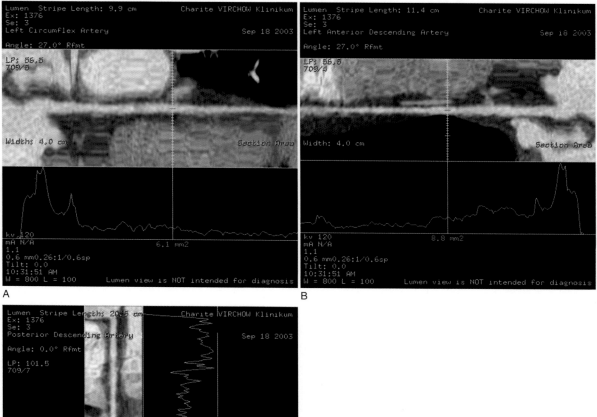

Fig. 6-9 A, The curved reformat of the circumflex branch of the left coronary artery documents a patent and unobstructed course of the entire vessel in a single image. **B,** The curved reformat of the right coronary artery documents a patent and unobstructed course of the entire vessel in a single image. **C,** The curved reformat of the LAD documents a patent and unobstructed course of the entire vessel in a single image.

has been less encouraging. The problem with CT angiography of stent implants is that the metal implant may cause severe image artifacts, and the small lumen of the stent requires a very high spatial resolution of the CT system. With the 3-mm slice thickness of the C150 EBCT system, it was clearly not possible to evaluate the stent lumen directly. Even with a slice thickness of 0.75 mm, the diagnosis remains limited to the detection of complete stent occlusion.[23]

Since patients with established obstructive coronary disease can be expected to display a significant amount of coronary calcification, it may be very difficult or impossible to rule out obstructive lesions at sites other than the stent implant.

Special Case: Patients after Bypass Surgery

Evidence from EBCT investigations of bypass patency suggests that bypass occlusion can be detected reliably by CT, although the detection of high-grade bypass stenosis remains problematic.[24] With improved spatial resolution of 16-row

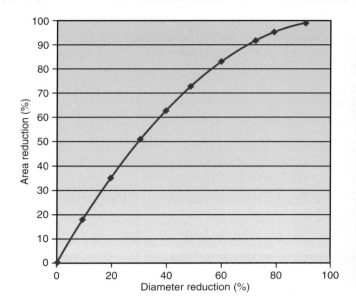

Fig. 6-10 Relation of coronary luminal diameter and area reductions. Note that with a diameter reduction of 40%, more than 60% of the luminal area is obstructed.

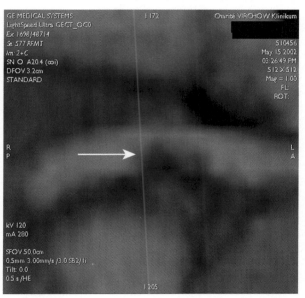

Fig. 6-12 Longitudinal reconstruction of a noncalcified, lipid-rich, eccentric LAD plaque with luminal obstruction as the suggested CT correlate of a vulnerable plaque (arrow).

most cases to minimize the time required for a breath hold.

Special Case: Imaging of the Atherosclerotic Plaque

With the ability of CT systems to provide spatially accurate renderings of the coronary artery wall transection, recent improvements in spatial resolution have led to new insights into coronary artery wall morphology.

Pathological studies in patients with myocardial infarction and other acute coronary syndromes suggest that a combination of a large body of lipid enclosures in the coronary artery wall, a thin fibrous cover, macrophage activity, and enzymatic activity at the site of the atherosclerotic plaque cap predispose to plaque rupture and coronary thrombosis.[25,26] To prevent plaque rupture, early detection would be a critical accomplishment, and early data suggest that CT features of coronary plaque may help detect plaques that are prone to rupture.[27] In particular, there is early evidence that calcified plaque can be differentiated from noncalcified plaque on the basis of the CT attenuation, and that lipid-rich noncalcified plaques have a lower attenuation than predominantly fibrotic noncalcified plaque.[28] However, the differentiation between the latter two may still be equivocal (Figure 6-12). In a

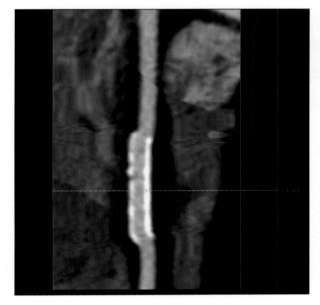

Fig. 6-11 Coronary CTA of a stent implant in the right coronary artery from a 64-row MSCT unit. In the curved reformat, the patency of the stent lumen is clearly documented, and artifacts from the metal stent implant do not preclude the diagnosis.

MSCT, an improved diagnostic accuracy for assessing bypass stenoses may be expected. For a bypass study, however, the scan length is greater than in normal coronary angiography, and a slice thickness of 1.25 mm is deemed appropriate in

direct comparison of CT features with intracoronary ultrasound images, the sensitivity of MSCT for detecting noncalcified plaque was only 53% in non-stenotic segments, and MSCT underestimated the plaque volume significantly.[29]

The potential clinical consequence of CT findings indicative of a vulnerable coronary plaque is primarily statin treatment. Presently, features of plaque instability can be detected by intracoronary ultrasound only, and researchers plan to elaborate on imaging features with this technique.[30]

The clinical potential of this approach remains unproven. Consequently, it is subject to further research and has no role in clinical practice today.

Special Case: Functional Assessment

Since the retrospectively EKG-gated helical data set contains image data from throughout the cardiac cycle, images at different time points can be reconstructed in retrospect (Figure 6-13). Thus, ventric-

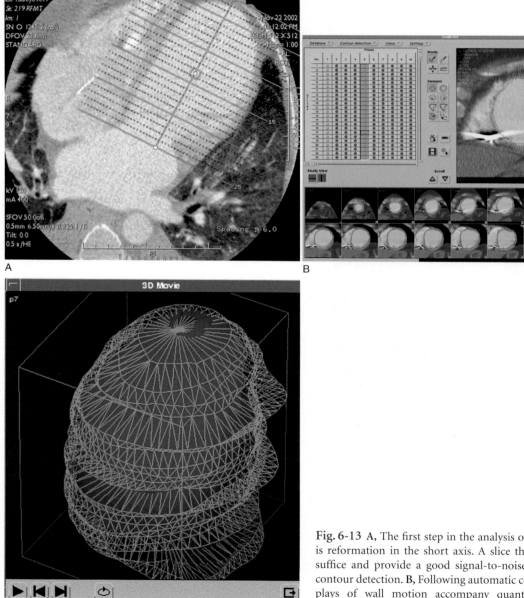

Fig. 6-13 A, The first step in the analysis of cardiac wall motion is reformation in the short axis. A slice thickness of 6 mm will suffice and provide a good signal-to-noise ratio for automatic contour detection. **B,** Following automatic contour detection, displays of wall motion accompany quantitative computation. **C,** Three-dimensional display of wall motion from a cine loop.

ular volume, left ventricular myocardial mass, myocardial thickening, and segmental wall motion can be derived.

Although wall motion analysis by CT is feasible, it does not constitute a common reason to perform a cardiac CT examination, since similar functional information can be obtained from echocardiography without any associated radiation or contrast use. Also, the limited temporal resolution of MSCT causes an underestimation of wall motion, especially at heart rates greater than 60 bpm. This method has been useful, however, in patients with end-stage heart failure in whom surgical resection of a ventricular aneurysm is contemplated. In this case, the cardiac surgeon prefers an image documentation of the exact extent of the aneurysm that is independent of the operator performing the exam.

Special Case: Pediatric Cardiac MSCT

For the pediatric cardiology patient, dose considerations are of special interest. Since many patients present with heart rates of more than 70 bpm and may not tolerate beta blocker treatment, most examinations are acquired without EKG synchronization. This accelerates the scan acquisition to a degree that even small children who cannot cooperate in a breath hold maneuver can be examined with good image quality. Typical indications for performing the scan are the assessment of aortic coarctation or pulmonary artery stenosis. The examination protocol is fine-tuned according to the question at hand and usually requires a much closer rapport with the pediatric cardiologist or cardiac surgeon than the standardized coronary protocol in adults (Table 6-4). Interest is often focused on the

Table 6-4   Pediatric Cardiac MSCT Protocol

Indication	Patient with known congenital heart disease, morphological assessment to plan further surgery or other treatment
Protocol designed for (scanner type)	LightSpeed 16 pro
Patient preparation	No coffee or smoking before the exam; patient fills out cardiac questionnaire before exam; breath hold trained before scan.
Oral contrast	—
IV contrast administration	2 ml/kg body weight iomeprol, 400 mg iodine/ml, 3 ml/s, scan delay depends on age and clinical history
Tube settings	kV 120 mA 320 (adjusted to patient age)
Gantry speed (sec)	0.4
Table speed (mm/sec)	18.75 mm/rotation
Slice thickness (mm)	16*1.25
Anatomical coverage	Entire chest
Reconstruction kernel	Standard
Breath hold	Inspiration
Window settings	900/80
Postprocessing	Interactive volume-rendering technique
Other	No EKG synchronization
Typical dose	CTDI = 12.77 mGy, DLP = 420 mGycm at 300 mm scan length

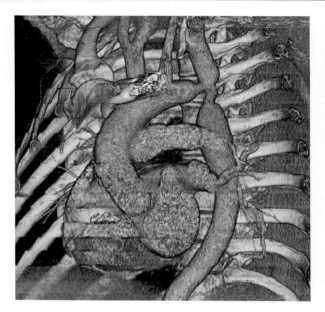

Fig. 6-14 Volume-rendered MSCT scan after surgery for aortic coarctation displaying two residual areas of stenosis at the typical location.

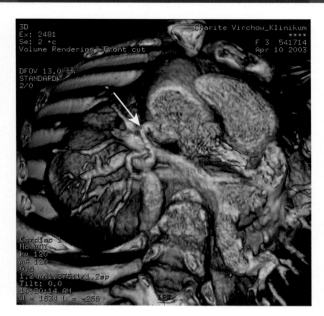

Fig. 6-15 Volume-rendering technique reconstruction from an MSCT scan of a 3-year-old female after surgical correction of Fallot's tetralogy. The right pulmonary artery had been treated with a stent, but pulmonary perfusion was still insufficient. The CT reconstruction displays a stenotic left pulmonary artery (arrow), whereas the pulmonary artery stent on the right side is patent.

great vessels or conduits. Such conduits include those from the superior vena cava to the right pulmonary artery (Glenn shunt) in patients with tricuspid atresia or pulmonary atresia, and the Blalock-Taussig (BT) shunt from the subclavian artery to the pulmonary artery. For an assessment of shunt function and further surgical planning, the demonstration of aberrant pulmonary arteries arising from the descending aorta is another important task.

To achieve satisfactory vascular contrast, the contrast injection protocol needs to be adapted to the target vessel and to patient size (Figures 6-14 to 6-16). In the smallest pediatric patients, maximum contrast injection rate may be as low as 0.5 ml/s, and a dose of 2 ml/kg body weight is generally sought. In patients less than 12 years old, the examination is started upon completion of contrast injection.

LIMITATIONS

Image Artifacts

As evidenced by the evaluable case rates published in the literature and the percentage of patients in

whom all coronary segments could be assessed, a significant proportion of patients could not be explored fully even with fast-rotating 16-row MSCT. In a failure mode and effects analysis, only a few major types of artifacts are encountered. This type of analysis is an engineering tool designed to detect the most important sources of defects and to guide future improvements.[31] One such defect is the beam-hardening artifact that appears as a shadow next to severe calcifications of coronary arteries. Since such calcifications are much more common in advanced coronary atherosclerosis, coronary CTA may be more severely limited by this effect in patients with known coronary disease. Such beam-hardening artifacts are generally reduced at a thinner slice thickness, and the introduction of sub-millimeter MSCT systems has made it possible to evaluate lesions that could not be assessed with earlier systems.

The other major limitation remains the appearance of motion artifacts (Figure 6-17). Motion artifacts appear as a distortion of anatomical details within the axial image plane or as a mismatch of

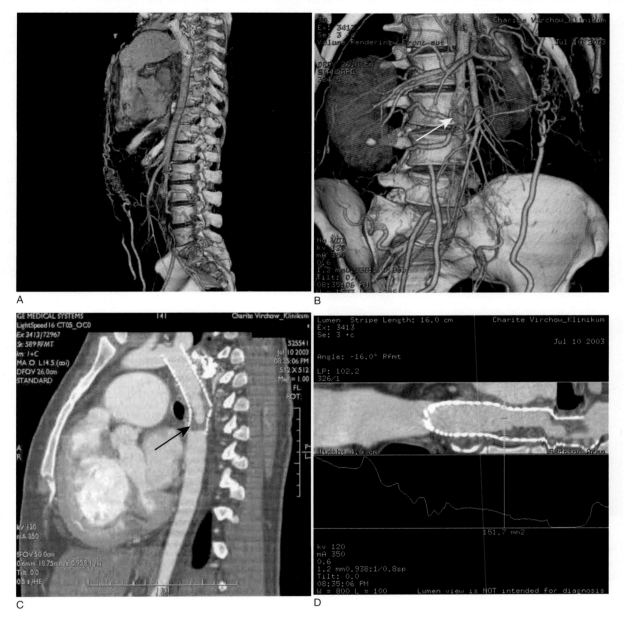

Fig. 6-16 A, VRT reconstruction of the aorta from a 22-year-old patient with a history of ventricular septal defect and Eisenmenger's syndrome. The patient had received a stent implant for treatment of aortic coarctation and now presented with severe back pain. The reconstruction displays the stent position. The abdominal aorta is occluded, and extensive collaterals supply the lower extremities. **B,** Occlusion of the abdominal aorta *(arrow)* as seen anteriorly. **C,** A sagittal reformat revealed thrombosis *(arrow)* of the aortic stent. **D,** On a curved reformat, however, residual lumen could be discerned. Symptoms resolved with anticoagulation.

two adjacent slice positions, which is most readily noted on three-dimensional reconstructions.

The cause for in-plane anatomical distortion is insufficient temporal resolution of the imaging system, and improvements of temporal resolution have the potential to resolve this type of artifact: an increase in gantry speed or use of an electron-beam type of radiation source would increase temporal resolution directly. As a postprocessing tool, image data segmentation is an alternative, and although this method is theoretically promising, clinical applications are limited by the physiological sinus

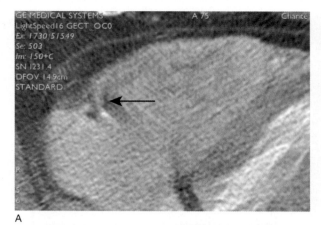

A

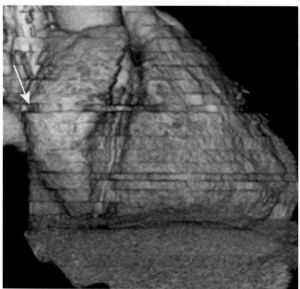

B

Fig. 6-17 **A,** Motion artifact of the right coronary artery transsection in an axial image. The coronary cross-section is distorted into a multi-tailed ellipsoid *(arrow).* **B,** Image mismatch artifacts in a three-dimensional volume-rendering technique. The discrepancy in anatomical position between adjacent slices is apparent as a stair-step artifact *(arrow).*

arrhythmia of the human heart and beat-to-beat variations in cardiac preload. Another approach is the attempt to reduce the patient's heart rate (e.g., by intravenous beta blockers). However, this necessitates a detailed review of the patient's other medications and clinical history. The success of such treatment is also quite variable.

The cause for image mismatch in the z-direction lies in the fact that image data are collected from several consecutive heart beats, and the exact spatial orientation of small anatomical objects such as a coronary artery segment typically vary slightly from one heart beat to another, caused by physiological sinus arrhythmia and beat-to-beat variation in cardiac load. Such artifacts could be avoided if the entire image data set were acquired within a single heart beat, as with a 12-cm area detector.

Patient Dose

As with all CT examinations, cardiac MSCT applications are associated with significant patient exposure to ionizing radiation.[32] In retrospectively EKG-gated helical scan acquisitions, the table speed is typically slow enough to allow for reconstruction of multiple image data sets at different time points in the cardiac cycle. With this technique, radiation exposure is much higher than with prospectively EKG-triggered series on an EBCT scanner. The estimated effective dose is also higher than the radiation dose associated with coronary angiography. To reduce this radiation dose, manufacturers have devised EKG-based tube current modulation, which reduces tube current during systole to as little as 20% of the diastolic tube current. Although some estimates have cited a 50% dose savings,[33] patients with heart rates of more than 60 bpm will encounter smaller dose benefits, and at a heart rate of more than 70 bpm, the net dose effect may be less than 20%.

THE FUTURE OF CORONARY CT

Technical developments have dictated a fast pace in the development of coronary CT applications. It is not hard to foresee that future innovations will produce larger area detectors with more z-axis coverage and the potential for even thinner slices. Some prototypes have already been on display at trade fairs in the last 2 years. An extension of such developments is the use of digital area detectors, similar to those in clinical use for radiography today, for CT applications. Such systems would capture the entire heart within a single-slice rotation and thus eliminate image artifacts caused by beat-to-beat data mismatch. At the same time, spatial resolution can be significantly improved. Early research indicates that the spatial resolution of conventional coronary angiography can be matched by such systems[34] (Figure 6-18).

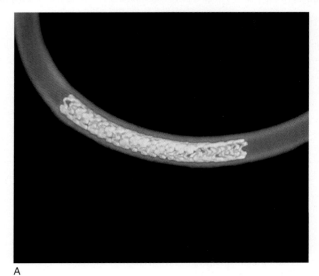

A

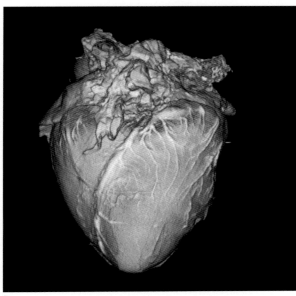

B

Fig. 6-18 A, Flat panel CT image of a coronary stent in vitro, acquired with a spatial resolution of 50 μm during a single detector rotation (VCT, GE Corporate Research). **B,** VCT image of porcine heart (same object as in Figure 6-1).

Another trend has been the increasing gantry speed in recent years, which is close to the physical limits of a mechanically rotating tube. With faster gantry speed, the tube capacity needs to increase to provide a sufficient photon density on the detector side, thus necessitating a heavier tube, which, in turn, makes it even harder to increase gantry speed. At this time, it is difficult to foresee if gantry rota-

tion times of less than 0.3 seconds will be feasible in a clinical system. It is also difficult to predict if electron beam technology will regain importance in this field, because the technology is focused on dedicated cardiac systems and is still more costly than a conventional MSCT unit.

REFERENCES

1. Wexler L, Brundage B, Crouse J, et al: Coronary artery calcification: pathophysiology, epidemiology, imaging methods, and clinical implications, *Circulation* 94:1175-1192, 1996.
2. O'Rourke RA, Brundage BH, Froelicher VF, et al: American College of Cardiology/American Heart Association consensus document on electron-beam computed tomography for the diagnosis and prognosis of coronary artery disease, *Circulation* 102:126-140, 2000.
3. Smith SC, Greenland P, Grundy SM: Prevention Conference V Executive Summary, *Circulation* 101:111-116, 2000.
4. DeBacker G, Ambrosioni E, Borch-Johnsen K, et al: European guidelines on cardiovascular disease prevention in clinical practice, *Eur Heart J* 24:1601-1610, 2003.
5. Greenland P, LaBree L, Azen SP, et al: Coronary artery calcium score combined with Framingham score for risk prediction in asymptomatic individuals, *JAMA* 291:210-215, 2004.
6. Budoff MJ, Oudiz RJ, Zalace CP, et al: Intravenous three-dimensional coronary angiography using contrast enhanced electron beam computed tomography, *Am J Cardiol* 83:840-845, 1999.
7. Nieman K, Oudkerk M, Rensing BJ, et al: Coronary angiography with multi-slice computed tomography, *Lancet* 357:599-603, 2001.
8. Scanlon PJ, Faxon DP: ACC/AHA guidelines for coronary angiography, *J Am Coll Cardiol* 33:1756-1824, 1999.
9. Ulzheimer S, Kalender WA: Assessment of calcium scoring performance in cardiac computed tomography, *Eur Radiol* 13:484-497, 2003.
10. Rumberger JA, Kaufman L: A Rosetta stone for coronary risk stratification, *Am J Roentgenol* 181:743-748, 2003.
11. Knollmann FD, Helmig K, Kapell S, et al: Coronary artery calcium scoring: diagnostic accuracy of different software implementations, *Invest Radiol* 38(12):761-768, 2003.
12. Knollmann F, Yankah CA, Kaisers U, et al: In vitro coronary artery imaging with sixteen-slice helical computed tomography, *Acta Radiol* 45:159-163, 2004.
13. Knollmann FD, Cangoz T, Cesmeli E, et al: Gauging effective spatial resolution in multirow helical cardiac computed tomography with a dynamic phantom, *Invest Radiol* 39(1):13-19, 2004.
14. Raggi P, Callister TC, Cooil B, et al: Identification of patients at increased risk of first unheralded acute myocardial infarction by electron-beam computed tomography, *Circulation* 101:850-856, 2000.
15. Vogl TJ, Abolmaali ND, Diebold T, et al: Techniques for the detection of coronary atherosclerosis: multi-detector row CT coronary angiography, *Radiology* 223:212-220, 2002.
16. Eusterman JH, Achor RWP, Kincaid OW, et al: Atherosclerotic disease of coronary arteries: a pathologic-radiologic correlative study, *Circulation* 26:1288-1295, 1962.

17. Gray CR, Hoffman HA, Hammond WS, et al: Correlation of arteriographic and pathologic findings in the coronary arteries in man, *Circulation* 26:494-499, 1962.

18. Isner JM, Kishel J, Kent KM, et al: Accuracy of angiographic determination of left main coronary arterial narrowing, *Circulation* 63:1056-1064, 1981.

19. Kastrati A, Mehilli J, Dirschinger J, et al: Restenosis after coronary placement of various stent types, *Am J Cardiol* 87:34-39, 2001.

20. Ruygrok PN, Webster MWI, de Valk V, et al: Clinical and angiographic factors associated with asymptomatic restenosis after percutaneous coronary intervention, *Circulation* 104:2289-2294, 2002.

21. Pump H, Möhlenkamp S, Sennert CA, et al: Coronary arterial stent patency: assessment with electron-beam CT, *Radiology* 214:447-452, 2000.

22. Pump H, Moehlenkamp S, Sehnert C, et al: Electron-beam CT in the noninvasive assessment of coronary stent patency, *Acad Radiol* 5:858-862, 1998.

23. Nieman K, Cademartiri F, Raaijmakers R, et al: Noninvasive angiographic evaluation of coronary stents with multislice spiral computed tomography, *Herz* 28:136-142, 2003.

24. Achenbach S, Moshage W, Ropers D, et al: Noninvasive, three-dimensional visualization of coronary artery bypass grafts by electron beam tomography, *Am J Cardiol* 79:856-861, 1997.

25. Davies MJ: Stability and instability: two faces of coronary atherosclerosis, *Circulation* 94:2013-2022, 1996.

26. Maseri A, Fuster V: Is there a vulnerable plaque? *Circulation* 107(16):2068-2071, 2003.

27. Schroeder S, Kopp AF, Baumbach A, et al: Noninvasive detection and evaluation of atherosclerotic coronary plaques with multislice computed tomography, *J Am Coll Cardiol* 37:1430-1435, 2001.

28. Becker CR, Nikolaou K, Muders M, et al: Ex vivo coronary atherosclerotic plaque characterization with multidetector-row CT, *Eur Radiol* 13:2094-2098, 2003.

29. Achenbach S, Moselewski F, Ropers D, et al: Detection of calcified and noncalcified coronary atherosclerotic plaque by contrast-enhanced, submillimeter multidetector spiral computed tomography, *Circulation* 109:14-17, 2004.

30. Association for Eradication of Heart Attack. www.vp.org.

31. Breyfogle FW III: *Implementing six sigma—smarter solutions usng statistical methods,* New York, 1999, John Wiley & Sons, pp. 256-274.

32. Morin RL, Gerber TC, McCollough CH: Radiation dose in computed tomography of the heart, *Circulation* 107:917-922, 2003.

33. Jakobs TE, Becker CR, Ohnesorge B, et al: Multislice helical CT of the heart with retrospective ECG gating: reduction of radiation exposure by ECG-controlled tube current modulation, *Eur Radiol* 12:1081-1086, 2002.

34. Knollmann F, Pfoh A: Coronary artery imaging with flat-panel computed tomography, *Circulation* 107:1209, 2003.

CHAPTER 7

Multislice Computed Tomography of the Hepatobiliary System

Afia Umber
Fergus V. Coakley

The emergence of multislice (i.e., multidetector row) CT (MSCT) in 1998 was a technological breakthrough that has resulted in major advances in hepatobiliary imaging. Multiphasic scanning of the liver can now be performed routinely and with near isotropic resolution (isotropic resolution refers to equal resolution in the x, y, and z axes, so that voxels are cubic in shape), allowing generation of exquisitely detailed three-dimensional volumetric reconstructions (Figure 7-1). Three-dimensional data sets, narrow collimation, and multiphasic imaging provide improved lesion detection, multiplanar capability, and the ability to perform high-quality CT angiography (Figure 7-2). However, this new technology, which continues to evolve, also poses significant challenges for hepatobiliary imaging. The major challenge is the vast quantity of image data generated. This remains an unsolved problem that will require the development of innovative image processing and viewing strategies. The traditional paradigm of reviewing tomographic slices may be replaced by a primarily volumetric approach. The rapidity with which the liver can be imaged with MSCT also requires new thinking with respect to the rate of intravenous contrast

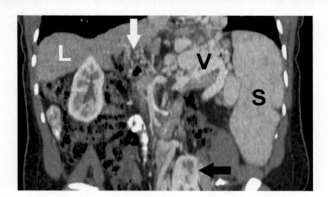

Fig. 7-1 Curved planar reconstruction in a 71-year-old man with cirrhosis illustrating how multiple findings can be demonstrated on a single reformatted image. The liver *(L)* is small and shrunken as a result of cirrhosis. The portal vein *(white arrow)* shows cavernous transformation. Large varices *(V)* are visible in the left upper quadrant. The spleen *(S)* is enlarged. A pelvic left kidney *(black arrow)* is present as an incidental finding.

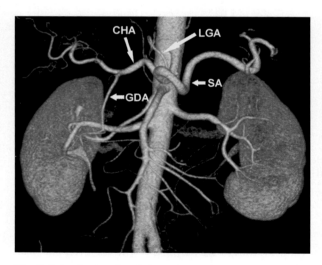

Fig. 7-2 Surface-rendered view of a CT arteriogram obtained using MSCT technology. The information provided by such high-quality CT angiography is competitive with the detail provided by conventional catheter angiography. The common hepatic *(CHA),* left gastric *(LGA),* gastroduodenal *(GDA),* and splenic *(SA)* arteries can be seen clearly arising from the upper abdominal aorta via the celiac axis.

administration, contrast injection duration, contrast bolus volume, and scan delays. With scanning times as short as 10 seconds, smaller contrast volumes injected at a faster rate may be more appropriate. Although narrow collimation may seem intuitively advantageous, it does increase

image noise and may reduce the geometric efficiency of the detectors. Finally, the radiation dose is increased with MSCT (unless other factors are adjusted), which may be compounded by multiphasic imaging. Careful attention must be paid to technical parameters during scanning, and the dose needs to be tailored to the specific clinical situation. Use of commercially available dose-modifying software may help. The aim of this chapter is to review the MSCT strategies for hepatobiliary imaging and to provide evidence-based guidelines for the performance and interpretation of these studies.

TERMINOLOGY FOR MULTIPHASE MSCT OF THE LIVER

Phases of Enhancement

MSCT allows breath-hold imaging of the liver during the rapid administration of an intravenous contrast medium bolus. Scanning may be performed at different and repeated times from the initiation of the contrast injection. There is no standard or universal terminology for the different phases of enhancement that are seen at different periods subsequent to intravenous contrast injection, although common and logical use would suggest the following nomenclature:

1. *Early arterial (or arteriographic) phase.* Typically acquired after a scan delay of 20 seconds. The arterial system is well opacified without significant parenchymal enhancement (Figure 7-3, *A*), allowing for optimal arteriographic imaging. The phase can be acquired after a fixed scan delay or after an individualized delay determined by a test bolus or by bolus-tracking software.

2. *Late arterial phase.* Typically acquired after a scan delay of 40 to 45 seconds. Rapidly enhancing structures such as hypervascular tumors and the renal cortex are well opacified (Figure 7-3, *B*) and are optimally imaged against the background of relatively unenhanced adjacent parenchyma. This phase is used for detection of hypervascular tumors such as early enhancing hemangioma, hepatocellular carcinoma, neuroendocrine tumor, focal nodular hyperplasia, and hepatic adenoma.

3. *Portal (or hepatic) venous phase.* Typically acquired after a scan delay of 60 to 110 seconds.

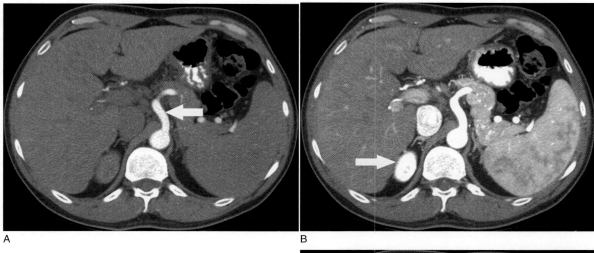

Fig. 7-3 A, Axial CT image obtained in the early arterial (arterial graphic) phase shows that the arteries, such as the caliac artery *(arrow)*, are well opacified, whereas the parenchyma of the liver, spleen, and other viscera does not demonstrate significant enhancement. Such images are typically obtained after a scan delay of approximately 20 seconds. **B,** Axial CT image obtained in the late arterial phase. Rapidly enhancing structures such as the renal cortex *(arrow)* are well opacified. The pancreas also enhances early and is well opacified. The spleen shows heterogeneous early enhancement, whereas the liver parenchyma shows only minimal enhancement. Such images are typically obtained after a scan delay of approximately 40 to 45 seconds. **C,** Axial CT image obtained in the portal (or hepatic) venous phase. The hepatic parenchyma is well opacified, and contrast is clearly visualized in the portal vein *(arrow)*. Such images are typically acquired after a scan delay of 60 to 110 seconds.

The hepatic parenchyma is well opacified, with contrast visible in both the portal and hepatic venous systems (Figure 7-3, *C*). This is the phase used for routine abdominal imaging and best depicts hypovascular hepatic tumors (which account for the majority of clinically important lesions).

4. *Delayed (or equilibrium) phase.* The scan delay for delayed imaging is variable and can range from 2 to 15 minutes or even longer. Such images may be helpful for showing centripetal enhancement in hepatic hemangiomas or to depict delayed enhancement in cholangiocarcinoma or in the central scar of focal nodular hyperplasia (Figure 7-4).

Several important details regarding these phases merit specific mention. These phases are not rigidly separated by objective criteria, but rather are descriptive terms that represent arbitrary divisions of what is a continuum of changes in vascular and parenchymal densities after a contrast bolus. The terms *early* and *late* arterial phases only entered common usage after the advent of MSCT. Although single-slice spiral CT was a considerable advance, it was not fast enough to temporally resolve these phases. Older studies referring to *arterial phase* in isolation are usually referring to the later arterial phase. Precontrast or noncontrast images can also be acquired and may be helpful in the definitive determination of enhancement or the demonstration of calcification. Noncontrast images can also contribute to the diagnosis of fatty liver. The role of noncontrast images in the detection of hepatic metastases will be discussed in detail later. Strictly speaking, precontrast images should not be regarded as a "phase" of enhancement, since the

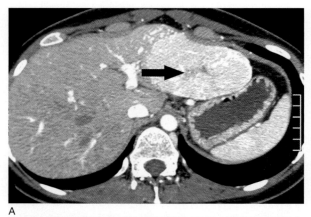

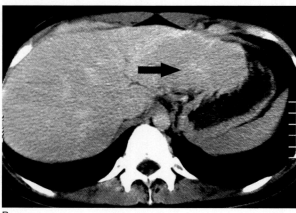

Fig. 7-4 A, Axial CT image obtained in the arterial phase in a patient with focal nodular hyperplasia in the lateral segment of the left hepatic lobe. The lesion is hypervascular and well demarcated against the less-enhanced hepatic parenchyma in this phase. Note the presence of a hypovascular central scar *(arrow)*. **B,** Axial CT image obtained in the delayed phase of enhancement at the same level seen in **A**. Note that the central scar *(arrow)* demonstrates delayed enhancement. This is a critical finding in the distinction of the central scar of focal nodular hyperplasia from the central scar of fibrolamellar hepatocellular carcinoma and illustrates how images obtained in the delayed phase of enhancement can assist in the characterization of focal hepatic masses.

term *phase of enhancement* only has meaning after contrast has been given.[1]

Multiphase Terminology

As noted above, the terminology for naming the various phases of enhancement after intravenous contrast medium administration is not standardized. The terminology for multiphasic studies that combine two or more of these phases is even more confusing. The term *biphasic* or *dual phase* CT is probably most commonly used to refer to combined (late) arterial and portal venous phase images, but it is also used to refer to combinations of precontrast and portal venous phase images, early and late arterial phase images, or portal venous and delayed phase images. Similar, if not greater, confusion exists regarding the use of the terms *triple* and *quadruple* phase studies.[1,2] Until a universal terminology is established, it is probably best to avoid unclear terms such as *dual, triple,* or *quadruple* and instead refer explicitly to the phases that have been acquired.

Hypovascular and Hypervascular Liver Tumors

In our experience, the terminology and pathophysiology related to the classification of hepatic tumors as hypovascular or hypervascular is another source of confusion. To clarify, a tumor is *hypovascular* if the tumor is less dense than the surrounding hepatic parenchyma and *hypervascular* if it is denser than the surrounding hepatic parenchyma. A tumor that is of equal density to the surrounding parenchyma is *isovascular*, but such a tumor can only be seen if it has mass effect or has a contrast difference with the parenchyma on another phase. As such, the classification of a hepatic tumor as hypovascular or hypervascular is phase dependent; that is, a tumor such as focal nodular hyperplasia might be hypervascular on the arterial phase, but it might be hypovascular on the portal venous phase. Tumors can also be of mixed vascularity, with some parts of the tumor being hypervascular and other parts being hypovascular. Conversely, a tumor such as a hemangioma might be hypovascular on the arterial phase but hypervascular on the portal venous phase. However, hypovascular tumors are commonly understood as those that have a lower density than the parenchyma in both arterial and portal venous phases, whereas hypervascular tumors are those that have a higher density than the parenchyma in the arterial phase. Common hypervascular tumors include hepatocellular carcinoma, neuroendocrine and other hypervascular metastases, small (early-enhancing) hemangiomas, focal nodular hyperplasia, and adenomas (Figure 7-5). These tumors have a brisk blood supply and enhance at an earlier time and to a greater degree than the adjacent tissues. The distinction of hypovascular and hypervascular tumors is important because hypervascular tumors

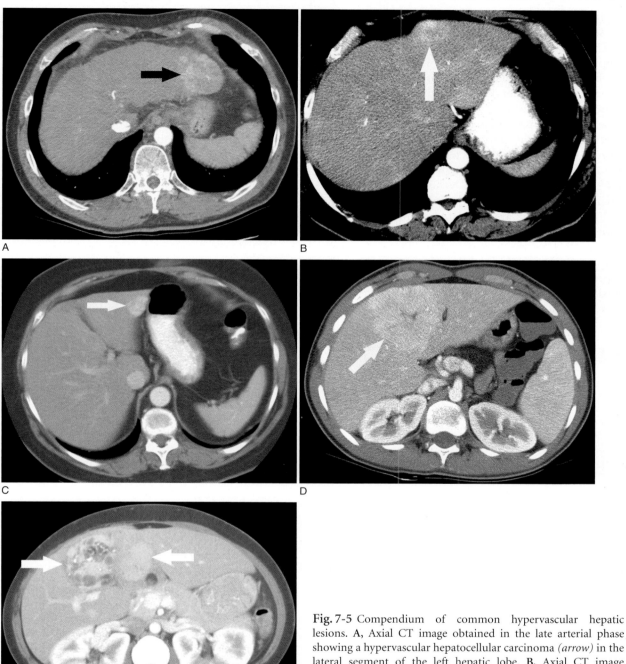

Fig. 7-5 Compendium of common hypervascular hepatic lesions. **A,** Axial CT image obtained in the late arterial phase showing a hypervascular hepatocellular carcinoma *(arrow)* in the lateral segment of the left hepatic lobe. **B,** Axial CT image obtained in the later arterial phase shows multiple hypervascular metastases from neuroendocrine carcinoma, with the dominant lesion *(arrow)* lying anteriorly in the left hepatic lobe. **C.** Axial CT image showing a small (early enhancing) hemangioma *(arrow)* in the tip of the left hepatic lobe. **D,** Axial CT image obtained in the late arterial phase showing the typical appearance of focal nodular hyperplasia *(arrow)* in the medial segment of the left hepatic lobe. The lesion is hypervascular with a hypovascular central scar. Delayed phase images (not shown) showed delayed enhancement in the central scar. **E,** Axial CT image in the late arterial phase in a patient with von Gierke's disease. Two hypervascular adenomas *(arrows)* are visible. One of the lesions contains small nodules of microscopic fat, which is one of the recognized findings in hepatic adenoma.

are frequently most conspicuous during the arterial phase of imaging.

The liver is unusual because it has a dual blood supply, with approximately 30% delivered from the hepatic artery and 70% from the portal vein. Hepatic tumors generally receive their blood supply from the hepatic artery. As a result, hepatic tumors appear hypodense when contrast is administered selectively into the portal vein, as in CT arterioportography (contrast injected into the superior mesenteric artery passes through the gut and opacifies the liver through portal venous passage). It is crucial to understand that the terms *hypovascular* and *hypervascular* are unrelated to blood supply; both hypovascular and hypervascular tumors are supplied by the hepatic artery. The difference is in the briskness of blood flow. Hypovascular and hypervascular tumors are both supplied by the hepatic artery and both will appear hypovascular on CT arterioportography.

INTRAVENOUS CONTRAST ADMINISTRATION FOR HEPATOBILIARY MSCT

General Comments

Optimal delivery of intravenous contrast medium is a complex and critical issue for MSCT of the hepatobiliary system, both for optimal CT angiography and for optimal arterial phase imaging of hypervascular hepatic masses. Controlling the level and time course of arterial enhancement and correctly synchronizing CT acquisition relative to arterial enhancement becomes more difficult and less forgiving with MSCT acquisition times for the entire liver in the range of 5 to 10 seconds. A basic understanding of contrast medium dynamics is crucial for the rational design of contrast medium injection technique. Intravenous contrast travels sequentially from the arm vein to the right heart, the lungs, and the left heart before entering the arterial system for systemic distribution. The degree of arterial enhancement following the same intravenous contrast medium injection varies greatly among individuals. The key physiological parameters affecting individual arterial enhancement are cardiac output and the central blood volume. Cardiac output is inversely related to the degree of arterial enhance-

ment.[3] If more blood is ejected per unit of time, the contrast medium injected per unit of time will be more diluted. Therefore, arterial enhancement is weaker in patients with high cardiac output but stronger in patients with low cardiac output (despite the increased contrast medium transit time in the latter).[3] Blood volume is also inversely related to arterial enhancement but presumably affects recirculation rather than the first-pass effect. Blood volume is correlated with body weight.

Practical Aspects of Contrast Injection

The thickest antecubital vein is usually the most favorable site for contrast medium delivery. Flushing the delivery system with saline immediately after the contrast medium injection pushes the contrast medium column from the arm veins into the bloodstream, where it contributes to arterial enhancement and produces a "tighter" bolus, thus reducing the required contrast medium volume. Dual-chamber power injectors are now available that allow an automated saline flush to rapidly follow the contrast bolus. They are especially helpful if small total volumes, short injection durations, or high iodine concentration contrast media are used. Recently, automatic devices for the local detection of extravasation have been developed to avoid the leakage of significant amounts of contrast, which is a particular concern at higher injection rates.

Contrast Injection Rate

According to Bae et al.,[3] an increase in the injection rate above 2 ml/sec does not substantially increase hepatic peak parenchymal enhancement. Rather, it is beneficial in increasing the magnitude of arterial enhancement and temporally separating the arterial and venous phase of enhancement for multiphase studies. Therefore, rapid injection rates (i.e., 4 to 5 ml/sec) should be used for multiphase examinations in the liver, because in comparison with lower injection rates, they provide increased vascular enhancement and longer separation between the arterial and portal venous enhancement phases. With a securely placed intravenous line, injection rates of up to 10 ml/sec of nonionic contrast medium have been well tolerated.[11]

Contrast Volume

Contrast medium volume, injection rate, and injection duration have interrelated effects on the time course of arterial enhancement.[4] Biphasic or multiphasic injections (an initial period of high injection flow rate followed by one or more periods of lower injection flow rates) lead to more uniform arterial enhancement than uniphasic injections.[8,81] If CT arteriography is combined with parenchymal imaging, such as in multiphasic MSCT of the liver, the total contrast medium volume is chosen independently of the acquisition speed of the scanner but according to the needs for the parenchymal phases of the study (e.g., 150 ml of standard 300 mg I/ml contrast medium). If total contrast medium volumes are chosen relative to body weight, then 1.5 to 2.0 ml/kg body weight is a reasonable quantity for CT arteriography. Preliminary results with high osmolar contrast medium suggest that a lower contrast volume can be used with similar hepatic enhancement to conventional contrast protocols, which could lead to cost-saving. The degree of hepatic arterial enhancement is largely dependent on the rate of iodine delivery and the timing of the bolus, whereas venous hepatic enhancement is most dependent on the total iodine dose delivered.[5]

Iodine Concentration

Arterial enhancement is correlated with the number of iodine molecules administered per unit of time. This iodine administration rate can be heightened by increasing either the injection flow rate or the iodine concentration of the contrast medium. A number of studies have shown that there is significantly greater arterial enhancement with high-concentration (370 mg/ml) contrast media over conventional contrast, regardless of whether the contrast volume is equal to or decreased to administer a similar total iodine dose.[6,7] High iodine administration rates are desirable for CT arteriography and for certain nonvascular imaging applications, such as the detection of hypervascular liver lesions and for organ perfusion studies. Conversely, low concentration contrast media have the advantage of causing less perivenous streak artifacts at the level of the brachiocephalic veins and the superior vena cava in thoracic CT, particularly if saline flushing of the veins is not performed.

Optimizing the Scan Delay for Arterial Phase MSCT

Optimal timing of the arterial phase remains controversial (Table 7-1). Various authors[8,9] recommend a scan delay of 20 to 30 seconds after the initiation of intravenous injection of the bolus of contrast medium, with an injection rate of 4 to 5 ml/sec. However, such a fixed scan delay may lead to inconsistent results because of differences in variables such as patient size and cardiovascular status. Administering a dose of contrast medium based on patient weight (e.g., 2 ml/kg) helps minimize patient size as a variable, but circulatory function remains an unknown factor. This can be overcome by individualizing the arterial phase scan delay, by either using a test bolus or commercially available bolus-tracking technology. A study using bolus tracking found the optimal scan delay for the early arterial phase was 14 to 36 seconds (mean, 19 seconds); the optimal scan delay for the later arterial phase was 30 to 52 seconds (mean, 35 seconds).[10] The variability of the scan delay in this and other studies[11] suggests that individualized scan delays are preferable to fixed scan delays, if such an approach is logistically and practically possible.

Table 7-1   Variability of optimal scan delays for arterial phase CT of the liver

Reference	n	Dose of contrast (ml)	Time to peak hepatic enhancement after end of injection (sec)	
			Median	Range
Harmon et al[81]	50	160	23	20-26
Chambers et al[82]	14	126-132	35.5	34-37
Bree et al[83]	902	100-175	25	8-42
Silverman et al[84]	56	150	30	30

CHOOSING SLICE THICKNESS FOR HEPATOBILIARY MSCT

Effect of Slice Thickness on Detection of Focal Liver Lesions

For dynamic CT with a single-detector helical CT scanner, a section thickness (collimation) of 7 to 10 mm has been commonly used.[9,12-18] The advent of MSCT scanners allows the acquisition of images of thin sections through large areas of anatomy without concern for breathing artifacts or x-ray tube-cooling problems. Reconstruction of thin sections (1.25 to 2.5 mm) is essential for good quality CT angiography,[19,20] but the optimal collimation and reconstruction interval for detection of focal hepatic lesions is less well established. Spiral CT reconstructed with 50% overlap increases reader confidence and overall detection rate of focal liver lesions. The additional images provide information that supports the use of smaller interscan spacing in the appropriate clinical setting, especially since the extra images can be generated without an additional dose of radiation to the patient or an increase in scanning time. The most significant benefit is improved confidence in the evaluation of smaller lesions. Web et al.[21] used a dual-detector CT scanner to study the usefulness of thin collimation for evaluating small (diameter < 10 mm) liver lesions, primarily hypovascular metastases. These researchers detected more lesions on images obtained with a 2.5-mm collimation than on those obtained with a 5-, 7.5-, or 10-mm collimation. Using MSCT, other investigators have described findings regarding the detection rate for focal hepatic lesions that conflict in terms of optimal slice thickness.[22,23] The value of a relatively thin (4 to 7 mm) collimation has been well documented for detection of most hypovascular focal liver lesions. Kawata et al.[24] studied the effect of slice thickness on the detection of 87 hypervascular hepatocellular carcinomas in 43 patients and found no difference in the area under the receiver operating characteristic curve when comparing 2.5 mm (A_z = 0.79), 5 mm (A_z = 0.80), and 7.5 mm (A_z = 0.78) slice thickness.

Prognostic Importance of Small Hypoattenuating Hepatic Lesions

The improved detection of smaller hypoattenuating hepatic lesions with thinner slices raises an obvious question: Do such lesions matter? Small ($\leq$15 mm in diameter) hypoattenuating hepatic lesions are a common incidental finding on contrast-enhanced CT of the abdomen,[25] particularly with the increasing use of thinner collimation caused by the advent of helical and MSCT.[26] Such small hypoattenuating hepatic lesions are often described as "too small to characterize," because attenuation measurements are unreliable because of partial volume averaging and pseudo-enhancement.[27,28] The inability to positively characterize these lesions is particularly problematic in patients with cancer, since the differential diagnosis is frequently considered to include metastases. One study using serial CT suggested that, in breast cancer patients, up to 22% of hypoattenuating hepatic lesions of 10 mm or less in diameter are metastases.[29] However, this study did not address the key clinical question: What is the relative risk of subsequently developing hepatic metastases for a patient in whom the only hepatic finding at CT is one or more small hypoattenuating hepatic lesions? A recent study by Krakora et al.[30] showed that in patients with breast cancer, small hypoattenuating hepatic lesions without other evidence of hepatic metastases at baseline CT are not associated with an increased risk of subsequently developing hepatic metastases (Figure 7-6). Some of the conflicting results of these studies may be due to the possibility that small metastases are less detectable on CT, even with thin collimation, because they may be isoattenuating. This is supported by a study of 31 patients with hepatic metastases (30 from colorectal carcinoma and 1 from gastrointestinal stromal tumor) in whom preoperative CT showed 88 small hypoattenuating hepatic lesions.[26] Twenty-five of these lesions were metastases. Thinner collimation (2.5 mm versus 5 mm) improved overall lesion detection but did not increase detection of these small metastases. If small metastases were isoattenuating, thinner collimation would not improve lesion detection. Partial volume averaging would also tend to obscure visualization of small metastases that are only slightly different in attenuation to the adjacent hepatic parenchyma, whereas small cysts are more likely to be seen because of greater attenuation difference between fluid and hepatic

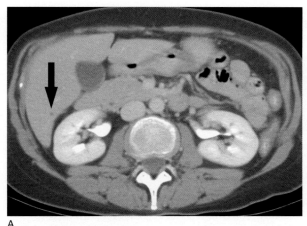

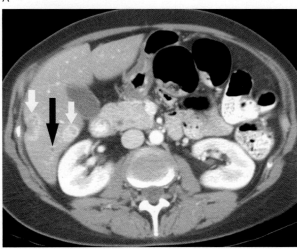

Fig. 7-6 A, Axial CT image in a 54-year-old woman with breast cancer. A small hyperattenuating hepatic lesion *(arrow)* is visible in the inferior right hepatic lobe. **B,** Axial CT image obtained in the same patient 2 years after the image shown in **A.** Two metastases *(white arrows)* are now visible, although the small hyperattenuating lesion *(black arrow)* is unchanged. This illustrates that even in patients who develop metastases, small hypoattenuating hepatic lesions seen on the baseline study are likely tiny cysts, and therefore the use of increasingly thin collimation to detect such lesions is questionable.

parenchyma. An analogy can be made with the traditional teaching that a small nodule visible on chest x-ray is probably calcified and benign, because a malignant soft-tissue nodule of the same size would be invisible[31]; the fact that a small hepatic lesion is visible at CT may inherently suggest the lesion is cystic. These considerations also suggest that the pursuit of small hypoattenuating lesions with thinner and thinner slices may be inappropriate. For

daily practice, review of abdominal CT images of 5 mm in thickness appears to be adequate.

WHICH PROTOCOL SHOULD BE USED? MATCHING PHASES TO PATIENTS

General Comments

The ability to rapidly acquire precontrast and postcontrast images in multiple phases raises an obvious question: Should all phases be acquired in all patients, or should phases be matched to patients? The notion that all phases should be acquired in all patients is clearly untenable; such an approach would result in unacceptably high radiation doses, tube loading, and data storage demands. Furthermore, the rapid injection rates used in multiphase imaging require placement of a larger bore needle than that required for portal venous phase imaging alone. This increases patient discomfort and can be extremely difficult or impossible in patients with poor venous access (e.g., oncologic patients with a history of prior intravenous chemotherapy administration or intravenous drug users). Accordingly, phases of enhancement should be chosen according to the clinical setting. Indications for acquisition of noncontrast and different postcontrast phase images are shown in Table 7-2 and are reviewed in detail in the following sections.

Non-Enhanced CT for the Diagnosis of Fatty Liver

Fatty liver can be seen with obesity, excessive alcohol ingestion, diabetes, Cushing's syndrome, malnutrition, parenteral hyperalimentation, certain toxins such as carbon tetrachloride, chemotherapy, and radiation.[32,36] Non-alcoholic fatty liver disease (NAFLD) is not always a benign condition; it may be associated with necroinflammatory change, in which case it is known as non-alcoholic steatohepatitis (NASH). NASH is increasingly recognized as an important cause of end-stage liver disease and is becoming more frequent because of the current obesity epidemic. Accordingly, the diagnosis of fatty liver, which was the focus of several reports in the early CT era, is once again topical and of clinical interest. Fatty liver is also important to recognize

Table 7-2 Indications for acquisition of noncontrast and multiphase postcontrast images

Phase	Indications
Noncontrast	Diagnosis of fatty liver Diagnosis of hemorrhage Baseline for detection of calcification or confirmation of enhancement
Early arterial (arteriographic) 20-second delay	CT arteriogram for arterial anatomy Detection of hypervascular liver tumors
Late arterial (parenchymal arterial) 40-second delay	Detection of hypervascular liver tumors Characterization of small lesions
Portal venous 60-110-second delay	Routine study Liver metastases
Delayed (equilibrium) 2-15-minute delay	Diagnosis of cholangiocarcinoma, hemangioma

for radiological reasons, because fatty infiltration may reduce the conspicuousness of hypodense hepatic lesions such as metastases.[33,36] Three distinct criteria exist for the diagnosis of fatty liver:

- *NECT density criteria.* The liver normally measures several HU more than the spleen on NECT.[34,36] Fatty infiltration reduces the attenuation of the liver and may result in the liver being less dense than the spleen. The spleen is a useful and practical standard of reference for comparison with the liver because its attenuation is easily measured, the spleen is usually present on the same axial sections as the liver, and splenic attenuation is not affected by most diffuse pathological processes such as fatty infiltration.[34] Conditions that alter splenic attenuation are rare and usually easy to recognize. Examples include metastases, iron deposition, splenic vascular disruption, and posttraumatic hypotension.[35] Other confounding factors that can alter the hepatic attenuation include hemosiderosis, hemochromatosis, prior thorotrast administration, amiodarone usage, radiation therapy, hepatitis, cirrhosis, Wilson's disease, and glycogen storage disease.[36] Iron and fat have opposing effects on overall hepatic attenuation, such that iron deposition in a fatty liver may result in normal-appearing liver attenuation.[37] Thresholds for the NECT diagnosis of fatty liver have been suggested, based on a study including 126 patients, 23 with proven fatty liver[85] as shown in Table 7-3. In general, a hepatic density that is 10 HU (or more) less than the spleen is suggestive of fatty infiltration (Figure 7-7, *A*).

Table 7-3 Thresholds for the NECT diagnosis of fatty liver

L < S by	Sensitivity	Specificity
0 + HU	93%	88%
5 + HU	89%	97%
10 + HU[5]	84%	99%

- *CECT density criteria.* Many centers only acquire images in the portal venous phase for routine abdominal scans. A number of studies have investigated the density criteria for the diagnosis of fatty liver on such portal venous phase CECT studies[38,39] (Table 7-4). In general, a hepatic density that is 20 HU (or more) less than the spleen is suggestive of fatty infiltration (Figure 7-7, *B*).

- *Detection of fatty sparing.*[40] The recognition of areas of fatty sparing implies the remaining liver must be fatty, even if the liver does not meet the density criteria just described. The presence of sparing is highly specific for fatty infiltration and may be seen as geographic areas of subtle hyper-attenuation without mass effect around the porta hepatis, around the gallbladder fossa, or in the subcapsular portions of the liver (Figure 7-8).

NECT for the Detection of Hepatic Metastases

A number of studies have investigated whether NECT images are incrementally helpful in the

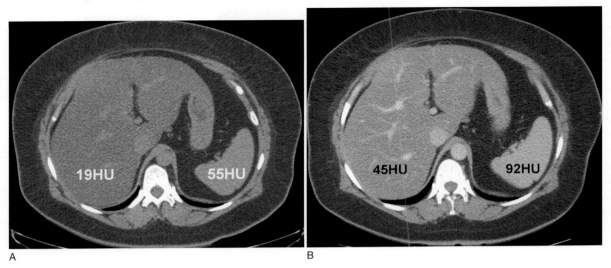

A

B

Fig. 7-7 A, A hepatic density that is 10 HU or more less than the splenic density on nonenhanced CT images is suggestive of diffuse fatty infiltration. **B,** A hepatic density that is 20 HU or more less than the splenic density is suggestive of diffuse fatty infiltration on portal venous phase contrast-enhanced CT images.

Table 7-4	Reported density thresholds[5] for the diagnosis of fatty liver on portal venous phase CECT			
L < S by	Sensitivity	Specificity	n	Reference number
L < S by 20+ HU	86%	87%	76 (18 fatty)	38
L < S by 20+ HU	87%	75%	126 (23 fatty)	5
L < S by 30+ HU	79%	94%	126 (23 fatty)	5
L < S	100%	4%	96 (16 fatty)	39
L < muscle	25%	100%	96 (16 fatty)	39

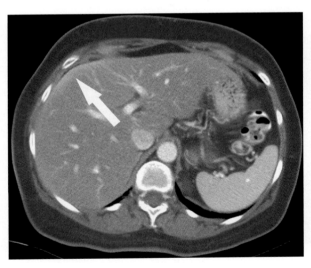

Fig. 7-8 Regardless of whether density criteria for the diagnosis of diffuse fatty infiltration are present, the finding of focal fatty sparing is indicative of diffuse fatty infiltration. Areas of fatty sparing may be seen at the porta hepatis or in a subcapsular location *(arrow).*

detection of metastases, based on the realization that some metastases may be isoattenuating on CECT but hypoattenuating on NECT—particularly vascular metastases that enhance in parallel with the liver parenchyma. Bresler et al.[41] reported 11 (39%) of 28 patients with hypervascular liver metastases (from carcinoid tumor, islet cell neoplasm, pheochromocytoma, and renal cell carcinoma) had tumors that were not apparent on portal venous phase images but rather were seen as low-attenuation foci on the unenhanced CT images. Oliver et al.[42] reported that in patients with hepatocellular carcinoma, unenhanced CT images depicted 17% (47 of 276 tumors) additional tumor foci not seen on portal venous phase images. In 3% (2 out of 81) of these patients, the NECT images were the only images to depict any tumor. Patten et al.[42a] showed that even though unenhanced CT images may show additional hypervascular metastatic lesions, portal venous phase images reveal some evidence of hepatic metastatic disease in most patients. Frederick et al.[43] reported on the added benefit of multiphase helical CT in evaluating hepatic metastases in patients with breast carcinoma, but the rate of injection in that study was low (2 ml/sec), which appears to limit the sensitivity of arterial phase images, according to the growing clinical experience of many investigators. Oliver et al.[44] showed that both arterial phase and unenhanced CT images depict additional hypervascular tumors within the liver not seen on portal venous phase images. However, unlike previous reports for hepatocellular carcinoma, unenhanced images depicted significantly more additional lesions than arterial phase images (28% versus 13% additional lesions, respectively). Arguably, it may be justified to perform all three phases (unenhanced, arterial phase, and portal venous phase) during the first CT examination to optimally screen the liver for metastatic disease and to assess the vascularity of the former foci to determine which sequence should be used for follow-up CT. In summary, there is some evidence that NECT images may occasionally help in the detection of hepatic masses (Figure 7-9), particularly in those that are typically hypervascular. Whether this is of sufficient magnitude to justify obtaining NECT images in all such patients is a more problematic issue and ultimately depends on an individual's professional judgment and evaluation of the available evidence.

Early Arterial Phase CT for Hepatic Arteriography

Hepatic CT arteriography is usually performed to define the hepatic arterial anatomy before surgical or therapeutic intervention (Figure 7-10). Examples include definition of hepatic arterial anatomy for vascular variations before right hepatic lobe resection for living-related donor transplantation, before chemoembolization of hepatocellular carcinoma, or before hepatic arterial chemotherapy pump placement for treatment of metastatic colorectal cancer. Occasional indications for CT angiography of the hepatic venous system include cirrhosis, suspected vascular malformations, and planning of transjugular intrahepatic portosystemic shunt (TIPS) placement (Reference Smith et al.,[44a] dual phase CT with 3D volume rendering).

Early Arterial Phase CT for Detection of Hypervascular Masses

The advent of MSCT and the ability to perform two acquisitions rather than one during the arterial phase raises the question of whether the early arterial phase (which is primarily used for CT arteriography) is incrementally useful in detecting hypervascular masses. Three studies have addressed

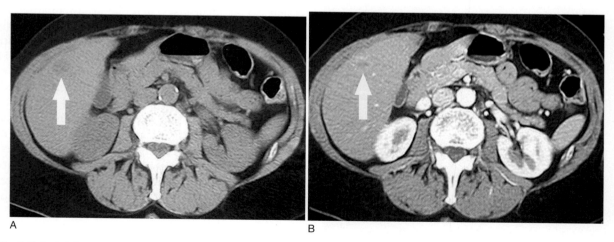

A   B

Fig. 7-9 A, Axial nonenhanced CT image in a patient with a large hepatocellular carcinoma (not shown) elsewhere in the liver. A small well-circumscribed hypodense lesion is visible *(arrow)*. **B,** Axial contrast-enhanced CT image at the same level seen in A, showing that the lesion *(arrow)* seen on nonenhanced images is only barely visible on these post-contrast images. Nonenhanced CT is occasionally useful in the detection of enhancing tumors such as hepatocellular carcinoma and neuroendocrine metastases, because such lesions can be relatively isodense after contrast administration.

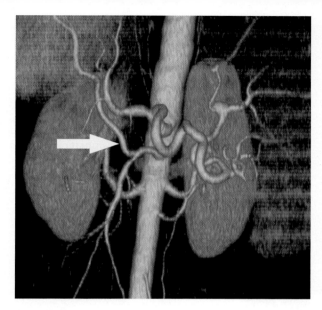

Fig. 7-10 Three-dimensional reformation of an abdominal CT arteriogram in a patient being considered as a potential right hepatic lobe liver donor. The right hepatic artery *(arrow)* is seen to have an aberrant origin from the superior mesenteric artery. The presence of such an arterial variant is a relative contraindication to right lobe harvest.

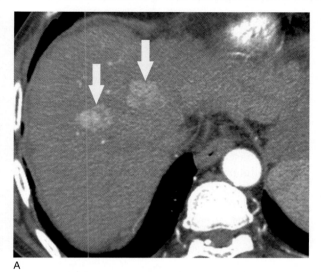

A

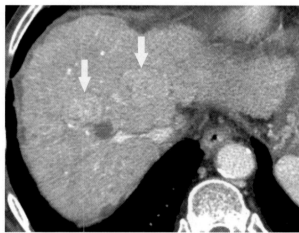

B

Fig. 7-11 A, Axial contrast-enhanced CT image obtained in the early arterial phase in a 68-year-old man with long-standing cirrhosis. Two foci of hypervascular hepatocellular carcinoma *(arrows)* are clearly visible. **B,** Axial contrast-enhanced CT image obtained in the late arterial phase at the same level as the image seen in **A.** The contrast between the very briskly enhancing tumor *(arrows)* in the adjacent hepatic parenchyma is less marked in this phase. Occasionally, markedly hypervascular tumors may be better detected on early arterial phase imaging. However, this situation is uncommon, and most hypervascular masses are best seen on the late arterial phase.

this issue, and all examined the effect on the area under the receiver operating characteristic curve (A_z) of adding the early arterial phase to the late arterial phase in the detection of hepatocellular carcinoma. In a study of 96 patients, the addition of early arterial phase images significantly increased A_z (0.80 with both phases versus 0.71 for late phase only, p less than 0.05).[45] However, in two additional studies of 78 and 33 patients, the addition of early arterial phase images did not significantly increase A_z (0.98 versus 0.98 and 0.97 versus 0.98, respectively).[46,47] In analyzing these data, it should be noted that the study by Murakami et al.[45] included the largest number of patients and that the studies by Ichikawa et al.[46] present unusually high accuracy for hepatocellular carcinoma detection by arterial phase CT (0.98 in both studies). In view of these considerations, it would appear reasonable to conclude that the use of early arterial phase images may occasionally help detect hepatocellular carcinoma (Figure 7-11) and should probably be included in an MSCT scanning protocol for patients in whom hepatocellular carcinoma is a concern.

Late Arterial Phase CT for Detection of Hypervascular Masses

Arterial phase imaging has been shown to improve detection of hypervascular neoplasms, especially hepatocellular carcinoma[14,15,48] and metastatic neuroendocrine cancer.[15,42,49] In a study by Paulson et al.[49] of 23 patients with 206 hepatic metastases from carcinoid tumors, 72 (35%) lesions were best seen on noncontrast images, 72 (35%) were best seen on arterial phase images, and 62 (30%) were best seen on portal venous phase images. Six of 206 (3%) lesions were seen only on noncontrast images, 28 (14%) were seen only on arterial phase images, and 6 (3%) were seen only on portal venous phase images. Oliver et al.[42] confirmed the benefits of arterial phase imaging in detecting hypervascular hepatocellular carcinoma. In a study group of 42 patients with 157 foci of hepatocellular carcinoma, 127 (81%) of the lesions were visible on portal venous phase images, 98 (62%) were visible on unenhanced images, and 120 (76%) were visible on arterial phase images. Of the 30 lesions not seen on portal venous phase images, 9 were seen on both unenhanced and arterial phase, 3 were seen on unenhanced images only, and 18 were seen on arterial phase images only. A similar study by Baron et al.[15] evaluated biphasic contrast-enhanced CT in 66 patients with 326 foci of hepatocellular carcinoma. Arterial phase images depicted 309 foci (95%) and portal venous phase images 268 (82%). In seven patients, (11%) tumor was visible only on arterial phase images (Figure 7-12). There is some evidence that arterial phase imaging may also help detect liver metastases from renal cell carcinoma and melanoma.[50,51] In a study of 72 liver metastases from renal cell carcinoma in 16 patients, 7 lesions were not seen on portal venous phase image. Six of these potentially missed lesions were seen on

arterial phase images[50] (Figure 7-13). A study done by Blake et al.[51] on 13 patients with metastatic melanoma to the liver showed a total of 57 liver lesions on CT: 48 on arterial phase, 49 on portal venous phase, and 30 on delayed phase images. Of 8 lesions (14%) overlooked on portal venous phase, 6 were seen on nonenhanced images and 6 were seen on arterial phase images (Figure 7-14). Twenty-eight lesions were graded as more conspicuous on portal venous phase, and 10 were more conspicuous on arterial phase imaging.

It is evident from this discussion that arterial phase is helpful in detecting additional tumor foci

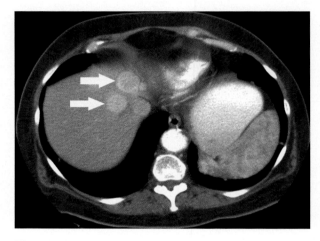

Fig. 7-13 Axial CT image obtained in the arterial phase in a patient with renal cell carcinoma. Hypervascular metastases *(arrows)* are visible.

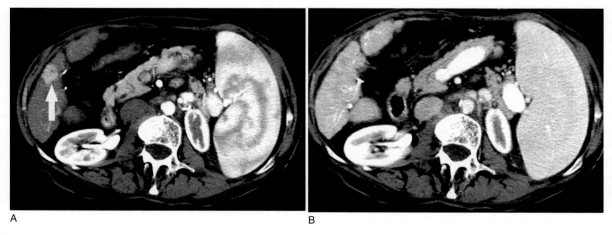

Fig. 7-12 **A,** Axial CT image obtained in the arterial phase in a patient with long-standing cirrhosis, showing a focus of hypervascular hepatocellular carcinoma *(arrow).* **B,** Axial contrast-enhanced CT image obtained at the same level as **A** in the portal venous phase. The tumor is not visible. In approximately 11% of patients with hepatocellular carcinoma, the tumor will only be visible on arterial phase images. Multiphase imaging is therefore crucial in patients suspected of having hepatocellular carcinoma.

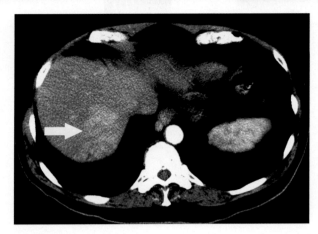

Fig. 7-14 Axial contrast-enhanced CT image obtained in the arterial phase in a patient with melanoma. Hypervascular metastases (arrow) are visible.

in hepatocellular and neuroendocrine carcinoma, and possibly in metastatic melanoma and renal cell carcinoma. Conversely, the available data do not support the use of arterial phase imaging to detect liver metastases from breast cancer.[10,43] Frederick et al.[43] studied 44 patients with 46 breast cancer metastases to the liver. Portal venous phase images depicted 39 (85%) lesions, arterial phase images depicted 27 (59%) lesions, and noncon-trast images depicted 28 (61%) lesions. Two malignant lesions were seen only on arterial phase, 3 only on noncontrast phase, and 10 only on portal venous phase. In this breast cancer patient population, portal venous phase was found to be superior to noncontrast and arterial phase images for liver metastasis detection. In 79 patients with 387 liver metastases from breast carcinoma, Sheafor et al.[10] found 364 were detected on portal venous phase images, 319 on arterial phase images, and 348 on noncontrast images. More lesions were identified on portal venous phase than either hepatic arterial or unenhanced images. Thus, the routine use of all three phases in patients with breast carcinoma does not seem warranted. Arteriographic images are helpful in colorectal metastases to the liver before surgical exploration, since accessory or aberrant arteries might require ligation before placement of a hepatic artery chemotherapy infusion pump in patients with unresectable disease. Late arterial phase images probably do not increase lesion detection[12,13] but may be performed for completeness in presurgical cases.

Late Arterial Phase CECT for Characterization of Small Hypoattenuating Lesions

Although the available data do not strongly support the use of (late) arterial phase imaging for the detection of traditionally hypovascular masses (e.g., colorectal and breast cancer metastases to the liver), it has been suggested that arterial phase imaging may improve the characterization of small hypoattenuating metastases because these lesions may have a hyperemic rim in the arterial phase that is not seen with small cysts[52] (Figure 7-15). It is possible that such a hyperemic rim represents the viable "growing edge" of the tumor.[53-56]

Portal Venous Phase CECT

Portal venous phase is the backbone of routine hepatic CT and the best phase for detection of most metastases and masses. Portal phase imaging (usually after 70 seconds) is always mandatory[2] because it shows the organ during higher parenchymal enhancement and consequently allows depiction of most lesions with greater lesion-to-liver conspicuousness when compared to other phases. Frederick et al.[43] reported that 85% of metastases to liver from breast carcinoma were detected on portal venous phase images, 59% on arterial phase images, and 61% on noncontrast images. In addition, 10 lesions were only found on portal venous phase. Sheafor et al.[10] also demonstrated the same results in 300 patients and showed that more lesions were detected on portal venous phase than on either arterial or unenhanced images.

Delayed Phase CECT

The scan delay for delayed imaging is variable and can range from 2 to 15 minutes or even longer. Such images may be helpful for showing centripetal enhancement in hepatic hemangiomas or to depict delayed enhancement in cholangiocarcinoma or in the central scar of focal nodular hyperplasia. Hepatic hemangiomas are present in up to 7.3% of the population,[57] and therefore the CT appearances merit specific attention. Focal nodular, globular, or flame-shaped peripheral enhancement during portal venous phase imaging is a characteristic finding (Figure 7-16, A). In one study, 32 of 34 (94%) lesions with this appearance were hemangiomas.[58] In this study, the other 2 lesions were both

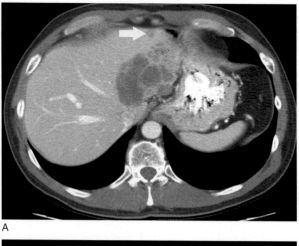

A

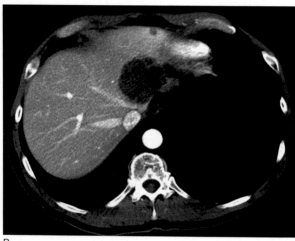

B

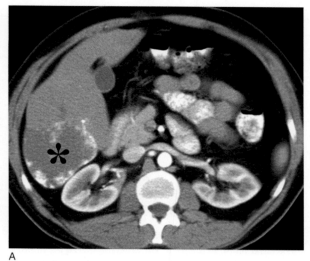

A

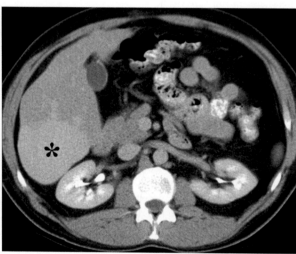

B

Fig. 7-15 A, Axial contrast-enhanced portal venous phase CT image of a small hypoattenuating lesion *(arrow)* in the anterior aspect of the left lateral segment in a patient with colon cancer. The lesion is too small to accurately characterize. A large metastasis is visible more posteriorly in the left lobe. **B,** Axial contrast-enhanced arterial phase CT image, showing that the small hypoattenuating lesion has a hyperdense perilesional rim. The presence of such a hyperdense rim is said to be suggestive of reactive hyperemia and indicates that such a small lesion is a metastasis rather than a cyst. In this way, arterial phase images may assist characterization of small hypoattenuating lesions.

Fig. 7-16 A, Axial contrast-enhanced CT image obtained in a patient with a large hemangioma *(asterisk)*. The lesion demonstrates characteristic focal nodular globular peripheral enhancement. **B,** Contrast-enhanced CT image obtained in the delayed phase at the same level as the image in **A.** The hemangioma *(asterisk)* demonstrates centripetal enhancement. Such progressive centripetal enhancement is an additional characteristic of hemangiomas.

colorectal liver metastases, and 5 additional hemangiomas did not demonstrate the typical pattern of peripheral enhancement. A more recent trial reported that globular enhancement on single-phase CT has a sensitivity of 88% and specificity of 84% to 100% in differentiating hepatic hemangiomas from hypervascular metastases.[59] The other classical CT finding in hemangiomas is progressive cen-

tripetal enhancement[60,61] (Figure 7-16, *B*). The rate of enhancement may vary from essentially immediate ("early enhancing" or "flash-filling" hemangiomas) to up to 60 minutes after contrast injection. Arterial-phase CT may help characterize early enhancing hemangiomas but does not appear to increase sensitivity.[24] Enhancement that is isodense to the aorta has also been described as a useful sign for the CT diagnosis of hemangioma, but this is more controversial.[62,63] In summary, although arterial and delayed images may be of some use, portal venous phase images are the cornerstone in the CT diagnosis of hemangiomas.

The role of delayed CT in the detection of cholangiocarcinoma has been highlighted in recent literature (Figure 7-17). The primary radiological finding is biliary and vascular obstruction. Liver atrophy is suggestive, but not specific.[64,65] The

frequency with which a mass is directly visualized varies between studies, with a range of 60% to 91%.[18,66] Delayed enhancement has been reported in 36% to 74% of tumors.[66,67] In one study, 3 of 47 tumors were seen only on delayed CT.[67] The optimal time for acquisition of delayed images is 10 to 20 minutes after contrast media injection.[66]

MSCT CHOLANGIOGRAPHY

General Comments

Two convergent developments have rekindled interest in the use of intravenous cholangiographic contrast media to opacify the biliary system—the excellent three-dimensional capability and resolution of MSCT and the need to define the second-order biliary branches in potential right hepatic lobe donors (Figure 7-18). Living-related liver donation is increasingly performed because of the nationwide shortage of cadaveric liver transplants. Preoperative

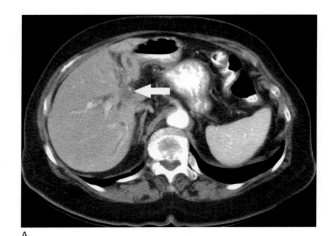

A

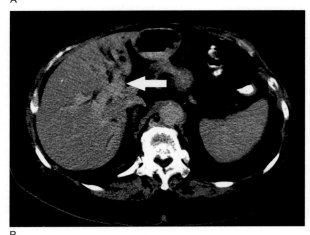

B

Fig. 7-17 A, Axial contrast-enhanced CT image obtained in the portal venous phase in a 71-year-old man with cholangiocarcinoma *(arrow).* The tumor is infiltrative, hypovascular, and associated with biliary dilation. **B,** Axial contrast-enhanced CT image obtained at the same level as **A** in the delayed phase of enhancement (15-minute delay). The tumor *(arrow)* demonstrates delayed enhancement. Although such delayed enhancement is reportedly common in cholangiocarcinoma, a very small minority of such tumors are visible only in the delayed phase.

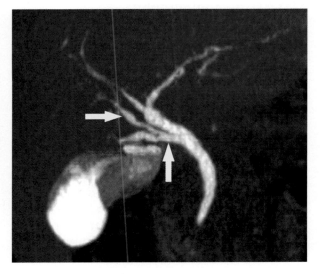

Fig. 7-18 Three-dimensional reformation of a CT cholangiogram in a patient being evaluated for potential right hepatic lobe harvest. The right posterior duct *(horizontal arrow)* can be seen draining into the cystic duct *(vertical arrow).* Such aberrant biliary anatomy represents relative contraindications for right lobe harvest and is a crucial component in the preoperative evaluation of such potential right lobe donors.

evaluation of biliary tract anatomy is of great importance in potential liver donors, because variant anatomy, particularly of the second order ducts, is seen in up to 45% of the population and can affect surgical approaches and biliary anastomotic techniques.[68-70] Several recent publications have suggested CT cholangiography (CT performed after intravenous administration of a radiographic biliary contrast medium) is a safe technique for the noninvasive evaluation of biliary anatomy and that it is more accurate than MR cholangiography.[71,72]

Yeh et al.[71] conducted a study to compare biliary tract depiction in living potential liver donors at conventional MR, mangafodipir trisodium-enhanced excretory MR, and MSCT cholangiography. In the evaluation of living liver donors, MSCT cholangiography enables significantly better biliary tract visualization than conventional or mangafodipir trisodium-enhanced excretory MR cholangiography either alone or in combination. In this study, nine patients proceeded to liver donation, and the intraoperative finding of biliary tract anatomy matched those at preoperative imaging in five (83%) of six patients for CT cholangiography.

Technique and Safety of MSCT Cholangiography

Our protocol for CT cholangiography involves administration of an intravenous biliary contrast agent, iodipamide meglumine (Cholografin; Bracco Diagnostics, Princeton, New Jersey), as a 30-minute infusion of 20 ml of the contrast medium diluted with 80 ml of normal saline. Images are obtained 15 to 45 minutes after infusion with 0.6 mm collimation; 50% overlap; and reconstruction of multiplanar, maximum intensity projection, and surface-rendered images. The incident of reaction is less than 1% (0.2% to 1%). These are usually minor reactions, mainly urticaria and rashes. A literature review of more than 2000 patients reported incidents of 3% minor, 0.3% moderate, and 0.2% severe reactions. Caoili et al.[73] evaluated feasibility and image quality of a few noninvasive biliary imaging techniques, such as helical CT cholangiography with three-dimensional volume rendering using an oral biliary contrast agent and concluded that it is a feasible noninvasive method for revealing biliary anatomy. However, visualization of the biliary tree was suboptimal in 36% of patients. This represents a substantial limitation of CT cholangiography based on an oral biliary contrast medium.

Application of MSCT Cholangiography

Polkowski et al.[73a] evaluated helical CT cholangiography and endosonography in nonjaundiced patients with suspected bile duct stones and reported 85% sensitivity, 88% specificity, and 86% accuracy in detecting bile duct stones in nonjaundiced patients. However, unenhanced HCT is significantly less sensitive and less accurate compared with endoscopic ultrasound (91% sensitivity, 100% specificity, and 94% accuracy). Fleischmann et al.[73b] reported that spiral CT cholangiography allows accurate assessment of the biliary system in patients with suspected obstructive biliary disease. They reported that CT cholangiography correctly depicted biliary obstruction in 14 of 27 patients with no false-positive or false-negative cases. Kwon et al.[74] recommended this technique for patients undergoing endoscopic cholecystectomy to avoid surgical injury to the bile ducts.

CONCLUSION

MSCT offers several major technical advantages in hepatobiliary evaluation, including improved three-dimensional CT reconstruction of hepatic anatomy[75,76] and rapid scanning of the liver and hepatic vasculature during peak contrast enhancement, which allows the use of lesser amounts of intravenous contrast material.[77-80] Our current protocols for MSCT of the liver and biliary system are shown in Table 7-5. As much as possible, these protocols have been evidence-based, using the results of scientific studies described earlier in this chapter. The pace of change continues to accelerate, and 32- and 64-slice scanners are already becoming available. Accordingly, these protocols will require revision as newer technology becomes available. The development of faster workstations with friendlier user interfaces coupled with faster acquisition and near isotropic imaging translates into improved diagnosis and better patient care. However, with great power comes great responsibility, and optimal use of hepatobiliary MSCT requires rational, evidence-based practice with matching of phases to patients and careful collimation. CT cholangiography is a promising modality for noninvasive biliary imaging.

Table 7-5 Sample Protocols for MSCT of the Liver and Biliary System on a 16-slice CT Scanner

Protocol	IV contrast rate	Scan delay	Collimation	Slice thickness and increment	Pitch	Rotation time	kV	mA
Routine liver	3 ml/s	80 s	16 × 1.5	5 mm/5 mm	0.9	0.75 s	120	240*
Multiphase liver	N/A	Pre-contrast	16 × 1.5	5 mm/5 mm	0.9	0.75 s	120	240*
	5 ml/s	40 s	16 × 1.5	5 mm/5 mm	0.9	0.75 s	120	240*
		80 s	16 × 1.5	5 mm/5 mm	0.9	0.75 s	120	240*
		180 s (PRN)	16 × 1.5	5 mm/5 mm	0.9	0.75 s	120	240*
CT cholangiography	20 ml Cholografin in 80 ml saline over 30 min	15 min after completion of Cholografin infusion	16 × 0.75	2 mm/1 mm	0.9	0.75 s	120	Max (225)

Or use dose-reduction software, if available.

REFERENCES

1. Silverman PM, Kalender WA, Hazle JD: Common terminology for single and multislice helical CT *(commentary)*, *Am J Roentgenol* 176:1135-1136, 2001.
2. Catalano O, Dodd G: Proper terminology for multiple-phase helical CT of the liver, *Am J Roentgenol* 176:547-548, 2001.
3. Bae K, Heiken J, Brink J: Aortic and hepatic peak enhancement at CT: effect of contrast medium injection rate—pharmacokinetic analysis and experimental porcine model, *Radiology* 206:455-464, 1998.
4. Fleischmann D: Use of high concentration contrast media: principles and rationale–vascular district, *Eur Radiol* 45: S88-S93, 2003.
5. Spielmann A: Liver imaging with MDCT and high concentration contrast media, *Eur Radiol* S50-S52, 2003.
6. Tsurusaki M, Sugimoto K, Fukuda T, et al: Effect of concentration of intravenous material on hepatic enhancement at multidetector-row CT (abstract), *Radiology* 221(P):105, 2001.
7. Fenchel S, Fleiter TR: Effect of iodine concentration on contrast enhancement, *RSNA*, 2001.
8. Van Leeuwen MS, Noordzij J, Feldberg MAM, et al: Focal liver lesions: characterization with triphasic spiral CT, *Radiology* 201:327-336, 1996.
9. Hollett MD, Jeffrey RB, Nino-Muricia M, et al: Dual-phase helical CT of the liver: value of arterial phase scans in the detection of small (≤1.5 cm) malignant hepatic neoplasms, *Am J Roentgenol* 164:879-884, 1995.
10. Sheafor D, Frederick M, Paulson E: Comparison of unenhanced, hepatic arterial-dominant, and portal venous-dominant phase helical CT for the detection of liver metastases in women with breast carcinoma, *Am J Roentgenol* 172, 1999.
11. Tello R, Seltzer S, Polger M: A contrast agent delivery nomogram for hepatic spiral CT, *J Comput Assist Tomogr* 21(2): 236-245, 1997.
12. Merine D, Takayasu K, Wakao F: Detection of hepatocellular carcinoma: comparison of CT during arterial portography with CT after intraarterial injection of iodized oil, *Radiology* 175:707-710, 1990.
13. Yoshimatsu S, Inoue Y, Ibukuro K, et al: Hypovascular hepatocellular carcinoma undetected at angiography and CT with iodized oil, *Radiology* 171:343-347, 1989.
14. Ohashi I, Hanafusa K, Yoshida T: Small hepatocellular carcinomas: two-phase dynamic incremental CT in detection and evaluation, *Radiology* 189:851-855, 1993.
15. Baron RL, Oliver JH III, Dobb GD III, et al: Hepatocellular carcinoma: evaluation with biphasic, contrast-enhanced, helical CT, *Radiology* 199:505-511, 1996.
16. Kim T, Murakami T, Oi H, et al: Detection of hypervascular hepatocellular carcinoma by dynamic MRI and dynamic spiral CT, *J Comput Assist Tomogr* 19:948-954, 1995.
17. Oi H, Murakami T, Kim T, et al: Dynamic MR imaging and early-phase helical CT for detecting small intrahepatic metastases of hepatocellular carcinoma, *Am J Roentgenol* 166:369-374, 1996.
18. Yamashita Y, Misuzaki K, Yi T, et al: Small hepatocellular carcinoma in patients with chronic liver damage: prospective comparison of detection with dynamic MR imaging and helical CT of the whole liver, *Radiology* 200:79-84, 1996.
19. Foley WD, Mallisee TA, Hohenwalter MD, et al: Multiphase hepatic CT with a multirow detector CT scanner, *Am J Roentgenol* 175:679-685, 2000.
20. Takahashi S, Murakami T, Kim T, et al: Multi-detector row helical CT angiography of the hepatic vessel: separate depiction of hepatic arterial, portal, and venous anatomy (abstract), *Radiology* 213(P):126, 1999.
21. Web N, Scheer MR, Gabor MP: Liver lesions: improved detection with dual-detector-array CT and routine 2.5-mm thin collimation, *Radiology* 209:417-426, 1998.
22. Kopka L, Rodenwaldt J, Hamm BK: Biphasic multislice helical CT of the liver: intraindividual comparison of different slice thickness for the detection and characterization

of focal liver lesion (abstract), *Radiology* 217(P):367-368, 2000.

23. Basilico R, Filippone A, Ricciardi M, et al: Impact of slice thickness on the detection of liver lesions with multislice CT (abstract), *Radiology* 217(P):368, 2000.

24. Kawata S, Murakami T, Kim T: Multidetector CT: Diagnostic impact of slice thickness on detection of hypervascular hepatocellular carcinoma, *Am J Roentgenol* 179:61-66, 2002.

25. Jones EC, Chezmar JL, Nelson RC, et al: The frequency and significance of small hepatic lesions (<15 mm) detected by CT, *Am J Roentgenol* 158:535-539, 1992.

26. Haider MA, Amitai MM, Rappaport DC, et al: Multidetector row helical CT in preoperative assessment of small (<1.5 cm) liver metastases: Is thinner collimation better? *Radiology* 225:137-142, 2002.

27. Birnbaum BA, Maki DD, Chakraborty DP, et al: Renal cyst pseudoenhancement: evaluation with an anthropomorphic body CT phantom, *Radiology* 225:83-90, 2002.

28. Maki DD, Birnbaum BA, Chakraborty DP, et al: Renal cyst pseudoenhancement: beam-hardening effects on CT numbers, *Radiology* 213:468-472, 1999.

29. Schwartz LH, Gandras EJ, Colangelo SM, et al: Prevalence and importance of small hepatic lesions found at CT in patients with cancer, *Radiology* 210:71-74, 1999.

30. Krakora G, Coakley F, Williams G, et al: Prognostic importance of small hypoattenuating hepatic lesions on CECT in patients with breast cancer. Presented at RSNA, 2003.

31. Ketai L, Malby M, Jordan K, et al: Small nodules detected on chest radiography: Does size predict calcification? *Chest* 118:610-614, 2000.

32. Leevy CM: Fatty liver: a study of 270 patients with biopsy proven fatty liver and a review of the literature, *Medicine* 41:249-276, 1962.

33. Bydder GM, Kreel L, Chapman RWG, et al: Accuracy of computed tomography in diagnosis of fatty liver, *Br Med J* 281:1042, 1980.

34. Piekarski J, Goldberg HI, Royal SA, et al: Difference between liver and spleen CT numbers in the normal adult: its usefulness in predicting the presence of diffuse liver disease, *Radiology* 137:727-729, 1980.

35. Berland LL, Van Dyke JA: Decreased splenic enhancement on CT in traumatized hypotensive patients, *Radiology* 156:469-471, 1985.

36. Baron RL: Liver: normal anatomy, imaging techniques, and diffuse diseases. In Haaga JR, Lanzieri CF, Sartoris DJ, Zerhouni EA, editors. *Computed tomography and magnetic resonance imaging of the whole body,* ed 3, St Louis, 1994, Mosby, pp. 945-977.

37. Wenzel DJ, Batist G: Implications of rapid uniform density changes on hepatic computed tomography, *J Comput Assist Tomogr* 7:209-214, 1983.

38. Jacobs J, Birnbaum B, Shapiro M, et al: Diagnostic criteria for fatty infiltration of the liver on contrast-enhanced helical CT, *Am J Roentgenol* 171:659-664, 1998.

39. Panicek, David M, Giess, et al: Qualitative assessment of liver for fatty infiltration on contrast-enhanced CT: is muscle a better standard of reference than spleen? *J Comput Assist Tomogr* 21(5):699-705, 1997.

40. Jacobs J et al: Presented at American Roentgen Ray Society annual meeting, San Diego, May 1996.

41. Bresler EL, Alpern MB, Glazer GM, et al: Hypervascular hepatic metastasis: CT evaluation, *Radiology* 162:49-51, 1987.

42. Oliver III JH, Baron RL, Federle MP, et al: Detecting hepatocellular carcinoma: value of unenhanced or arterial phase CT imaging or both used in conjunction with conventional portal venous phase contrast-enhanced CT imaging, *Am J Roentgenol* 167:71-77, 1996.

42a. Patten RM, Byun JY, Freeny PC: CT of hypervascular hepatic tumors: are unenhanced scans necessary for diagnosis? *AJR Am J Roentgenol* 161(5):979-984, 1993.

43. Frederick MG, Paulson EK, Nelson RC: Helical CT for detecting focal liver lesions in patients with breast carcinoma: comparison of noncontrast phase, hepatic arterial phase and portal venous phase, *J Comput Assist Tomogr* 21:229-235, 1997.

44. Oliver JH III, Baron RL, Federle MP, et al: Hypervascular liver metastases: do unenhanced and hepatic arterial phase CT images affect tumor detection?, *Radiology* 205:709-715, 1997.

44a. Smith PA, Klein AS, Heath DG, et al: Dual-phase spiral CT angiography with volumetric 3D rendering for preoperative liver transplant evaluation: preliminary observations. *J Comput Assist Tomogr* 22(6):868-874, 1998.

45. Murakami T, Kim T, Takamura M, et al: Hypervascular hepatocellular carcinoma: detection with double arterial phase multi-detector row helical CT, *Radiology* 218(3):763-767, 2001.

46. Ichikawa T, Kitamura T, Nakajima H: Hypervascular hepatocellular carcinoma: can double arterial phase imaging with multidetector CT improve tumor depiction in the cirrhotic liver? *Am J Roentgenol* 179:751-758, 2002.

47. Kwon K, Lim, Hoon L, et al: Detection of hepatocellular carcinoma: comparison of dynamic three-phase computed tomography images and four-phase computed tomography images using multidetector row helical computed tomography, *JCAT* 26(5):691-698, 2002.

48. Khihara Y, Tamura S, Yuki Y, et al: Optimal timing for delineation of hepatocellular carcinoma in dynamic CT, *J Comput Assist Tomogr* 17:719-722, 1993.

49. Paulson EK, McDermott VG, Keogan MT, et al: Carcinoid metastases to the liver: role of triple-phase helical CT, *Radiology* 206:143-150, 1998.

50. Raptopoulos VD, Blake SP, Weisinger K, et al: Multiphase contrast-enhanced helical CT of liver metastases from renal cell carcinoma, *Eur Radiol* 11:2504-2509, 2001.

51. Blake SP, Weisinger K, Atkins MB, et al: Liver metastases from melanoma: detection with multiphasic contrast-enhanced CT, *Radiology* 213:92-96, 1999.

52. Ch'en IY, Katz DS, Jeffrey RB Jr, et al: Do arterial phase helical CT images improve detection or characterization of colorectal liver metastases? *J Comput Assist Tomogr* 21:391-397, 1997.

53. Baron RL: Understanding and optimizing use of contrast material for CT of the liver, *Am J Roentgenol* 163:323-331, 1994.

54. Irie T, Takeshita K, Wada Y, et al: CT evaluation of hepatic tumors: comparison of CT with arterial portography, CT with infusion hepatic arteriography, and simultaneous use of both techniques, *Am J Roentgenol* 164:1407-1412, 1995.

55. Foley WD, Jochem RJ: Computed tomography: focal and diffuse liver disease, *Radiol Clin North Am* 29:1213-1233, 1991.

56. Moss AA, Dean PB, Axel L, et al: Dynamic CT of hepatic masses with intravenous and intraarterial contrast material, *Am J Roentgenol* 138:847-852, 1982.

57. Ishak KG, Rabin L: Benign tumors of the liver, *Med Clin North Am* 59:999-1013, 1975.

58. Quinn SF, Benjamin GG: Hepatic cavernous hemangiomas: simple diagnostic sign with dynamic bolus CT, *Radiology* 182:545-548, 1992.

59. Leslie DF, Johnson CD, MacCarty RL, et al: Single-pass CT of hepatic tumors: value of globular enhancement in distinguishing hemangiomas from hypervascular metastases, *Am J Roentgenol* 165:1403-1406, 1995.

60. Itai Y, Furui S, Araki T, et al: Computed tomography of cavernous hemangioma of the liver, *Radiology* 137:149-155, 1980.

61. Freeny PC, Marks WM: Hepatic hemangioma: dynamic bolus CT, *Am J Roentgenol* 147:711-719, 1986.

62. Kim T, Federle MP, Baron RL, et al: Discrimination of small hepatic hemangiomas from hypervascular malignant tumors smaller than 3 cm with three-phase helical CT, *Radiology* 219:699-706, 2001.

63. Leslie DF, Johnson CD, Johnson CM, et al: Distinction between cavernous hemangiomas of the liver and hepatic metastases on CT: value of contrast enhancement patterns, *Am J Roentgenol* 164:625-629, 1995.

64. Sans N, Fajadet P, Galy-Fourcade D, et al: Is capsular retraction a specific CT sign of malignant liver tumor? *Eur Radiol* 9:1543-1545, 1999.

65. Keogan MT, Seabourn JT, Paulson EK, et al: Contrast-enhanced CT of intrahepatic and hilar cholangiocarcinoma: delay time for optimal imaging, *Am J Roentgenol* 169:1493-1499, 1997.

66. Feydy A, Vilgrain V, Denys A, et al: Helical CT assessment in hilar cholangiocarcinoma: correlation with surgical and pathologic findings, *Am J Roentgenol* 172:73-77, 1999.

67. Lacomis JM, Baron RL, Oliver JH III, et al: Cholangiocarcinoma: delayed CT contrast enhancement patterns, *Radiology* 203:98-104, 1997.

68. Puente SG, Bannura GC: Radiological anatomy of the biliary tract: variations and congenital abnormalities, *World J Surg* 7:271-276, 1983.

69. Russell E, Yrizzary JM, Montalvo BM, et al: Left hepatic duct anatomy: implications, *Radiology* 174:353-356, 1990.

70. Marcos A, Ham JM, Fisher RA, et al: Surgical management of anatomical variations of the right lobe in living donor liver transplantation, *Annals Surg* 231:824-831, 2000.

71. Yeh BM, Breiman RS, Taouli B, et al: Biliary tract depiction in living potential liver donors: comparison of conventional MR, mangafodipir trisodium-enhanced excretory MR, and multi-detector row CT cholangiography—initial experience, *Radiology* 230:645-651, 2004.

72. Stockberger SM, Wass JL, Sherman S, et al: Intravenous cholangiography with helical CT: comparison with endoscopic retrograde cholangiography, *Radiology* 192:675-680, 1994.

73. Caoili, EM, Paulson EK, Heyneman LE, et al: Helical CT cholangiography with three-dimensional volume rendering using an oral biliary contrast agent: feasibility of a novel technique, *Am J Roentgenol* 174:487-492, 2000.

73a. Polkowski M, Palucki J, Regula J, et al: Helical computed tomographic cholangiography versus endosonography for suspected bile duct stones: a prospective blinded study in non-jaundiced patients. *Gut* 45(5):744-749, 1996.

73b. Fleischmann D, Ringl H, Schofl R, et al: Three-dimensional spiral CT cholangiography in patients with suspected obstructive biliary disease: comparison with endoscopic retrograde cholangiography. *Radiology* 198(3):861-868, 1996.

74. Kwon A, Uetsuji S, Ogura T: Spiral computed tomography scanning after intravenous infusion cholangiography for biliary duct anomalies, *Am J Surg* 174:396-402, 1997.

75. Vock P, Jung H, Kalender WA, et al: Single-breath-hold volumetric CT of the hepatobiliary system (abstract), *Radiology* 173(P):377, 1989.

76. Wunderlich AP, Lenz M, Gmeinwieser J, et al: Color-coded three-dimensional reconstruction of abdominal organs and vessels (abstract), *Radiology* 181(P):261, 1991.

77. Zwicker C, Langer MF, Langer R, et al: Spiral CT of hypervascular liver tumors and liver transplants (abstract), *Radiology* 181(P):95, 1991.

78. Bautz W, Strotzer M, Lenz M, et al: Perioperative evaluation of the vessels of the uppper abdomen with spiral CT: comparison with conventional CT and arterial DSA (abstract), *Radiology* 181(P):261, 1991.

79. Costello P, Dupuy DE, Ecker CP, et al: Spiral CT of the thorax with reduced volume of contrast material: a comparative study, *Radiology* 183:663-666, 1992.

80. Costello P, Ecker CP, Tello R, et al: Assessment of the thoracic aorta by spiral CT, *Am J Roentgenol* 158:1127-1133, 1992.

81. Harmon BH, Berland LL, Lee JY: Effect of varying rates of low-osmolarity contrast media injection for hepatic CT: correlation with indocyanine green transit time, *Radiology* 184:379-382, 1992.

82. Chambers TP, Baron RL, Lush RM, et al: Hepatic CT enhancement: comparison of ionic and nonionic contrast agents in the same patients, *Radiology* 190:721-725, 1994.

83. Bree RL, Parisky YR, Bernardino ME, et al: Cost-effective use of low-osmolality contrast media for CT of the liver: evaluation of liver enhancement provided by various doses of iohexol, *Am J Roentgenol* 163:579-583, 1994.

84. Silverman PM, Cooper C, Trock B, et al: The optimal temporal window for CT of the liver using a time-density analysis: implications for helical (spiral) CT, *J Comput Assist Tomogr* 19:73-79, 1995.

8

Investigating the Pancreas

Marc Zins

The advent of spiral acquisition in the early 1990s was the first major stride toward returning computed tomography (CT) to prominence as a tool for investigating the pancreas.[1,2] In several European centers, endosonography was a strong candidate for the investigation of patients with pancreatic disorders. Advances related to volume acquisition by spiral scanning restored credibility to CT, most notably in the assessment of pancreatic tumors.[3-5] Multislice CT (MSCT), which produces approximately 1-mm sections of the entire pancreas, thus considerably improving both longitudinal spatial resolution and quality of multiplanar reconstructions, is a recent refinement that will undoubtedly increase CT's usefulness.[6] This chapter will describe the CT acquisition technique used at our center and will indicate how MSCT benefits the evaluation of specific pancreatic disorders.

TECHNICAL CONSIDERATIONS

The technical rules for single-slice row spiral CT also apply to multislice row spiral CT. Thus, there is general agreement that acquisition at the "pancreatic" phase, starting 45 to 50 seconds after injection of 2 ml/kg of contrast agent at a flow rate of 3 ml/sec, is preferable over acquisition at the strictly arterial phase, which starts within the first 30 seconds, or at the "parenchymatous" phase, which starts 70 seconds after injection.[7-10] A key advantage of the arterioportal or "pancreatic" spiral is improved enhancement of the superior mesenteric vein at a time when the arteries are still substantially enhanced, so that a comprehensive evaluation of vascular tumor spread can be performed. Another valuable advantage is that the density gradient between the tumor and the normal pancreatic tissue is greater at the pancreatic phase than at the arterial or parenchymatous phase, making the pancreatic spiral more sensitive for tumor detection.[8,10] This last point has been confirmed by a MSCT study providing the first comparative data on adenocarcinoma detection at the arterial, pancreatic, and parenchymatous phases.[11]

Because MSCT scanners decrease both the acquisition time and the nominal slice thickness, they should ensure optimal imaging of the pancreas and other supracolic structures at all three phases (arterial, pancreatic, and parenchymatous). Although routinely adding the arterial phase to the classically indicated pancreatic and parenchymatous phases has not been proven to benefit the detection or staging of pancreatic adenocarcinoma,[11] the arterial phase may be helpful in patients with hypervascular tumors or arterial disorders. In everyday practice at our center, we reserve the strictly arterial phase to patients with clinical and/or laboratory test findings suggesting an endocrine tumor or an arterial disorder (pseudoaneurysm); in this situation, we examine the entire liver and pancreas for hypervascular lesions. Comparative studies are needed to determine whether this strategy is warranted; indeed, a study of MSCT for detecting hepatocellular carcinoma nodules opens up the possibility that the arterioportal phase may be more sensitive than the strictly arterial phase for detecting hypervascular pancreatic tumors.[12,13]

The protocol used in our center with a 4-row MSCT to investigate the pancreas in all other situations is outlined in Table 8-1.

The patient is asked to swallow 500 ml of water within 15 minutes before scanning to ensure easy identification of the stomach and duodenum.

1. Spiral CT without contrast injection: investigation of the entire supracolic space.

   Collimation, 2.5 mm; slab thickness, 5 mm; pitch, 1.5; mean spiral duration, 10 seconds. Tube voltage is 120 kV, and tube current is 170 mA.

   Note: This spiral is used for three purposes: to detect pancreatic calcifications, to look for a focus of spontaneously increased density consistent with bleeding, and to obtain an accurate measure of pancreatic height in order to optimally adjust the pancreatic spiral, thereby reducing radiation exposure.

2. Pancreatic spiral: investigation is focused on the pancreas but including the origins of the celiac and superior mesenteric arteries (field of view is 20 to 25 cm).

   Collimation, 1.25 mm; slab thickness, 2.5 mm; pitch, 0.75 or 1.5; spiral duration, 10 to 20 seconds. Tube voltage is 120 kV or 140 kV, and tube current 180 to 220 mA, according to body mass and pitch (with a pitch factor of 0.75, the voltage and current must be kept low in order to minimize radiation exposure).

   Note: This spiral is used to obtain detailed images of the pancreas and peripancreatic area; it serves as the basis for multiplanar reconstruction (see next section).

3. Parenchymatous spiral: investigation of the liver and entire abdomen and pelvic space.

   Collimation, 2.5 mm; slab thickness, 5 mm; pitch, 1.5; mean spiral duration, 15 seconds. Tube voltage is 120 kV, and tube current is 180 to 220 mA according to body mass.

On average, the pancreatic spiral starts 45 seconds after injection of 2 ml/kg of iodinated contrast agent at a rate of 3 ml/sec. A bolus-tracking device may be useful but is not indispensable in everyday practice. The parenchymatous spiral starts, on average, 70 to 80 seconds after the injection. The use of slabs that are thicker than the acquired images is helpful in reducing the number of images that must be reproduced on film if needed. Pancreatic spiral images visualized initially with 2.5-mm thickness are reconstructed in a sequence of 1.25-mm images with a 50% overlap. After transfer to the postprocessing console, a series comprising 200 images on

Table 8-1   CT Protocol Sample

Pancreas

Indication:	Suspicion of pancreatic disease: jaundice, epigastralgia
Protocol designed for (scanner type):	LightSpeed plus (4 Row)
Patient preparation:	No coffee or smoking before the exam

First Series   Detection of pancreatic calcification or bleeding

Oral contrast:	—	
IV contrast administration:	—	
Tube settings	kV	120
	mA	170
Gantry speed (sec)	0.8	
Table speed (mm/sec)	15	
Slice thickness (mm):	5	
Anatomic coverage:	Supracolic space	
Recon kernel:	Standard	
Breath hold:	Inspiration	
Window settings:		
Postprocessing:		
Other:		

Second Series: Pancreatic Phase

Oral contrast:	Water: 500 ml	
IV contrast administration	Iomeprol, 350 mg I/ml	
Volume/injection rate/delay	1.120/3/50	
Tube settings	kV	120
	mA	200
Gantry speed (sec)	0.8	
Table speed (mm/sec)	3.75 or 7.5	
Slice thickness:	1.25 mm	
Anatomic coverage:	From the origin of the celiac axis to the third duodenum, focused on the pancreas (FOV: 25 cm)	
Recon kernel:	Standard	
Breath hold:	Inspiration	
Window settings:	400/40	
Postprocessing:	—Image reconstruction 1.25/0.6 mm	
	—Review of axials	
	—MPR	
	—MIP for vessel analysis	
	—minIP for biliary and pancreatic ducts analysis	
Other:		

Third Series: Parenchymatous Phase

Oral contrast:	Water: 500 ml	
IV contrast administration	Iomeprol, 350 mg I/ml	
Volume/injection rate/delay	1.120/3/80	
Tube settings	kV	120
	mA	180
Gantry speed (sec)	0.8	
Table speed (mm/sec)	15	
Slice thickness:	2.5 mm	
Anatomic coverage:	Abdomen and pelvis	
Recon kernel:	Standard	
Breath hold:	Inspiration	
Window settings:	400/40	
Postprocessing:		
Other:		

average is used for two- and three-dimensional multiplanar reconstruction. The very thin slices result in high-quality reconstructions, and the low noise level makes the reconstructions suitable as a basis for interpretation, if needed.

Investigation of the pancreas usually requires multiplanar reconstruction with thick-slab maximum intensity projections (MIPs) for evaluating the peripancreatic vessels and hypervascular tumors (Figure 8-1).[14] Reconstructions with minimum intensity projections (min-IPs) are very useful for investigating the pancreatic and bile ducts (Figure 8-1).[15-17] Curved reconstructions along the axis of the pancreatic and bile ducts or the celiac and mesenteric vessels visualize the entire length of a structure but do not provide an anatomical evaluation (Figure 8-1).[17]

At our center, we routinely use interactive cine display of axial images, which has been shown to improve the evaluation of ducts by single-row spiral CT.[18] In our experience, interactive cine display substantially improves image interpretation. In addition, it guides the selection of the multiplanar reconstructions performed on the postprocessing console.

RESULTS

Adenocarcinoma

CT of the pancreas is used as the investigation of reference for the diagnosis and staging of pancreatic cancer.

Diagnosis

CT has proved effective for diagnosing pancreatic cancer, with sensitivities greater than 90% in most of the studies that used single-row or two-row spiral CT scanners.[5,19,20] Because this detection rate

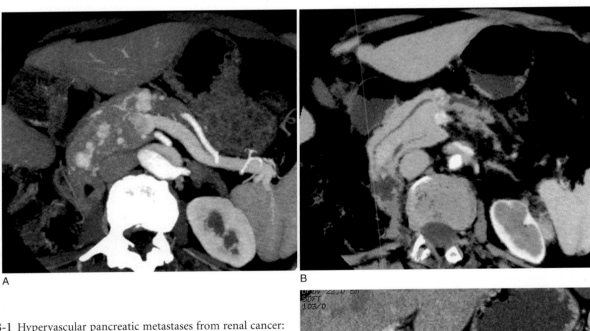

A

B

C

Fig. 8-1 Hypervascular pancreatic metastases from renal cancer: contribution of multiplanar reconstruction with maximal intensity projections (MIPs) and minimal intensity projections (min-IPs). Thick-slab axial oblique reconstruction with MIP (**A**) and min-IP (**B**), providing accurate information not only on the tumor (multiple hypervascular nodules 5 to 10 mm in diameter), but also on the ducts (pancreas divisum with dilation of the main duct of the left pancreas contrasting with the normal slender appearance of the ducts in the right pancreas). **C,** Curved reconstruction along the axis of the main pancreatic duct.

is high, obtaining further improvements with multislice spiral CT will be difficult. Tumors that are less than 2 cm in diameter and isodense to the pancreas remain difficult to detect; they contribute to 5% to 20% of pancreatic cancers.[19,21] Careful attention should be given to indirect signs (dilation of the pancreatic and bile ducts, segmental atrophy, vascular involvement), which may be isolated and should lead to a suspicion of pancreatic cancer, even in the absence of direct signs of pancreatic tumor.[22]

Staging

Vascular Involvement The main case-series evaluating the performance of spiral CT for detecting vascular spread of pancreatic cancer produced consistent results: sensitivity ranged from 80% to 91%, specificity was 89% to 100%, overall precision was 89% to 93%, and performance was better for detecting arterial than venous spread.[20,23,24] Because spiral CT is highly specific, it is valuable for identifying patients with unresectable vascular lesions. Evaluation of the axial images is crucial and provides a detailed analysis of the superior mesenteric vessels. Recent series evaluated the performance of first-generation MSCT scanners (with four sections per rotation). They showed that specificity ranged from 82% to 100%,[25,26] sensitivity ranged from 83% to 100%,[25,26] and negative predictive value for vascular involvement was 100% in a study using curved vascular reconstructions.[27]

The contribution of multiplanar reconstruction to the diagnosis of vascular spread has been evaluated using single-row CT scanners, with conflicting results.[20,28,29] Nevertheless, the findings establish that moderate stenosis of the splenoportal junction is difficult to spot on original axial images and that multiplanar volume rendering improves the visibility of these lesions.[28,29] Thus, MSCT scanners should noticeably benefit the detection of vascular involvement; in particular, the marked improvement in longitudinal resolution can be expected to ensure visualization of vascular stenoses along the coronal or sagittal axis (Figure 8-2). Multi-planar reconstruction of MSCT images may also improve the assessment of arterial involvement, most notably in patients with partial arterial encasement (Figure 8-3).

Involvement of the Lymph Nodes, Peritoneum, and Liver The performance of spiral CT in detecting lymph node and peritoneal involvement is fair, with sensitivity rates of 60% and 75%, respectively.[5,20] Multislice spiral CT can be expected to show better

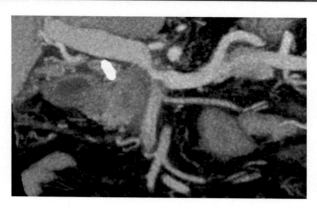

Fig. 8-2 Adenocarcinoma of the head of the pancreas with involvement of the splenic-mesenteric-portal vein confluence. Thick-slab coronal reconstruction with MIP providing a clear image of the stenosis at the venous confluence. Note the clearly visualized anatomic variant in which the inferior mesenteric vein empties into the right edge of the superior mesenteric vein.

sensitivity for detecting involved lymph nodes, most notably in the peripancreatic area (Figure 8-4); however, this improved sensitivity may come at the price of reduced specificity if visible nodes less than 1 cm in diameter are considered positive. A helpful approach may consist of using the lymph node data obtained by CT to map out the surgical procedure. Detecting tiny liver metastases or incipient peritoneal carcinomatosis will remain difficult. However, peritoneal involvement rarely occurs in isolation. Most patients also have vascular involvement, which is easier to detect with spiral CT scanning.

Multislice Spiral CT versus MRI and Endosonography

There is general agreement that spiral CT is the second-line investigation of reference and should be performed immediately after ultrasonography in patients with suspected pancreatic tumors.[4,5]

Role for MRI Studies comparing first-generation spiral CT to MRI for the diagnosis and staging of pancreatic cancer found no significant superiority of MRI. The main theoretical advantage of MRI is its "all-in-one" nature: in a single session, MRI provides information on the lesion, its effects on the ducts (magnetic resonance cholangiopancreatography), and tumor spread, most notably to the blood vessels (magnetic resonance angiography).[30] The introduction of MSCT scanners will affect the balance between CT and MRI. Indeed, the sub-

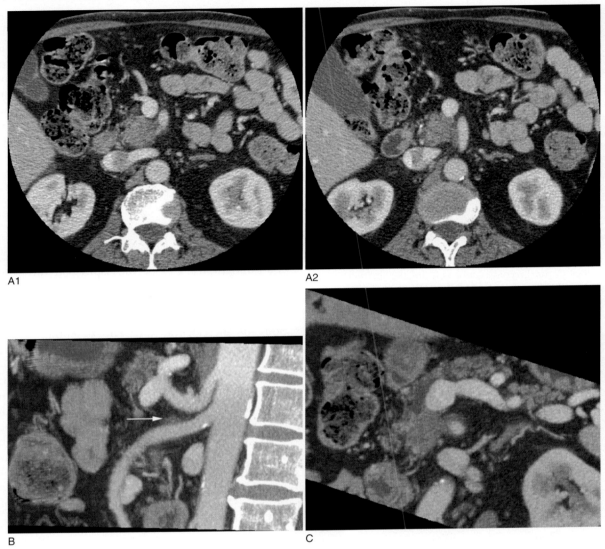

Fig. 8-3 Adenocarcinoma of the uncus of the pancreas with involvement of the superior mesenteric artery. **A,** The original axial images (**A1, A2**) show that the lesion is in contact with the superior mesenteric artery but do not provide definite evidence of arterial involvement. **B,** On the sagittal reconstruction, the tumor is seen to form a bridge over the artery *(arrow),* but encasement is not greater than 180 degrees. **C,** The oblique axial reconstruction, in contrast, clearly shows encasement of the superior mesenteric artery by the tumor along more than 180 degrees, indicating that the artery is involved.

stantial improvement in spatial resolution provided by multislice spiral CT, even in the coronal and sagittal planes, translates into vascular reconstructions (MIP) of far better quality than those obtained with MRI (see Figure 8-2). In addition, duct reconstructions (min-IP) allow detailed analysis of bile and pancreatic duct obstructions at or near the ampulla (Figure 8-5). Thus, CT is also an "all-in-one" investigation but offers the considerable

advantage over MRI of thinner sections and, therefore, better spatial resolution.

Role for Endosonography Endosonography is an invasive investigation that requires general anesthesia. Because of this major disadvantage, endosonography should not be performed until a CT scan is obtained. The main advantage of endosonography is its ability to directly visualize tumors smaller than 2 cm in diameter, whereas CT detection rests on

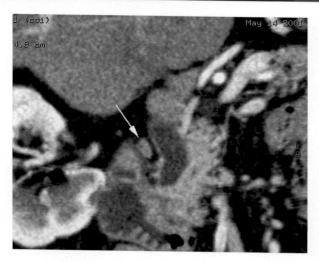

Fig. 8-4 Staging of cholangiocarcinoma of the distal main bile duct. Coronal reconstruction showing the obstruction of the main bile duct near the ampulla; a 5-mm lymph node is visible *(arrow)* in contact with the duodenal wall.

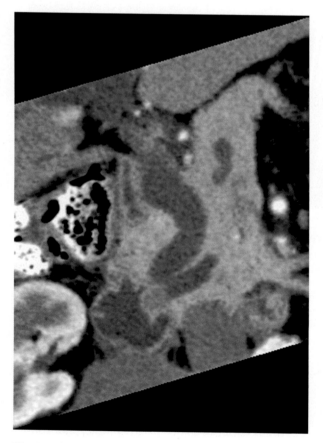

Fig. 8-5 Ampullar pseudotumor with dilation of both ducts upstream from pseudotumoral hypertrophy of the papilla. Thick-slab coronal oblique reconstruction with min-IP providing a detailed evaluation of the duodenal wall.

indirect signs when a small tumor is isodense to the pancreas. Thus, endosonography should be reserved for the few patients in whom CT fails to establish the diagnosis of pancreatic cancer. First-generation spiral CT is at least as effective as endosonography in detecting vascular involvement.[5] Thus, the development of multislice scanners should further establish CT as a key investigational tool for the staging of pancreatic adenocarcinoma.

Cystic Tumors

Cystic Adenoma

The diagnosis of cystic adenoma is based on CT, endosonography, and needle aspiration for histological and biochemical studies.[31,32] The main CT studies for the diagnosis of serous or mucinous cystic adenoma of the pancreas are early investigations of incremental CT. The potential benefits provided by spiral acquisition and multislice systems have not been evaluated. In all likelihood, multislice spiral CT will improve diagnostic accuracy in patients with small serous microcystic adenomas, by providing clearer images of the microcystic component. In addition, it will produce more accurate information about the location of the lesion, particularly as it relates to the bile and pancreatic ducts, which are well visualized on min-IP reconstructions. This last point is valuable when limited resection of a cephalic lesion is being considered (Figure 8-6).

Intraductal Papillary Mucinous Tumor of the Pancreas (IPMTP)

The imaging diagnosis of IPMTP is based on converging evidence obtained by CT, MRI, and endosonography.[32] The usefulness of spiral CT in establishing the diagnosis, determining the type of involvement (main duct, branch duct, or mixed), and evaluating tumor spread within the pancreatic gland has been convincingly demonstrated, although the diagnosis of malignant transformation may be difficult to establish.[33] The additional advantage of multislice spiral CT stems from improved spatial resolution, which ensures the diagnosis of cystic branch duct dilation, visualization of the entire main duct, and accurate mapping of lesions in preparation for limited resection (Figure 8-7).[17]

MRI is the main rival of MSCT as a tool for investigating IPMTP. The high contrast resolution offered by MRI provides accurate information on the bile and pancreatic ducts on magnetic resonance cholangiopancreatography sequences.

Pancreatitis

Despite the considerable progress made in the field of MRI, CT remains the key investigation for the diagnosis and prognosis of acute pancreatitis. The additional benefits provided by MSCT include detection of vascular complications, most notably arterial pseudoaneurysms, and detection of main bile duct lithiasis or pancreas divisum as the cause of acute pancreatitis (Figure 8-8). Duct

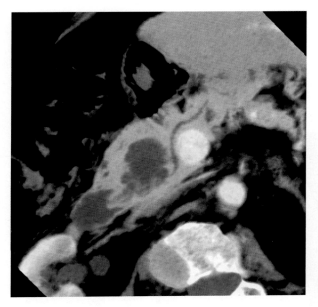

Fig. 8-6 Cystic adenoma of the pancreas. Thick-slab coronal oblique reconstruction with min-IP clearly showing close contact between the lesion and the main pancreatic duct, which precludes partial resection.

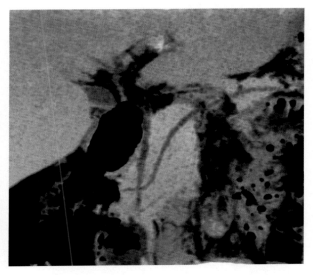

Fig. 8-8 Recurrent acute pancreatitis (etiological evaluation). Thick-slab axial oblique reconstruction with min-IP giving a clear image of pancreas divisum with the crossing sign.

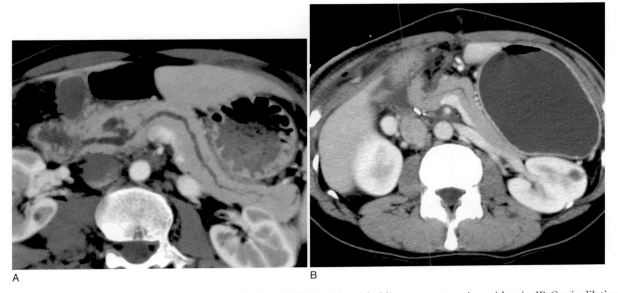

A   B

Fig. 8-7 TIPMP in the distribution of the Santorini duct. **A,** Thick-slab axial oblique reconstruction with min-IP. Cystic dilation of the branch ducts and communication with the main duct are clearly visible. **B,** Follow-up after limited resection.

reconstructions using min-IP can even suggest a diagnosis of duct rupture, which is usually established only by endoscopic retrograde cholangiopancreatography or MRI (Figure 8-9).

In patients with chronic pancreatitis, MSCT visualizes pancreatic calcifications and shows their exact location; provides accurate details on alterations in pancreatic and bile ducts (Figures 8-10 and 8-11); shows the exact location of duodenal pseudocysts or cystic dystrophy of the duodenal wall in a heterotopic pancreas (Figure 8-11); and provides an accurate map of vascular abnormalities, particularly in patients with arterial pseudoaneurysms (Figure 8-12).

In the investigation of pancreatitis, the main choices are MSCT and MRI. MRI is more informative for evaluating the contents of necrotic areas and pseudocysts (e.g., detecting bleeding). However, for the time being, CT remains superior over MRI in patients with suspected vascular abnormalities.

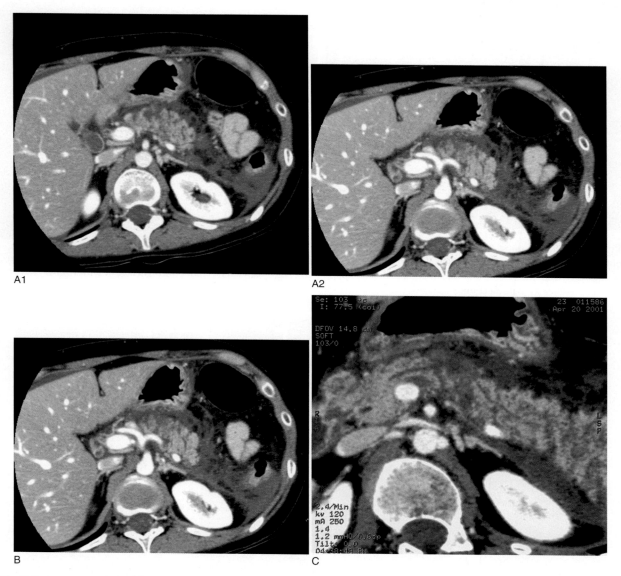

Fig. 8-9 Acute necrotizing biliary pancreatitis complicated by pancreatic duct rupture. A-B, Original axial images showing severe pancreatitis with a fluid collection anterior to the pancreas and absence of enhancement within the left pancreas. The Wirsung duct cannot be evaluated accurately. C, Thick-slab axial oblique reconstruction with min-IP showing a clearly visible breach in the pancreatic duct, indicating probable duct rupture.

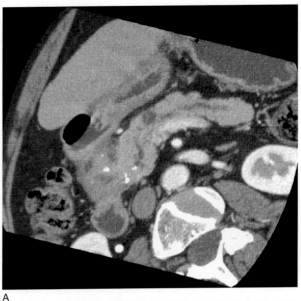

A

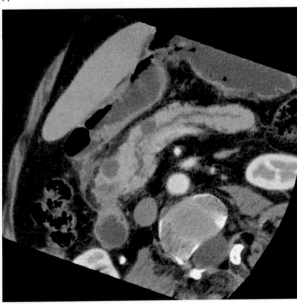

B

Fig. 8-10 Chronic calcifying pancreatitis. A-B, Axial oblique reconstructions with MIP and min-IP showing calcifications located within the ducts and dilation of the main pancreatic duct.

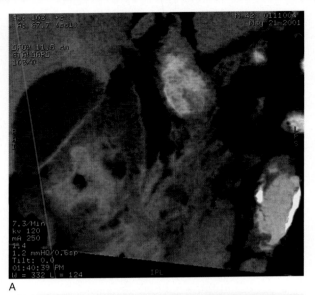

A

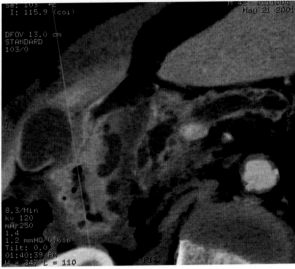

B

Fig. 8-11 Chronic pancreatitis with dilation of the bile ducts and pancreatic ducts. A, Coronal oblique reconstruction with min-IP along the axis of the bile and pancreatic ducts showing gradual stenosis of both duct systems upstream from a nodule of pancreatitis. B, Coronal oblique reconstruction showing thickening of the duodenal wall, which contains several small cysts, producing an overall picture highly suggestive of cystic dystrophy of the duodenal wall with heterotopic pancreas.

Lesions of the Ampulla

Accurate evaluation of the ampullar area is among the main benefits of MSCT. A prerequisite to a successful evaluation is adequate repletion of the duodenum by water. Intravenous injection of a spasmolytic agent (tiemonium) is recommended but does not ensure a 100% success rate.

In the evaluation of lesions located in or near the ampulla, multislice CT ensures easy identification of the main papilla, and of accessory papillae if present, even when there is no duct dilation (see

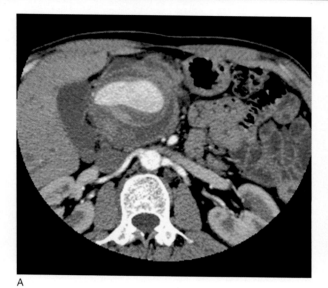

A

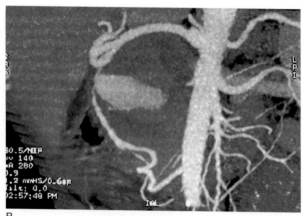

B

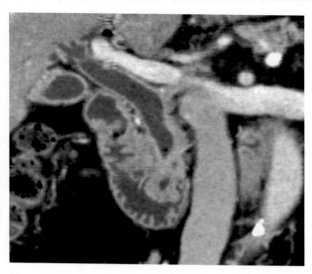

Fig. 8-13 Tumor of the ampulla. Coronal oblique reconstruction with min-IP along the axis of the main papilla–dilation of the main bile duct that stops opposite a nodular area of tissue thickening centered on the ampulla.

Fig. 8-12 Chronic pancreatitis complicated by pseudoaneurysm. **A,** The original axial section at the arterial phase shows the pseudoaneurysm but does not clearly indicate its origin. **B,** The thick-slab coronal oblique reconstruction with MIP shows that the pseudoaneurysm originates from the left edge of the gastroduodenal artery and is fed both by the common hepatic artery and by the superior mesenteric artery via the posterior-inferior pancreaticoduodenal artery.

Figure 8-8); accurate evaluation of duct alterations secondary to obstruction of the ampulla (see Figure 8-5); a detailed evaluation of the duodenal wall; and the diagnosis of ampullary adenoma when focal tissue thickening is found (Figure 8-13).[17]

In the evaluation of ampullar lesions, multislice spiral CT is in competition with endosonography, which is the imaging method of reference in this indication. However, CT must be obtained before endosonography, and the currently high false-negative rate with CT imaging can be expected to drop with the introduction of multislice scanners.

Endocrine Tumors and Rare Tumors

The reliability of MSCT for detecting and staging endocrine pancreatic tumors remains to be determined. At present, the diagnosis of small secreting tumors (insulinomas and gastrinomas) is usually based on converging evidence from endosonography and octreotide scans. MSCT should be capable of detecting small tumors (<10 mm) and of visualizing focal hypervascularity, which is a nearly consistent feature of endocrine pancreatic tumors. Similar features occur with a number of rare tumors, such as pancreatic metastases from renal cancer (see Figure 8-1).

MSCT should improve the detection rate of small peripancreatic lymph nodes and, perhaps, of intraduodenal nodules.

CONCLUSION

MSCT has been a considerable benefit to the evaluation of pancreatic lesions in everyday clinical practice. The greatest improvements concern the diagnosis of vessel and duct abnormalities. An exciting rivalry is developing between CT and other investigations (e.g., endosonography and MRI), some of which are also benefiting from significant technological advances. This rivalry will no doubt continue over the next few years and can be expected to improve patient management.

REFERENCES

1. Dupuy DE, Costello P, Ecker CP: Spiral CT of the pancreas, *Radiology* 183:815-818, 1992.
2. Wyatt SH, Fishman EK: Spiral CT of the pancreas, *Semin Ultrasound CT MR* 15:122-132, 1994.
3. Dufour B, Zins M, Vilgrain V, et al: Comparison between spiral x-ray computed tomography and endosonography in the diagnosis and staging of adenocarcinoma of the pancreas. Clinical preliminary study, *Gastroenterol Clin Biol* 21:124-130, 1997.
4. Howard TJ, Chin AC, Streib EW, et al: Value of helical computed tomography, angiography, and endoscopic ultrasound in determining resectability of periampullary carcinoma, *Am J Surg* 174:237-241, 1997.
5. Legmann P, Vignaux O, Dousset B, et al: Pancreatic tumors: comparison of dual-phase helical CT and endoscopic sonography, *Am J Roentgenol* 170:1315-1322, 1998.
6. Fishman EK, Horton KM, Urban BA: Multidetector CT angiography in the evaluation of pancreatic carcinoma: preliminary observations, *J Comput Assist Tomogr* 24:849-853, 2000.
7. Boland GW, O'Malley ME, Saez M, et al: Pancreatic-phase versus portal vein-phase helical CT of the pancreas: optimal temporal window for evaluation of pancreatic adenocarcinoma, *Am J Roentgenol* 172:605-608, 1999.
8. Graf O, Boland GW, Warshaw AL, et al: Arterial versus portal venous helical CT for revealing pancreatic adenocarcinoma: conspicuity of tumor and critical vascular anatomy, *Am J Roentgenol* 169:119-123, 1997.
9. Keogan MT, Mc Dermott VG, Paulson EK, et al: Pancreatic malignancy: effect of dual phase helical CT in tumor detection and vascular opacification, *Radiology* 205:513-518, 1997.
10. Lu DS, Vedantham S, Krasny RM, et al: Two-phase helical CT for pancreatic tumors: pancreatic versus hepatic phase enhancement of tumor, pancreas, and vascular structures, *Radiology* 199:697-701, 1996.
11. McNulty NJ, Francis IR, Platt JF, et al: Multidetector row helical CT of the pancreas: effect of contrast-enhanced multiphasic imaging on enhancement of the pancreas, peripancreatic vasculature, and pancreatic adenocarcinoma, *Radiology* 220:97-102, 2001.
12. Foley WD, Mallisee TA, Hohenwalter MD, et al: Multiphase hepatic CT with a multirow detector CT scanner, *Am J Roentgenol* 175:679-685, 2000.
13. Murakami T, Kim T, Takamura M, et al: Hypervascular hepatocellular carcinoma: detection with double arterial phase multi-detector row helical CT, *Radiology* 218:763-767, 2001.
14. Ibukuro K, Charnsangavej C, Chasen MH, et al: Helical CT angiography with multiplanar reformation: techniques and clinical applications, *Radiographics* 15:671-682, 1995.
15. Raptopoulos V, Prassopoulos P, Chuttani R, et al: Multiplanar CT pancreatography and distal cholangiography with minimum intensity projections, *Radiology* 207:317-324, 1998.
16. Takeshita K, Furui S, Yamauchi T, et al: Minimum intensity projection image and curved reformation image of the main pancreatic duct obtained by helical CT in patients with main pancreatic duct dilation, *Nippon Igaku Hoshasen Gakkai Zasshi* 59:146-148, 1999.
17. Nino-Murcia M, Jeffrey RB Jr, Beaulieu CF, et al: Multidetector CT of the pancreas and bile duct system: value of curved planar reformations, *Am J Roentgenol* 176:689-693, 2001.
18. Bonaldi VM, Bret PM, Atri M, et al: Helical CT of the pancreas: a comparison of cine display and film-based viewing, *Am J Roentgenol* 170:373-376, 1998.
19. Bluemke DA, Cameron JL, Hruban RH, et al: Potentially resectable pancreatic adenocarcinoma: spiral CT assessment with surgical and pathologic correlation, *Radiology* 197:381-385, 1995.
20. Diehl SJ, Lehmann KJ, Sadick M, et al: Pancreatic cancer: Value of dual-phase helical CT in assessing resectability, *Radiology* 206:373-378, 1998.
21. Müller MF, Meyenberger C, Bertschinger P, et al: Pancreatic tumors: evaluation with endoscopic US, CT, and MR imaging, *Radiology* 190:745-751, 1994.
22. Prokesch RW, Chow LC, Beaulieu CF, et al: Isoattenuating pancreatic adenocarcinoma at multi-detector row CT: secondary signs, *Radiology* 224:764-768, 2002.
23. Lu DS, Reber HA, Krasny RM, et al: Local staging of pancreatic cancer: criteria for unresectability of major vessels as revealed by pancreatic-phase, thin-section helical CT, *Am J Roentgenol* 168:1439-1443, 1997.
24. Zeman RK, Cooper C, Zeiberg AS, et al: TNM staging of pancreatic carcinoma using helical CT, *Am J Roentgenol* 169:459-464, 1997.
25. Fletcher J, Wiersema M, Farrell M, et al: Pancreatic malignancy: value of arterial, pancreatic, and hepatic phase imaging with multidetector row CT, *Radiology* 229:81-90, 2003.
26. Catalano C, Laghi A, Fraioli F, et al: Pancreatic carcinoma: the role of high-resolution multislice spiral CT in the diagnosis and assessment of resectability, *Eur Radiol* 13:149-156, 2003.
27. Vargas R, Nino-Murcia M, Trueblood W, et al: MSCT in pancreatic adenocarcinoma: prediction of vascular invasion and resectability using a multiphasic technique with curved planar reformations, *Am J Roentgenol* 182:419-425, 2004.
28. Raptopoulos V, Steer ML, Sheiman RG, et al: The use of helical CT and CT angiography to predict vascular involvement from pancreatic cancer: correlation with findings at surgery, *Am J Roentgenol* 168:971-977, 1997.
29. Zeman RK, Davros WJ, Berman P, et al: Three-dimensional models of the abdominal vasculature based on helical CT: usefulness in patients with pancreatic neoplasms, *Am J Roentgenol* 162:1425-1429, 1994.

30. Trede M, Rumstadt B, Wendl K, et al: Ultrafast magnetic resonance imaging improves the staging of pancreatic tumors, *Ann Surg* 226:393-407, 1997.

31. Mathieu D, Guigui B, Valette PJ, et al: Pancreatic cystic neoplasm, *Radiol Clin North Am* 27:163-176, 1989.

32. Vilgrain V, Mathieu D, Bruel JM, et al: Cystic tumors of the pancreas. In Baert AL, Delorme G, Van Hoe L, editors: *Radiology of the pancreas*, Berlin, 1999, Springer, pp. 235-257.

33. Taouli B, Vilgrain V, Vullierme MP, et al: Intraductal papillary mucinous tumors of the pancreas: helical CT with histopathologic correlation, *Radiology* 217:757-764, 2000.

9.

Virtual Colonoscopy

Andrea Laghi
Franco Iafrate
Roberto Passariello

Virtual colonoscopy (VC), also known as computed tomography colonography (CTC), is a novel imaging modality for the evaluation of the colonic mucosa in which thin-section spiral CT provides high-resolution, two-dimensional (2D) axial images; CT data sets are edited off-line to produce multiplanar reconstructions (coronal and sagittal images) as well as three-dimensional (3D) modeling, including endoscopic-like views. VC was first proposed by Vining et al.[1] in 1994; since then, enormous technical progress followed (computer power and dedicated software rapidly improved, with considerable reduction of both postprocessing and interpretation time) and wide popularity among patients (due to its enhanced compliance compared with more invasive modalities, such as conventional colonoscopy) and physicians (due to its ability to examine the entire colonic mucosa even in the presence of stenosing lesions). For all these reasons, VC is likely to become a useful tool for colorectal cancer disorders in the near future, obviating the need for invasive diagnostic colonoscopy.[2] A sample protocol for a colon study is presented in Table 9-1.

Table 9-1   CT Protocol Sample for a Colon Study

Indication	Unsuccessful colonoscopy; obstructing/stenosing tumor; surveillance; screening
Protocol designed for (scanner type)	Siemens volume zoom (4-slice)
Patient preparation	Low-fiber diet starting 3 days before the examination; colonic cleansing using cathartic drugs; air/CO_2 distention of the colonic lumen; spasmolytic
First series	Patient in prone position
Oral contrast	Iodinated contrast agent/none
IV contrast	—
Tube settings	
kV	120 (140 for ultra–low-dose examination)
mA	50-100 (10 for ultra–low-dose examination)
Gantry speed (sec)	0.5
Table speed (mm/sec)	17.5
Slice thickness (mm)	1.25-3
Anatomical coverage	Diaphragm–symphis pubis
Reconstruction kernel	b20f smooth
Breath hold	Inspiration
Window settings	Lung/abdominal
Postprocessing	Multiplanar reformation (MPR); volume rendering
Second series	Patient in supine position
Oral contrast	Iodinated contrast agent/none
IV contrast	Iodinated contrast agent (tumor/surveillance) None (screening/asymptomatic)
Volume/injection rate/delay	120-150/3.0/60-70
Tube settings	
kV	120 (140 for ultra–low-dose examination)
mA	50-100 (10 for ultra–low-dose examination) 165 (for contrast-enhanced scan)
Gantry speed (sec)	0.5
Table speed (mm/sec)	17.5
Slice thickness (mm)	1.25-3
Anatomical coverage	Diaphragm–symphis pubis
Reconstruction kernel	b20f smooth
Breath hold	Inspiration
Window settings	Lung/abdominal
Postprocessing	Multiplanar reformation (MPR); volume rendering

TECHNIQUE

The approach to a VC study can be didactically divided into four consecutive steps:
1. Bowel preparation
2. Patient preparation for scanning
3. Data acquisition
4. Image postprocessing and analysis

Bowel Preparation

Bowel preparation is critical. To obtain optimal image quality, the patient's bowel should be free of either stool or fluid residues. In fact, the presence of stool may mimic an endoluminal mass lesion inside the colon or may mask the presence of either a polyp or a colonic carcinoma (Figure 9-1). Fluid residues cover the colonic mucosa, leaving areas of

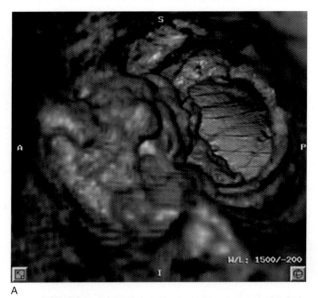

A

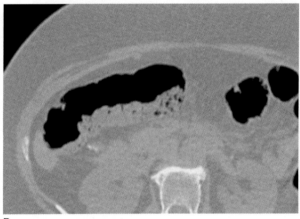

B

Fig. 9-1 A, Endoluminal 3D view showing a bulky pseudo-lesion. This finding, which may simulate an endoluminal vegetating neoplastic lesion, is the result of residual fecal material. **B,** Characterization of the pseudo-lesion as fecal residue can be obtained analyzing 2D axial slices, where nonhomogeneities resulting from multiple air bubbles are noted.

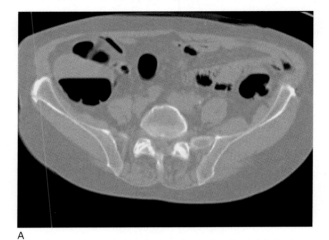

A

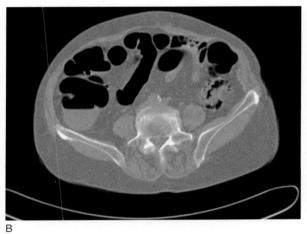

B

Fig. 9-2 A, On a patient scan in the prone position, fluid residue covers the anterior cecal wall, preventing the observer from assessing the presence of any abnormality. **B,** On a patient scan in the supine position, fluid moves and the anterior wall is well evaluated.

the internal surface unexplored. The negative effect of residual fluids can be minimized by the combined analysis of supine and prone scans. Turning patients from the prone to the supine position (or vice versa) will result in the shifting of residual fluids, allowing the operator to explore submerged colonic mucosa[3,4] (Figure 9-2).

The ideal colonic preparation is still under debate. It is generally agreed that patients should undergo a low-residue diet for 2 to 3 days before the examination and should ingest a cathartic agent the day before. The choice of the cathartic agent is also under discussion. Initially, based on the experience of conventional colonoscopy, most centers started using a standard colonoscopy preparation consisting of 4 liters of polyethylene glycol electrolyte solution with or without additional bisacodyl tablets; the major limitation of such an approach, apart from patient compliance, is the relatively large amount of residual fluids left inside the colonic lumen, which might affect the effectiveness of VC.[5] Subsequently, Macari et al. (2001)[6] reported that a phospho-soda preparation provides significantly less residual fluids than a polyethylene glycol electrolyte solution, which is more suitable for VC (the colon is "drier"). Due to contraindications to the use of phospho-soda (i.e., cardiac heart failure, chronic renal insufficiency) low-volume and low-sodium preparations (i.e., magnesium citrate) have been developed. The use of magnesium citrate in combination with nutritional support (providing a controlled, low-residue diet) seems to be a valid alternative to other bowel-cleansing protocols.[7]

To improve polyp detection and to reduce the number of false-positive examinations, "labeling" or "tagging" residual fluids, in combination with the administration of a cathartic agent, has been proposed.[8,9] It consists of the administration, before VC, of water-soluble iodinated contrast medium or diluted barium sulfate suspension. Such oral contrast agents are hyperattenuating to x-rays so that tagged residual bowel content appears hyperdense and is easily distinguished from true colonic lesions (Figure 9-3).

Because bowel cleansing is the most unpleasant and inconvenient aspect of colonic examination,[10] several attempts to reduce or eliminate the use of cathartic drugs are under development. This

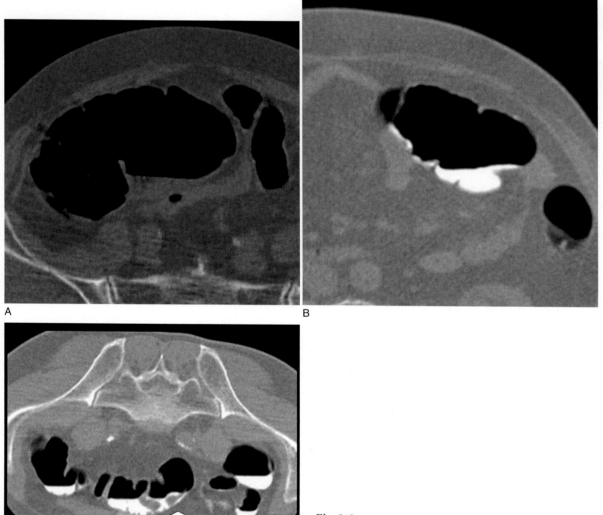

Fig. 9-3 A, Residual fluids present with soft-tissue density. **B,** Tagged fluids show high-density value caused by orally ingested iodinated or barium contrast agent. **C,** Tagged fluids make the identification of submerged polyps *(arrows)* possible due to a marked difference in density.

method, defined as "fecal tagging," includes the oral administration of barium sulfate with meals preceding the examination to completely tag colonic stools.[11,12]

If fluid tagging can be routinely implemented in clinical practice, fecal tagging is still under investigation, since optimal diet as well as the amount and dilution of tagging agent have not been established yet.

With both approaches, electronic cleansing of the bowel lumen using electronic stool subtraction software can be feasible, although artifacts at the air-fluid interface may still occur.[12,13] The availability of electronic cleansing, particularly in cases of fecal tagging, is mandatory if virtual navigation has to be perfomed[13] (Figure 9-4).

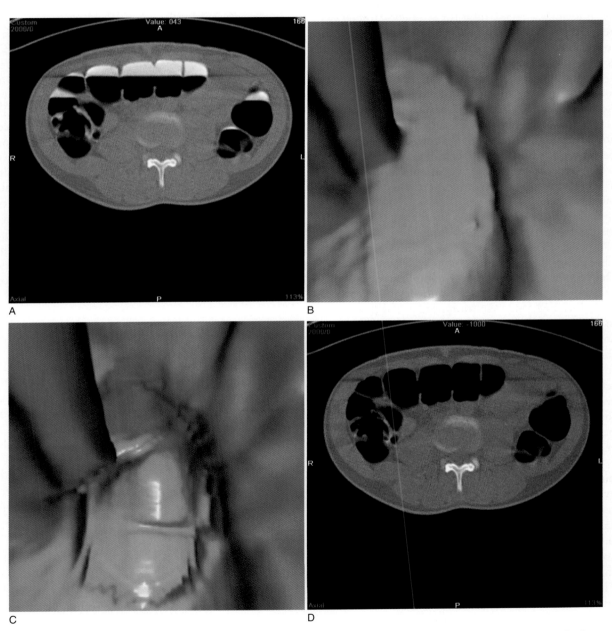

Fig. 9-4 Electronic cleansing. A, Distended colon with residual fluids tagged with iodinated oral contrast agent. B, Residual tagged fluids are electronically removed leaving the colonic lumen clean. C, 3D endoluminal view of an uncleansed colon, with air-fluid level. D, Following electronic cleansing, colon walls are completely assessable.

Patient Preparation for Scanning

Patient preparation includes gaseous distention of the colon, administration of an antiperistaltic drug, and intravenous injection of an iodinated contrast medium, depending on the individual centers and the clinical indication.

Gaseous distention is a critical step since collapsed bowel is a frequent cause of missed lesions at VC.[14] With the patient in the left lateral decubitus position, a rectal tube (or a Foley catheter) is inserted, and the colon is gently insufflated with room air to maximum patient tolerance; the patient is then turned to the prone position, and a standard CT scout film of the abdomen and pelvis is acquired to evaluate the adequacy of colonic distention. Additional air insufflation is performed, if needed.

The use of a rectal balloon catheter does not offer any advantage in terms of colonic distention compared with a thinner rubber tube (Foley catheter), which is best tolerated by patients[15]; the use of a rectal tube is reserved for patients with anal incontinence.

CO_2 represents a possible alternative to room air insufflation, because CO_2 diminishes discomfort following the procedure as a result of its quick resorption through the colon wall and blood.[16] Delivery of CO_2 is relatively complicated. For this reason, an automatic electronic device (Protocol TM; E-Z-EM, Inc. Westbury, New York) may be used. It provides better control of volume and pressure. At the time of this writing, trials comparing the efficacy of either air or CO_2 are still being performed. However, preliminary personal experience seems to confirm better patient compliance as well as optimal distention; the longer examination time compared with room air insufflation might be related to the operator's inexperience with the equipment.

The use of a spasmolytic agent (either hyoscine butylbromide or glucagon) is still questionable since evidence from studies is controversial. Glucagon seems not to be beneficial since it did not significantly improve polyp detection or colonic distention[17]; this evidence, combined with the known contraindications and the relatively high cost of the drug, prevent glucagon from routine use in VC. The effectiveness of hyoscine butylbromide (unlicensed in the United States), which has a better safety profile and is much less expensive, is not clear. In fact, some studies have shown that hyoscine butylbromide neither improves the overall adequacy of colonic distention nor the accuracy of polyp detection, but only provides a better distention of colonic segments proximal to diverticular disease.[18] A recent publication compared single-dose and double-dose hyoscine butylbromide with no spasmolytic administration in a population of 136 subjects undergoing VC. The study reported an improvement in colonic distention following a single dose of hyoscine butylbromide,[15] thus advocating its routine administration, if it is available.

The intravenous administration of iodine contrast medium is still under debate. It is generally agreed that it is certainly necessary in patients who have, or are suspected of having, colorectal cancer (for detection of extracolonic findings [i.e., liver metastases]). However, it does not add significant advantages to colonic evaluation, in terms of polyp detection. Morrin and Raptopoulos (2001)[19] reported an improvement in reader confidence, bowel wall conspicuity, and depiction of medium-size polyps after intravenous injection of iodinated contrast medium. This suggests its use in patients with a suboptimally prepared colon, which would account for less than 15% of scanned patients. Others[20] propose a routine use of iodine contrast medium injection, which is based on evidence that a variable degree of benign polyp and carcinoma enhancement might help in differentiating these solid lesions from residual colonic fluid. These data need further confirmation, however.

Data Acquisition

A prerequisite for VC is spiral CT technology, which allows a scan of the entire abdomen and pelvis within a single breath hold. The advent of multidetector technology has largely modified the acquisition protocols, which are shorter and at higher spatial resolution along the z-axis. It results in less motion artifacts (respiratory and peristaltic), especially in older adult patients, and higher quality of 3D reconstructions, with possible improvement in the lesion detection rate, especially small polyps and flat lesions.

Scanning Technique

The use of multidetector spiral CT equipment may provide different scanning techniques able to improve the longitudinal spatial resolution without the need for an excessively long breath hold. Different detector arrays, particularly 4-slice scanners, have many scanning protocols, from high-resolution to fast-scanning. There is no agreement about an optimal scanning technique on various equipments, and preliminary reports offer different study protocols regarding this topic. Gillams et al. (2002),[21] working on a 4-slice CT scanner with isotropic array, demonstrated an improved sensitivity and reader confidence for small polyps (<10 mm) when using a thin collimation (1 mm; effective slice width, 1.25 mm). In our personal in vitro experience,[22] performed on a colonic phantom with a 4-slice scanner with adaptive array matrix, three scanning protocols (high-resolution, intermediate, and fast-scanning) were tested using a different effective slice width (ranging from 1 to 5 mm) and a reconstruction index (ranging from 1 to 3 mm). In terms of lesion detection rate, a statistically significant difference was observed between high-resolution and fast-scanning protocols ($p < .05$), but not between 1- and 3-mm protocols.

A general consensus[23] of 3 mm was reached regarding the largest acceptable effective collimation, although some researchers still prefer using lower collimation (1 mm).

On 16-slice (and in the near future, 64-slice spiral CT scanners), additional longitudinal spatial resolution may be obtained with routine use of millimeter or submillimeter slice collimation and acquisition of an isotropic volume.[24] The major problem will be the excessive number of slices generated per patient (over 1000 per series), which will require updates of dedicated workstations and systems for image storage.

Dual Positioning

Typical imaging protocol includes two scans, with the patient scanned in supine and prone positions. Dual positioning helps discriminate between fluid or retained feces and fixed polyps.[3,4,25] The degree of distention of individual colonic segments is influenced by patient position. The transverse colon is more effectively evaluated on supine scans; the rectum is more effectively evaluated on prone scans. If the patient is unable to lie prone, a lateral decubitus position can be effectively used.[26]

Low-Dose Protocols

The high radiation exposure associated with VC prevents its use in screening programs for patients at risk for colorectal carcinoma. There are three reasons for the high radiation dose. First, the technique is usually performed in the prone and supine positions, which doubles the radiation dose. Second, VC examinations are currently performed with multislice CT scanners, which tend to have a higher effective dose level than single-slice equipment. This is especially true for 4-slice scanners, because of their geometric inefficiency. Third, there is a trend in several centers to use narrower collimations (1.0 or 1.25 mm instead of 2.5 or 5.0 mm); this offers the significant advantage of near isotropic spatial resolution but also leads to an increase in effective dose. Indeed, in a recent study, van Gelder et al. (2002)[27] showed that the median effective dose for complete (i.e., prone and supine acquisitions combined) VC in 12 institutions is 8.8 mSv. VC at 8.8 mSv may result in a risk of up to 0.02% for inducing cancer in the over-50 population (who are currently considered the target population for colorectal cancer screening). Taking these factors into consideration, increased attention has been focused on the optimization of low-dose protocols for multislice VC. Recently, Hara et al. (2001)[28] took advantage of the faster data acquisition provided by multislice CT (MSCT) and demonstrated better bowel distention and fewer respiratory artifacts with a beam collimation (5.0 mm) and an effective radiation dose (4.7 mSv for men; 6.7 mSv for women). A different approach was proposed by Macari et al. (2002),[29] who used a thin-beam (i.e., 1.0 mm) collimation protocol to obtain images with near isotropic voxels but simultaneously decreased the effective mAs to 50 to keep the effective radiation dose to a level comparable to single-slice CT (SSCT) (5.0 mSv for men and 7.8 mSv for women). Such a protocol provided excellent sensitivity for detection of polyps 10 mm in diameter or larger and improved differentiation of colorectal polyps from residual stool and hypertrophied folds (with a resulting reduction of false-positive diagnoses). A study by van Gelder et al. (2002)[27] used a 2.5-mm beam collimation protocol and demonstrated that, despite a perceptible decline in image quality, the sensitivity for detection of polyps was equal at 100, 50, and 30 effective mAs. These results indicated that multi-slice VC can be performed reliably with an effective dose of 3.6 mSv. In our experience,[30] we used an effective mAs value of 10, demonstrating that MSCT technology can achieve a further, substantial radiation dose reduction for VC with a complete (i.e., prone and supine acquisitions combined) effective dose of 1.8 mSv for men and 2.4 mSv for women. These values are substantially lower than previously published data for SSCT and MSCT. They are also lower than that of a barium enema (Table 9-2). This technical approach (defined as "ultra–low-dose" technique) was subsequently validated in a large population of patients, with results comparable to full-dose imaging protocols.[31] A potential problem with an ultra–low-dose mAs protocol is its poor assessment of low-contrast structures, such as the liver, pancreas, kidneys, and lymph nodes. This can be expected because the quality of low-contrast structures is affected more by noise than that of high-contrast structures (i.e., colonic mucosa-air interface) (Figure 9-5). Thus, this imaging protocol will prevent the detection of extracolonic findings, unless denoising filters are implemented.[32] A second problem with an ultra–low-dose mAs protocol is the potential inability to image obese patients. This issue has yet to be well evaluated.

Image Postprocessing and Analysis

Image postprocessing is performed on dedicated off-line workstations, suitable for 3D data management and reconstruction. Minimum requirements for the analysis of a VC study include the simulta-

Table 9-2 Dose exposure in different VC protocols		
	Male	**Female**
Ultra—low-dose MSCT[30]	1.8	2.4 mSv
MSCT[6]	5.0	7.8 mSv
MSCT[28]	4.7	6.7 mSv
SSCT[28]	4.4	6.7 mSv
DCBE[31a]		3-7 mSv
Natural radiation × yr	2.6 mSv	

MSCT, Multislice CT; SSCT, single slice CT; DCBE, double-contrast barium enema.

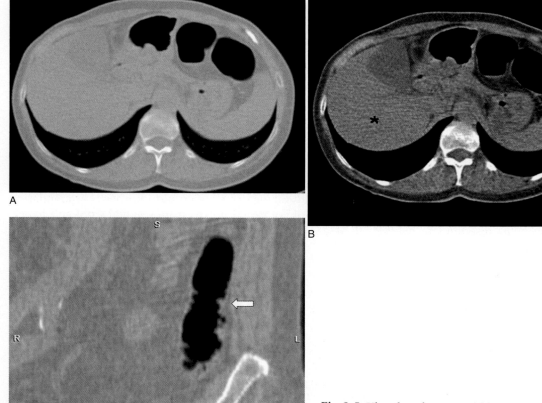

Fig. 9-5 Ultra–low-dose acquisition protocol. A, On lung window, an optimal evaluation of colonic lumen is obtained. B, On abdominal window, noise is evident, preventing a successful evaluation of abdominal parenchymatous organs (asterisk). C, Detection of a polyp (arrow), even if small, is adequate.

neous display of axial slices, reformatted sagittal and coronal planes (sometimes oblique reformations may also be available), and endoluminal view (Figure 9-6). Other complementary projections, such as "virtual double-contrast enema" (or tissue transition projection [TTP])[33] (Figure 9-7), and the so-called magic cube may be available (Figure 9-8).

Data analysis can be performed with the primary 2D or primary 3D approach. There is general agreement that scrolling through 2D axial images on the workstations and using a 3D endoluminal view for problem-solving is the most time-efficient method for analyzing VC datasets (primary 2D approach), with a mean interpretation time of around 10 minutes per case (if no major findings are detected).[34-36] A similar diagnostic performance was demonstrated by abdominal radiologists in polyp detection among 2D multiplanar reformation and 3D display techniques, although individual cases showed improved characterization with 3D display techniques.[37]

However, recent development of software able to automatically calculate a 3D fly-through pathway makes the "primary 3D approach" more time efficient.[38] Recent results seem to demonstrate how the primary 3D approach might positively affect the performance of VC.[39]

Following the renovated interest in 3D endoluminal views, researchers started to develop alternative views that might obviate the limitations of a classic antegrade and retrograde fly-through (i.e., polyps hidden behind a colonic fold). Differ-

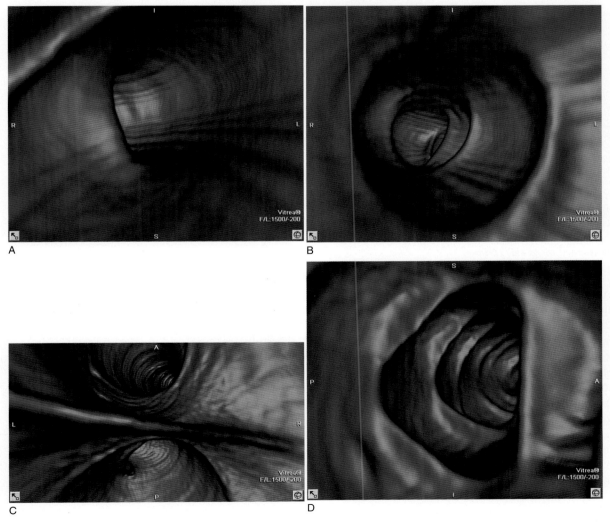

A   B   C   D

Fig. 9-6 Colon anatomy. Endoluminal views showing rectum (**A**), sigmoid colon (**B**), splenic flexure (**C**), and transverse colon (**D**).

Continued

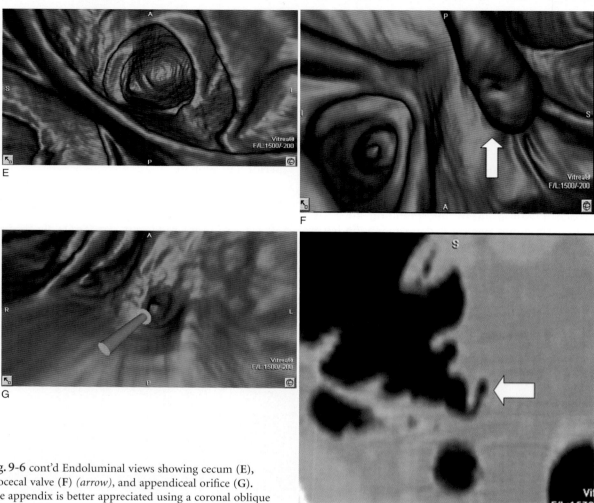

Fig. 9-6 cont'd Endoluminal views showing cecum (E), ileocecal valve (F) *(arrow)*, and appendiceal orifice (G). The appendix is better appreciated using a coronal oblique reformatted image (H) *(arrow)*.

ent display methods are therefore under evaluation, such as the unfolded cube display, which improves time efficiency and higher surface visibility compared with traditional fly-through.[40] Other authors developed displays that simulate gross anatomical pathological views of the colon ("virtual dissection"), such as the colon sliced lengthwise and laid open for en face inspection[41] (Figure 9-9). The advantage of such an approach in terms of polyp detection or easier and faster data analysis is still unclear.

Further development is represented by software able to automatically detect polyps (computer-assisted diagnosis [CAD]). The software identifies polyps using classification strategies based on colonic surface shape and attenuation values.[42] CAD is under research investigation, and it has been recently tested not only on phantoms, but also on human colonic data sets, showing good results in terms of sensitivity for detection of clinically significant polyps (greater than 10 mm); specificity is still poor.[43] For this reason, today CAD may serve successfully as a second reader, helping radiologists to "highlight" possible polyps. The advantage is twofold: the time required for VC reporting is reduced, and interobserver agreement is minimized.[44]

PERFORMANCE

Several studies demonstrate VC's ability to detect colonic neoplastic lesions—not only large carcinomas, but also polyps[25,31,45-59] (Figures 9-10 and 9-11). Concerning sensitivity for polyp detection, this is optimal for lesions larger than 10 mm and progressively diminishes with a decrease in polyp size. A good demonstration of what can be expected

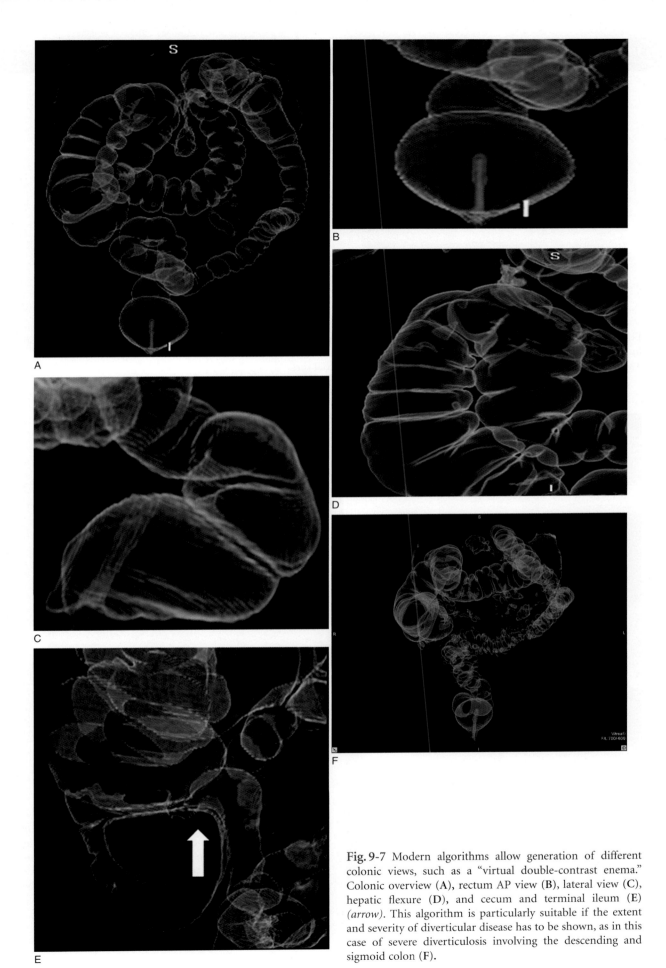

Fig. 9-7 Modern algorithms allow generation of different colonic views, such as a "virtual double-contrast enema." Colonic overview (**A**), rectum AP view (**B**), lateral view (**C**), hepatic flexure (**D**), and cecum and terminal ileum (**E**) *(arrow)*. This algorithm is particularly suitable if the extent and severity of diverticular disease has to be shown, as in this case of severe diverticulosis involving the descending and sigmoid colon (**F**).

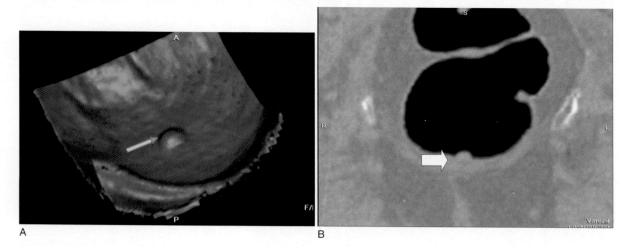

Fig. 9-8 The "magic cube" is another tool that enables the observer to define a sub-volume and to cut it and to show the endo-luminal aspect of the colonic wall of the selected region, without the need for a complete, virtual fly-through. **A,** "Magic cube" of a sessile polyp *(arrow)*. **B,** Same lesion *(arrow)* depicted on 2D axial slice.

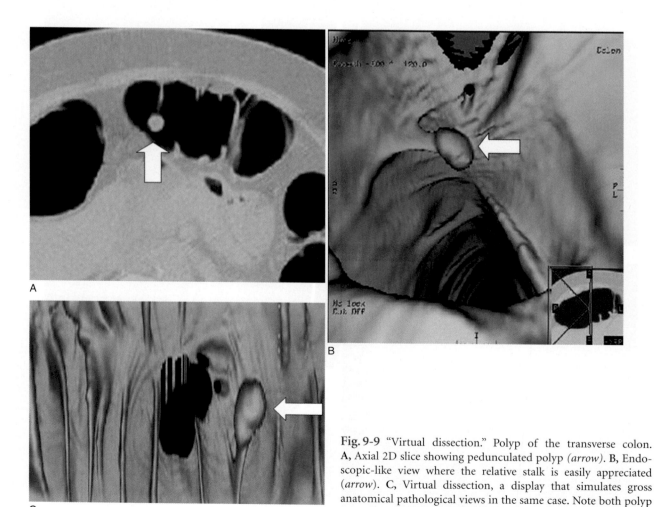

Fig. 9-9 "Virtual dissection." Polyp of the transverse colon. **A,** Axial 2D slice showing pedunculated polyp *(arrow)*. **B,** Endo-scopic-like view where the relative stalk is easily appreciated *(arrow)*. **C,** Virtual dissection, a display that simulates gross anatomical pathological views in the same case. Note both polyp *(arrow)* and folds, straightened by the electronic unfolding.

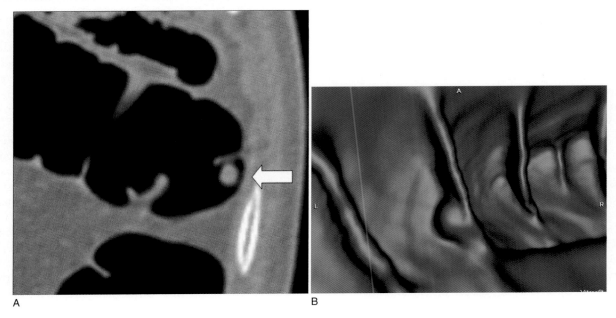

Fig. 9-10 **A,** Sessile polyp on axial 2D (**B**) *(arrow)* and endoluminal 3D images.

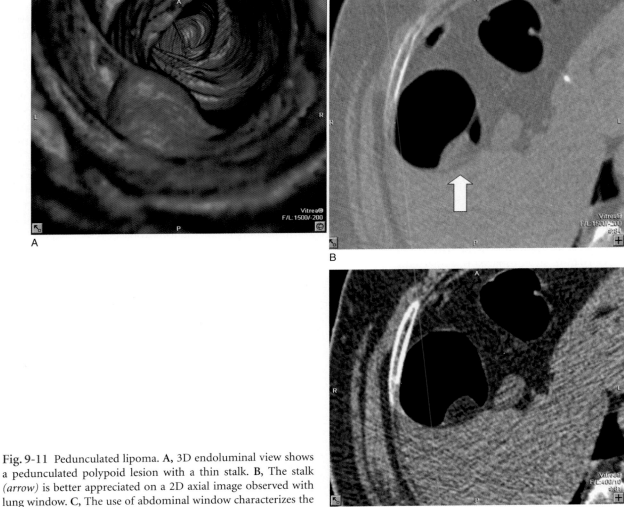

Fig. 9-11 Pedunculated lipoma. **A,** 3D endoluminal view shows a pedunculated polypoid lesion with a thin stalk. **B,** The stalk *(arrow)* is better appreciated on a 2D axial image observed with lung window. **C,** The use of abdominal window characterizes the lesion as a lipoma, because of fat density.

from VC is offered by a recently published meta-analysis considering 14 papers conducted between 1994 and 2002.[60] A total of 1324 patients and 1411 polyps were discussed. Patient sensitivity for polyps 10 mm or larger was 88% (CI, 0.84 to 0.93). For polyps between 6 and 9 mm, it was 84% (CI, 0.80 to 0.89), and for polyps 5 mm or smaller, it was 65% (CI, 0.57 to 0.73). Specificity was 95% (CI, 0.94 to 0.97).

In 2004, another more complex meta-analysis was presented.[61] It considered 24 studies from a total of 1398, with 4181 patients who had a prevalence of abnormality ranging between 14.7% and 72.2%. In regards to large polyps, meta-analysis of 2610 patients showed patient sensitivity of 92.5% (CI, 0.73 to 0.98) and specificity of 97.4% (CI, 0.95 to 0.98); if medium polyps were included, sensitivity was 86.4% (CI, 0.75 to 0.93) and specificity was 86.1% (CI, 0.75 to 0.92). Sensitivity for cancer was 95.9% (CI, 0.91 to 0.98).

These data confirm that the smaller the polyp size, the lower the sensitivity of VC; for this reason some operators do not even consider polyps smaller than 5 mm. However, exceptions to the results just described were recently reported in a multicenter study led by Cotton et al. (2004).[62] They performed a nonrandomized, evaluator-blinded, noninferiority study design of 615 participants 50 years or older who were referred for routine, clinically indicated colonoscopy in nine major hospital centers. VC study was performed by using multislice scanners immediately before standard colonoscopy; findings at colonoscopy were reported before and after segmental unblinding to the VC results. A total of 827 lesions were detected in 308 of 600 participants who underwent both procedures; 104 participants had lesions of at least 6 mm. Patient analysis showed a VC sensitivity of 39.0% with lesion sizes of at least 6 mm and 55.0% with lesion sizes of at least 10 mm. In comparison, sensitivities of 99.0% and 100%, respectively, were reported for conventional colonoscopy.

Variability of the results among different studies is probably the result of different examination techniques (especially in terms of slice collimation and image reconstruction thickness) and the experience level of the reader. Concerning this latter issue, a clear learning curve for VC was demonstrated by Spinzi et al. (2001),[51] who showed an increase in sensitivity from 32% to 92% from the first 25 cases to the last 75 cases of their series, respectively.

Results presented in the previous paragraph were obtained in so-called polyp-enriched populations, or those with a high prevalence of the disease, ranging between 14.7%[63] and 72.2%,[25] depending on the study. Thus, the results cannot be translated into a screening population, where the prevalence of the disease is much lower. At this time, only a few studies have been performed in a true screening population, and they have produced controversial results.

The first study based on a real screening population (asymptomatic subjects with no increased risk of cancer development) was published by Rex et al. (1999).[64] This study showed a very low sensitivity in the detection of clinically significant polyps (>1 cm), leading the authors to conclude that VC is not adequate as a colorectal cancer screening test. However, some limitations of the study should be recognized. First, although it was published in 1999, it reflects a very preliminary experience with VC (1995-1996). Most of the false-negative examinations can be attributed to perceptual errors (demonstrating reader inexperience and a learning curve of the technique). Second, poor colon preparation was another major cause of false-positive and false-negative studies. Third, poor colonic distention was recognized as a major limitation for a correct image interpretation.

In another study from the University of San Francisco, Yee et al. (2001)[65] reported the results of a series involving more than 300 patients who underwent both VC and conventional colonoscopy. Among these 300 patients, 96 were asymptomatic, thus representing a typical screening population. Data analysis showed similar results among the two patient populations (symptomatic patients and asymptomatic subjects), demonstrating no statistically significant differences. In particular, overall polyp sensitivity, independent of size and histology (hyperplastic or adenomatous polyps), was 69.0% and 69.7%, respectively. Similar results were demonstrated for individual patient sensitivity (88.0% and 82.0%, respectively, in symptomatic and asymptomatic subjects) and specificity (90.9% and 67%, respectively, in symptomatic and asymptomatic subjects). If considering only adenomatous polyps, which are the target lesions in screening, no statistically significant difference was demonstrated between symptomatic and asymptomatic subjects.

In another series of 703 asymptomatic subjects at higher-than-average risk for colorectal cancer who underwent a fecal occult blood test (FOBT), flexible sigmoidoscopy, colonoscopy, and double-read VC, Johnson et al. (2003)[63] showed disappointing results for VC, with a sensitivity for lesions

10 mm or larger ranging between 34% and 73%. Reasons for these results are unclear, although the study technique and reader fatigue might be two explanations. In fact, because of the low prevalence of adenomas larger than 1 cm (5%), a single observer could read more than 13,000 images before finding a single, 1-cm polyp.

Recently, a landmark study by Pickhardt et al. (2003)[39] increased interest in VC, reestablishing the view that it is now ready for widespread clinical use as an optional screening tool. They evaluated a total of 1233 asymptomatic adults (mean age, 57.8 years) who underwent same-day virtual and optical colonoscopy with segmental unblinding. The latter means that the colonoscopist is blinded to the VC results, but once he or she has cleared any colonic segment, a nurse or assistant will read the VC report for that segment. If any lesion was detected at VC, the scope is reintroduced and the segment is reevaluated. If no lesion is detected, the finding is false-positive; if a lesion is found, this is a false-negative of colonoscopy. Using this method, the sensitivity of the two techniques was compared. The sensitivity of virtual colonoscopy for adenomatous polyps was 93.8% for polyps at least 10 mm in diameter, 93.9% for polyps at least 8 mm in diameter, and 88.7% percent for polyps at least 6 mm in diameter. The sensitivity of optical colonoscopy for adenomatous polyps was 87.5%, 91.5%, and 92.3% for the three sizes of polyps, respectively. The specificity of virtual colonoscopy for adenomatous polyps was 96.0% for polyps at least 10 mm in diameter, 92.2% for polyps at least 8 mm in diameter, and 79.6% for polyps at least 6 mm in diameter.

INDICATIONS

Currently, the most widely accepted clinical indication for VC is incomplete or unsuccessful colonoscopy, which may be the result of redundant colon, patient intolerance to the procedure, spasm not resolving even with the use of spasmolytics, or obstructing colorectal cancer[66] (Figure 9-12). The major advantage of VC, also compared with barium enema, is that it can be performed on the same day of the colonoscopy without additional bowel preparation. VC can complete the examination in most of the cases, and it will also provide the cause for the endoscopic failure. In cases of occlusive carcinoma, VC can detect synchronous carcinomas,

occurring in 4.9% of cases; if intravenous injection of iodinated contrast medium is used, a complete staging of the patient can be performed.[67,68]

VC is also used to detect cancer in frail and immobile patients to avoid the sedation required for colonoscopy or to avoid the turning required during a barium enema.[69] The use of VC in patients under surveillance following colorectal cancer surgery was also investigated.[70,71] Additional studies are necessary to assess the cost-effectiveness of this approach.

Current uses of VC generally do not include the screening of asymptomatic persons, as suggested by the American Cancer Society[72] and the American Gastroenterological Association,[73] both of which decided that it should not yet be used for colorectal cancer screening, because data on true screening populations are missing. A practical approach is to consider VC as a credible alternative screening method and as a reasonable alternative to the other colorectal cancer screening tests when a patient is unable or unwilling to undergo conventional colonoscopy.[23]

OTHER CONSIDERATIONS FOR VIRTUAL COLONOSCOPY

Safety Profile

VC is inherently less invasive and safer than conventional colonoscopy, with no deaths related to the procedure ever reported. Recently, colonic perforations in two patients were reported, caused by over-inflation of air into an obstructed colon as a result of a lesion at the rectosigmoid junction in one case[74] and severe ulcerative colitis in an 81-year-old female in the second case.[75]

VC requires no sedation—a major advantage if dealing with older, unstable patients—or screening of asymptomatic subjects who would like to be able to return to work immediately after the procedure. In contrast, colonoscopy is associated with appreciable morbidity and even mortality, including significant cardiovascular effects related to sedation.[76]

If bowel preparation and distention are optimal, the success rate of VC is close to 100%, whereas up to 6% of conventional colonoscopy cannot reach the cecum.[77]

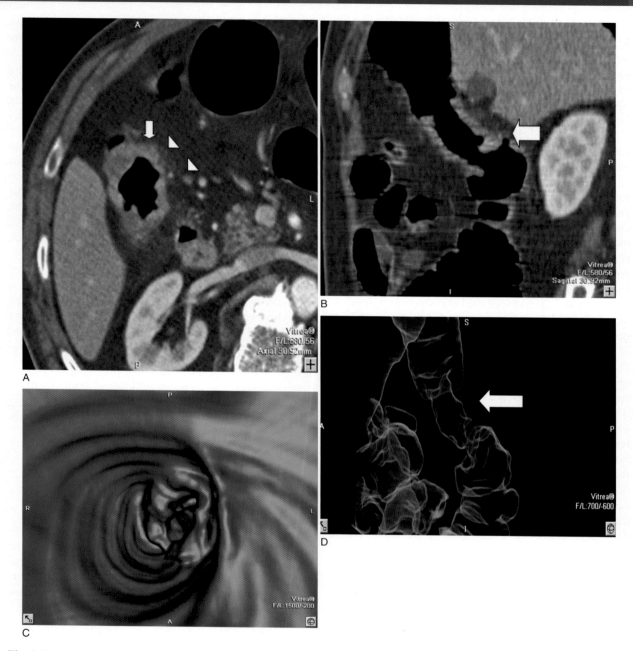

Fig. 9-12 Stenosing carcinoma of the hepatic flexure. **A,** Axial 2D slice shows annular thickening of the colonic wall with stranding into pericolonic fat tissue *(arrow)*; regional lymph nodes *(arrowheads)* are also observed. **B,** Coronal oblique reformatted image demonstrates longitudinal extension of a neoplastic lesion *(arrow)*. **C,** Endoluminal view of the stricture, with annular, irregular lesion and eccentric stenotic lumen. **D,** Virtual double contrast enema view demonstrates typical "apple-core" lesion *(arrows)*.

Patient Perspectives

From the patient's perspective, major advantages of VC include the very brief time required to perform the examination, the absence of barium contrast enemas, and the potential for same-day colonoscopy when polyps are detected. The latter issue requires a complex collaboration between endoscopy and radiology schedules, but it must be considered that in a screening setting, approximately 70% to 85% of colonoscopies identify no clinically significant pathology.[78] The theoretical rise in costs due to the 15% to 30% of patients who require polyp removal and who undergo a double colonic examination (VC and interventional colonoscopy) is counterbalanced by the avoidance of 70% to 85% of unnecessary diagnostic colonoscopy.

In terms of patient acceptability, mixed results have been reported. Some studies show a clear preference for conventional colonoscopy, whereas others demonstrate no real patient preference. Other studies indicate a clear preference for virtual colonoscopy.[79-81] The differences among these studies were the result of several factors: sedated or unsedated conventional colonoscopy, study population (i.e., symptomatic or asymptomatic subjects), scheduling of VC and conventional colonoscopy, patient awareness of the therapeutic capabilities of conventional colonoscopy, and the type of bowel preparation. If conventional colonoscopy is performed under sedation, the major limitation is represented by bowel preparation, independent of the cleansing agent. A significant advantage of VC will be realized when an examination without bowel cleansing is feasible.

Extracolonic Findings

A possible advocated advantage of VC is the detection of extracolonic findings. Findings are considered to be either minor, moderate, or major.[82] A minor finding (e.g., simple renal cyst, hepatic cyst, cholecystectomy) is of little or no clinical importance and deserves no further investigation. A finding of moderate importance (e.g., gallstones, splenomegalia, hiatal hernia) requires verification of patient history or clinical, radiological, or other follow-up. A major finding (e.g., lymphadenopathy, solid hepatic or renal masses, solid pancreatic mass) is a potentially life-threatening finding needing prompt patient evaluation (Figure 9-13).

The prevalence is still unknown, and it is reported to range between 11% and 23%[82-84] if only major findings are considered. If minor and moderate findings are also included, the prevalence is much higher, ranging between 15%[84] and 59%.[82] This discrepancy may be related to differences in patient selection, definitions, and reporting thresholds of extracolonic abnormalities. Thus, the proportion of patients with malignant disease, which may affect the frequency of extracolonic abnormalities, was not stated in these studies.[83,84] The major issue concerning extracolonic findings is the extra time necessary for reporting and the cost incurred by unnecessary investigation of common benign abnormalities. In a recent series of 681 patients who underwent VC, Gluecker et al. (2003)[85] calculated the cost incurred by the detection of extracolonic abnormalities to be $34 per patient.

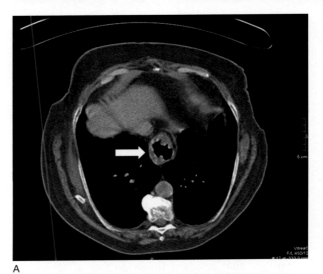

A

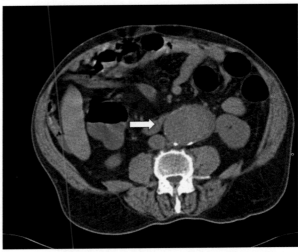

B

Fig. 9-13 Extracolonic findings. **A,** Hiatal hernia *(arrow).* **B,** Abdominal aortic aneurysm *(arrow).*

A secondary issue is the detection of extracolonic findings if a low-dose or an ultra–low-dose scanning technique is used. In these cases, the opportunity to evaluate the extracolonic solid organs will be reduced or lost as a result of poor image quality. Consequently, extracolonic evaluation might not be part of a VC study, solving the liability issue of the radiologist identifying and reporting extracolonic abnormalities. However, a general consensus about this issue has not been found yet.

Economic Analysis

A detailed economic analysis about the cost of VC has yet to be performed. Sonnenberg et al. (1999)[86] calculated that virtual colonoscopy must be 54%

less expensive than conventional colonoscopy and performed at 10-year intervals to equal the cost-effectiveness of conventional colonoscopy. However, this analysis did not consider the indirect costs of conventional colonoscopy, which is an important limitation. Moreover, technical advances (i.e., faster patient scanning, more powerful workstations, computer-assisted diagnosis) will reduce both examination and interpretation times, thus improving cost-effectiveness.

MR versus CT Virtual Colonoscopy

A virtual colonoscopy study can be successfully obtained with MR imaging.[87] Bowel preparation protocols are similar to CT, with the additional advantage that residual fluids do not affect image quality, since the colon is distended with a watery enema administered by way of a rectal tube. Fecal tagging techniques, without bowel preparation, are under development.[88,89]

There are two technical approaches, providing either a "bright" or a "dark" colonic lumen. A bright lumen is obtained with an enema of water spiked with gadolinium (1:100).[90] A dark lumen is the result of the administration of either water or air.[91,92] The dark lumen approach is the preferred technique, since it offers a better delineation of the enhancement of the colonic wall if intravenous contrast medium is given; moreover, it is also minimally affected by residual intraluminal air, avoiding the acquisition of dual scanning.

Technical requirements for generating MR virtual colonoscopy images include a high-field strength magnet with powerful gradients, a phased array multi-coil, and fast sequences. The need for a high-field strength magnet is due to the rather low intrinsic signal-to-noise ratio of 3D gradient echo sequences, which also require powerful gradients to implement short TR and TE values. To increase the signal-to-noise ratio, a phased-array multi-coil should be preferred; the use of a phased-array coil presents a limited field of view, which might result in incomplete coverage of the colon and a signal loss at the more cephalic and caudal sections in some patients.

Scanning protocol includes a 3D spoiled gradient echo (3.8/2.5, 40-degree flip angle) sequence acquired, if necessary, with patients in both the prone and supine positions. Each imaging sequence is performed in the coronal plane with a single breath hold less than 30 seconds. Imaging protocol also includes a 2D, single-shot fast spin-echo (SS-FSE or HASTE) (∞/64-90 ms [effective], 90-degree flip angle) pulse sequence and contrast-enhanced 2D or 3D spoiled gradient echo (177 ms/4.1 ms, 80-degree flip angle) sequence necessary to evaluate the extracolonic findings.[87]

Very few MR virtual colonoscopy studies have shown sensitivity and specificity approaching those obtained with CT for tumors and polypoid lesions larger than 10 mm[93,94] (Figure 9-14). However, reproducibility of MR data is still an issue since larger series and results by different research groups need to be assessed.

More debates about whether CT or MR is superior for colorectal cancer screening and detection are likely (Table 9-3). Advantages of CT over MR

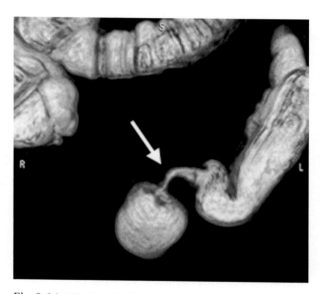

Fig. 9-14 MR virtual colonoscopy showing stenosing tumor *(arrow)* of the sigmoid colon.

Table 9-3 MR versus CT virtual colonoscopy

	MR	CT
Contraindications	Pacemaker, claustrophobia	None
Ionizing radiations	No	Yes
Contrast medium	Gd enema Air, barium	Air, CO_2
Artifacts	Metals, motion	Metals, motion
Spatial resolution	$2.5 \times 1.5 \times 1.2\,mm^3$	$0.6 \times 0.6 \times 1\,(0.8)\,mm^3$ (Multislice spiral CT)
Examination time	>30 min	15 min
Extracolonic findings	Yes	Yes

include fewer contraindications, shorter examination time, fewer imaging artifacts, and higher voxel resolution. MR imaging has absolute contraindications, such as implanted metallic devices (e.g., pacemakers, intracranial vascular clips), and requires sedation for patients with severe claustrophobia. When performed without intravenous administration of contrast media, CT virtual colonoscopy has virtually no contraindication.

Compared to CT, MR virtual colonoscopy requires longer examination times; with multislice CT, a single breath hold of approximately 10 to 20 seconds is necessary to acquire the entire data set, whereas a comprehensive MR study requires up to 10 minutes, because different sequences have to be performed for an exhaustive examination. The longer examination time of MR virtual colonoscopy indirectly affects image quality as antiperistaltic drug efficacy decreases in time, thus increasing the probability of artifacts related to colonic peristalsis. The higher voxel resolution inherent to CT results in a better quality of the endoluminal view. Thus, small polyps are better depicted with CT than with MR virtual colonoscopy, particularly when using a narrow collimation with MSCT. However, the impact of the higher spatial resolution on the detection of the larger lesions, which are regarded as clinically relevant, is still unclear.

The advantages of MR over CT include a lack of ionizing radiation, possibly better distention of the colon due to liquid filling, selective imaging of the colon without superposition of the small bowel, T2-weighted contrast, and sensitivity to intravenous contrast, when dynamic gradient echo imaging is performed.

The air used in CT as an enema is cleaner and less expensive than the liquid enema used in MR. However, air may result in more collapsed bowel loops than the liquid enema and, as in colonoscopy, requires a higher pressure for achieving and maintaining a colonic distention, which could be more painful than a liquid enema. New techniques using air distention at MR virtual colonoscopy are under development, although refinements are still needed.

Currently, MSCT appears to be more suitable for VC than MR, considering the speed of performing the examination, increased spatial resolution, and robustness in image quality.

CONCLUSION

VC is a reliable technique for detecting colonic disorders whose clinical role is evolving as more trial data become available. If performed well and interpreted by an experienced reader, VC is accurate, safe, and tolerated well by patients. It can safely replace double-contrast barium enema as a radiological tool for colonic evaluation. Current clinical indications include the evaluation of patients who have undergone unsuccessful or incomplete conventional colonoscopy, patients with obstructing colorectal cancer, and patients whose medical problems make them unsuitable for conventional colonoscopy. The use of VC as a colorectal cancer screening method cannot be recommended at this time. A practical approach is to consider VC as a currently credible alternative screening method and as a reasonable alternative to the other colorectal cancer screening tests when a patient is unable or unwilling to undergo conventional colonoscopy.

REFERENCES

1. Vining DJ, Gelfand DW, Bechtold RE, et al: Technical feasibility of colon imaging with helical CT and virtual reality, *Am J Roentgenol* 62 (suppl):104 (abstract), 1994.
2. Ferrucci JT: Virtual colonoscopy for colon cancer screening: further reflections on polyps and politics, *Am J Roentgenol* 181(3):795-797, 2003.
3. Chen SC, Lu DSK, Hecht JR, et al: CT colonography: value of scanning in both the supine and prone positions, *Am J Roentgenol* 172:595-599, 1999.
4. Yee J, Kumar NN, Hung RK, et al: Comparison of supine and prone scanning separately and in combination at CT colonography, *Radiology* 226:653-661, 2003.
5. Gryspeerdt S, Lefere P, Dewyspelaere J, et al: Optimisation of colon cleansing prior to computed tomographic colonography, *JBR-BTR* 85(6):289-296, 2002.
6. Macari M, Lavelle M, Pedrosa I, et al: Effect of different bowel preparations on residual fluid at CT colonography, *Radiology* 218:274-277, 2001.
7. Yee J: CT colonography: examination prerequisites, *Abdom Imaging* 27(3):244-252, 2002.
8. Lefere PA, Gryspeerdt SS, Dewyspelaere J, et al: Dietary fecal tagging as a cleansing method before CT colonography: initial results—polyp detection and patient acceptance, *Radiology* 224:393-403, 2002.
9. Thomeer M, Carbone I, Bosmans H, et al: Stool tagging applied in thin-slice multidetector computed tomography colonography, *J Comput Assist Tomogr* 27(2):132-139, 2003.
10. Gluecker TM, Johnson CD, Harmsen WS, et al: Colorectal cancer screening with CT colonography, colonoscopy, and double-contrast barium enema examination: prospective assessment of patient perceptions and preferences, *Radiology* 227:378-384, 2003.
11. Callstrom MR, Johnson CD, Fletcher JG, et al: CT colonography without cathartic preparation: feasibility study, *Radiology* 219(3):693-698, 2001.
12. Zalis ME, Hahn PF: Digital subtraction bowel cleansing in CT colonography, *Am J Roentgenol* 176:646-648, 2001.

13. Pickhardt PJ, Choi JH: Electronic cleansing and stool tagging in CT colonography: advantages and pitfalls with primary three-dimensional evaluation, *Am J Roentgenol* 181:799-805, 2003.

14. Rogalla P, Meiri N: CT colonography: data acquisition and patient preparation techniques, *Semin Ultrasound CT MR* 22:405-412, 2001.

15. Taylor SA, Halligan S, Goh V, et al: Optimizing colonic distention for multi-detector row CT colonography: effect of hyoscine butylbromide and rectal balloon catheter, *Radiology* 229(1):99-108, 2003.

16. Rogalla P, Schmidt E, Korvea M, et al: Optimal colonic distension for virtual colonoscopy: room air versus CO_2 insufflation, *Radiology* 213(P):341, 1999.

17. Yee J, Hung RK, Akerkar GA, et al: The usefulness of glucagons hydrochloride for colonic distension in CT colonography, *Am J Roentgenol* 173:169-172, 1999.

18. Bruzzi JF, Moss AC, Brennan DD, et al: Efficacy of IV Buscopan as a muscle relaxant in CT colonography, *Eur Radiol* 13(10):2264-2270, 2003.

19. Morrin MM, Raptopoulos V: Contrast-enhanced CT colonography, *Semin Ultrasound CT MR* 22(5):420-424, 2001.

20. Oto A, Gelebek V, Oguz BS, et al: CT attenuation of colorectal polypoid lesions: evaluation of contrast enhancement in CT colonography, *Eur Radiol* 13(7):1657-1663, 2003.

21. Gillams AR, Lees WR: What collimation is necessary for polyp detection at VC? Proceedings of the Third International Workshop on Multislice CT, 3D imaging, *Virtual Endoscopy*, June 5-8, 2002, Rome.

22. Laghi A, Iannaccone R, Mangiapane F, et al: Experimental colonic phantom for the evaluation of the optimal scanning technique for CT colonography using a multidetector spiral CT equipment, *Eur Radiol* 13:459-466, 2003.

23. Barish MA: Consensus statement. Proceedings of the Fourth International Symposium on Virtual Colonoscopy October 13-15, 2003, Boston.

24. Rottgen R, Schroder RJ, Lorenz M, et al: CT-colonography with the 16-slice CT for the diagnostic evaluation of colorectal neoplasms and inflammatory colon diseases, *Rofo Fortschr Geb Rontgenstr Neuen Bildgeb Verfahr* 175:1384-1391, 2003.

25. Fletcher JG, Johnson CD, Welch TJ, et al: Optimization of CT colonography technique: prospective trial in 180 patients, *Radiology* 216:704-711, 2000.

26. Gryspeerdt SS, Herman MJ, Baekelandt MA, et al: Supine/left decubitus scanning: a valuable alternative to supine/prone scanning in CT colonography, *Eur Radiol* 14(5):768-777, 2004.

27. van Gelder RE, Venema HW, Serlie IW, et al: CT colonography at different radiation dose levels: feasibility of dose reduction, *Radiology* 224:25-33, 2002.

28. Hara AK, Johnson CD, MacCarty RL: CT colonography: single- versus multi-detector row imaging, *Radiology* 219(2):461-465, 2001.

29. Macari M, Bini EJ, Xue X, et al: Colorectal neoplasms: prospective comparison of thin-section low-dose multidetector row CT colonography and conventional colonoscopy for detection, *Radiology* 224:383-392, 2002.

30. Iannaccone R, Laghi A, Catalano C, et al: Feasibility of ultra-low-dose multislice CT colonography for the detection of colorectal lesions: preliminary experience, *Eur Radiol* 13(6):1297-1302, 2003.

31. Iannaccone R, Laghi A, Catalano C, et al: Performance of lower dose multi-detector row helical CT colonography compared with conventional colonoscopy in the detection of colorectal lesions, *Radiology* 229(3):775-781, 2003.

31a. Huda W: Radiation dosimetry in diagnostic radiology. *AJR Am J Roentgenol* 169(6):1487-1488, 1997.

32. Rust GF, Reiser M: Virtual colonoscopy—chances for a screening procedure? *Radiology* 42(8):617-621, 2002.

33. Rogalla P, Bender A, Bick U, et al: Tissue transition projection (TTP) of the intestines, *Eur Radiol* 10:806-810, 2000.

34. Dachman AH, Kuniyoshi JK, Boyle CM, et al: CT colonography with three-dimensional problem solving for detection of colonic polyps, *Am J Roentgenol* 171:989-995, 1998.

35. Macari M, Milano A, Lavelle M, et al: Comparison of time-efficient CT colonography with two- and three-dimensional colonic evaluation for detecting colorectal polyps, *Am J Roentgenol* 174:1543-1549, 2000.

36. Bruzzi JF, Moss AC, Brennan DD, et al: Colonic surveillance by CT colonography using axial images only, *Eur Radiol* 14(5):763-767, 2004.

37. McFarland EG, Brink JA, Pilgram TK, et al: Spiral CT colonography: reader agreement and diagnostic performance with two- and three-dimensional image-display techniques, *Radiology* 218(2):375-383, 2001.

38. Pickhardt PJ: Three-dimensional endoluminal CT colonography (virtual colonoscopy): comparison of three commercially available systems, *Am J Roentgenol* 181:1599-1606, 2003.

39. Pickhardt PJ, Choi JR, Hwang I, et al: Computed tomographic virtual colonoscopy to screen for colorectal neoplasia in asymptomatic adults, *N Engl J Med* 349:2191-2200, 2003.

40. Vos FM, van Gelder RE, Serlie IW, et al: Three-dimensional display modes for CT colonography: conventional 3D virtual colonoscopy versus unfolded cube projection, *Radiology* 228(3):878-885, 2003.

41. Hoppe H, Quattropani C, Spreng A, et al: Virtual colon dissection with CT colonography compared with axial interpretation and conventional colonoscopy: preliminary results, *Am J Roentgenol* 182(5):1151-1158, 2004.

42. Yoshida H, Nappi J, MacEneaney P, et al: Computer-aided diagnosis scheme for detection of polyps at CT colonography, *Radiographics* 22:963-979, 2002.

43. Bogoni L, Jerebko A, Periaswamy S, et al: Automatic polyp detection: computer aided detection system performance, *Eur Radiol* 14 (suppl)6: N16, 2004.

44. Summers RM, Jerebko AK, Franaszek M, et al: Colonic polyps: complementary role of computer-aided detection in CT colonography, *Radiology* 225:391-399, 2002.

45. Hara AK, Johnson CD, Reed JE, et al: Detection of colorectal polyps with CT colography: initial assessment of sensitivity and specificity, *Radiology* 205:59-65, 1997.

46. Johnson CD, Hara AK, Reed JE: Computed tomographic colonography (virtual colonoscopy): a new method for detecting colorectal neoplasms, *Endoscopy* 29:454-461, 1997.

47. Fenlon HM, Nunes DP, Schroy PC, et al : A comparison of virtual and conventional colonoscopy for the detection of colorectal polyps, *N Engl J Med* 341:1496-1503, 1999.

48. Miao YM, Amin Z, Healy J et al: A prospective single centre study comparing computed tomography pneumocolon against colonoscopy in the detection of colorectal neoplasms, *Gut* 47:832-837, 2000.

49. Mendelson RM, Foster NM, Edwards JT, et al: Virtual colonoscopy compared with conventional colonoscopy: a developing technology, *Med J Aust* 173:472-475, 2000.

50. Pescatore P, Glucker T, Delarive J, et al: Diagnostic accuracy and inter-observer agreement of CT colonography (virtual colonoscopy), *Gut* 47:126-130, 2000.

51. Spinzi G, Belloni G, Martegani A, et al: Computer tomographic colonography and conventional colonoscopy for colon diseases: a prospective, blinded study, *Am J Gastroenterol* 96:394-400, 2001.

52. Laghi A, Di Giulio E, Iannaccone R, et al: Computed tomographic colonography (virtual colonoscopy): blinded prospective comparison with conventional colonoscopy for the detection of colorectal neoplasia, *Endoscopy* 34:1-6, 2002.

53. Laghi A, Iannaccone R, Carbone I, et al: Detection of colorectal lesions with virtual computed tomographic colonography: comparison with conventional colonoscopy in 165 patients, *Am J Surg* 183:124-131, 2002.

54. Gluecker T, Dorta G, Keller W, et al: Performance of multidetector computed tomography colonography compared with conventional colonoscopy, *Gut* 51:207-211, 2002.

55. Neri E, Giusti P, Battolla L, et al: Colorectal cancer: role of CT colonography in preoperative evaluation after incomplete colonoscopy, *Radiology* 223:615-619, 2002.

56. Pineau BC, Paskett ED, Chen GJ, et al : Virtual colonoscopy using oral contrast compared with colonoscopy for the detection of patients with colorectal polyps, *Gastroenterology* 125(2):304-310, 2003.

57. Gallo TM, Galatola G, Fracchia M, et al: Computer tomography colonography in routine clinical practice, *Eur J Gastroenterol Hepatol* 15:1323-1331, 2003.

58. Munikrishnan V, Gillams AR, Lees WR, et al: Prospective study comparing multislice CT colonography with colonoscopy in the detection of colorectal cancer and polyps, *Dis Colon Rectum* 46:1384-1390, 2003.

59. Ginnerup Pedersen B, Christiansen TE, Bjerregaard NC, et al: Colonoscopy and multidetector-array computed-tomograpic colonography: detection rates and feasibility, *Endoscopy* 35:736-742, 2003.

60. Sosna J, Morrin MM, Kruskal JB, et al: CT colonography of colorectal polyps: a metaanalysis, *Am J Roentgenol* 181:1593-1598, 2003.

61. Halligan S, Bartram C, Taylor S, et al: CT colonography for detection of colorectal neoplasia: meta-analysis, *Eur Radiol* 14 (suppl)6:N15, 2004.

62. Cotton PB, Durkalski VL, Pineau BC, et al: Computed tomographic colonography (virtual colonoscopy): a multicenter comparison with standard colonoscopy for detection of colorectal neoplasia, *JAMA* 291:1713-1719, 2004.

63. Johnson CD, Harmsen WS, Wilson LA, et al: Prospective blinded evaluation of computed tomographic colonography for screen detection of colorectal polyps, *Gastroenterology* 125(2):311-319, 2003.

64. Rex DK, Vining D, Kopecky KK: An initial experience with screening for colon polyps using spiral CT with and without CT colography, *Gastrointestinal Endosc* 50:309-313, 1999.

65. Yee J, Akerkar GA, Hung RK, et al: Colorectal neoplasia: performance characteristics of CT colonography for detection in 300 patients, *Radiology* 219:685-692, 2001.

66. Macari M, Berman P, Dicker M, et al: Usefulness of CT colonography in patients with incomplete colonoscopy, *Am J Roentgenol* 173:561-564, 1999.

67. Morrin MM, Farrell RJ, Raptopoulos V, et al: Role of virtual computed tomographic colonography in patients with colorectal cancers and obstructing colorectal lesions, *Dis Colon Rectum* 43:303-311, 2000.

68. Fenlon HM, McAneny DB, Nunes DP, et al: Occlusive colon carcinoma: virtual colonoscopy in the preoperative evaluation of the proximal colon, *Radiology* 210:423-428, 1999.

69. Burling D, Halligan S, Taylor SA, et al: CT colonography practice in the United Kingdom: a national survey, *Clin Rad* 59:39-43, 2004.

70. Laghi A, Iannaccone R, Bria E, et al: Contrast-enhanced computed tomographic colonography in the follow-up of colorectal cancer patients: a feasibility study, *Eur Radiol* 13:883-889, 2003.

71. Fletcher JG, Johnson CD, Krueger WR, et al: Contrast-enhanced CT colonography in recurrent colorectal carcinoma: feasibility of simultaneous evaluation for metastatic disease, local recurrence, and metachronous neoplasia in colorectal carcinoma, *Am J Roentgenol* 178(2):283-290, 2002.

72. Smith RA, Cokkinides V, Eyre HJ: American Cancer Society guidelines for the early detection of cancer, 2003, *CA Cancer J Clin* 53:27-43, 2003.

73. Winawer S, Fletcher R, Rex D, et al: Colorectal cancer screening and surveillance: clinical guidelines and rationale—update based on new evidence, *Gastroenterology* 124:544-560, 2003.

74. Kamar M, Portnoy O, Bar-Dayan A, et al: Actual colonic perforation in virtual colonoscopy: report of a case, *Dis Colon Rectum* 47(7):1242-1246, 2004.

75. Coady-Fariborzian L, Angel LP, Procaccino JA: Perforated colon secondary to virtual colonoscopy: report of a case, *Dis Colon Rectum* 47(7):1247-1249, 2004.

76. Taylor SA, Halligan S, O'Donnell C, et al: Cardiovascular effects at multi-detector row CT colonography compared with those at conventional endoscopy of the colon, *Radiology* 229(3):782-790, 2003.

77. Rex DK, Cutler CS, Lemmel GT, et al: Colonoscopic miss rates of adenomas determined by back-to-back colonoscopies, *Gastroenterology* 112:24-28, 1997.

78. Rex DK, Lehman GA, Ulbright TM, et al: Colonic neoplasia in asymptomatic persons with negative fecal occult blood tests: influence of age, gender and family history, *Am J Gastroenterol* 88:825-831, 1993.

79. Taylor SA, Halligan S, Saunders BP, et al: Acceptance by patients of multidetector CT colonography compared with barium enema examinations, flexible sigmoidoscopy, and colonoscopy, *Am J Roentgenol* 181:913-921, 2003.

80. Gluecker TM, Johnson CD, Harmsen WS, et al: Colorectal cancer screening with CT colonography, colonoscopy, and double-contrast barium enema examination: prospective assessment of patient perceptions and preferences, *Radiology* 227:378-384, 2003.

81. Ristvedt SL, McFarland EG, Weinstock LB, et al: Patient preferences for CT colonography, conventional colonoscopy, and bowel preparation, *Am J Gastroenterol* 98:578-585, 2003.

82. Hellstrom M, Svensson MH, Lasson A: Extracolonic and incidental findings on CT colonography (virtual colonoscopy), *Am J Roentgenol* 182(3):631-638, 2004.

83. Hara AK, Johnson CD, MacCarty RL, et al: Incidental extracolonic findings at CT colonography, *Radiology* 215:353-357, 2000.

84. Edwards JT, Wood CJ, Mendelson RM, et al: Extracolonic findings at virtual colonoscopy: implications for screening programs, *Am J Gastroenterol* 96:3009-3012, 2001.

85. Gluecker TM, Johnson CD, Wilson LA, et al: Extracolonic findings at CT colonography: evaluation of prevalence and cost in a screening population, *Gastroenterology* 124:911-916, 2003.

86. Sonnenberg A, Fabiola D, Bauerfeind P: Is virtual colonoscopy a cost-effective option to screen for colorectal cancer? *Am J Gastroenterol* 94:2268-2274, 1999.

87. Debatin JF, Schoenenberger AW, Luboldt W, et al: In vivo exoscopic and endoscopic MR imaging of the colon, *Am J Roentgenol* 69:1085-1088, 1997.

88. Weishaupt D, Patak MA, Froehlich J, et al: Faecal tagging to avoid colonic cleansing before MRI colonography, *Lancet* 354:835-836, 1999.

89. Lauenstein TC, Goehde SC, Ruehm SG, et al: MR colonography with barium-based fecal tagging: initial clinical experience, *Radiology* 223:248-254, 2002.

90. Luboldt W, Frohlich JM, Schneider N, et al: MR colonography: optimized enema composition, *Radiology* 212:265-269, 1999.

91. Morrin MM, Hochman MG, Farrell RJ, et al: MR colonography using colonic distention with air as the contrast material: work in progress, *Am J Roentgenol* 176:144-146, 2001.

92. Lomas DJ, Sood RR, Graves MJ, et al: Colon carcinoma: MR imaging with CO_2 enema–pilot study, *Radiology* 219:558-562, 2001.

93. Luboldt W, Bauerfeind P, Wildermuth S, et al: Colonic masses: detection with MR colonography, *Radiology* 216:383-388, 2000.

94. Pappalardo G, Polettini E, Frattaroli FM, et al: Magnetic resonance colonography versus conventional colonoscopy for the detection of colonic endoluminal lesions, *Gastroenterology* 119:300-304, 2000.

10.

Evidence-Based Principles and Protocols for Pediatric Body Multislice Computed Tomography

Donald P. Frush

Since its introduction more than 30 years ago, computed tomography (CT) has had a profound impact on the practice of medicine. Recent advances in CT technology, such as an increase in the number of detector rows for multislice CT (MSCT) together with submillimeter image thicknesses, have made CT a more versatile and powerful tool. This is due to the expansion of traditional applications, as well as the development of new applications.[1] For example, MSCT is now routine for common disorders such as appendicitis, nephrolithiasis and ureterolithiasis, and pulmonary thromboembolism. Imaging evaluation of these disorders virtually excluded CT just a decade ago. In addition, although single-slice helical technology provided many benefits for body CT in children,[2,3] multislice technology offers even greater application and potential for this group.

However, the increase in application has exceeded our ability to use the technology in an optimal or consistently appropriate fashion. Current standards of use for pediatric MSCT are based not only on performing adequate examinations from a diagnostic standpoint, but balancing the potential risks of computed tomography, namely radiation exposure.[4,5] In the pediatric population, radiologists tend to be much less familiar with body-imaging techniques. There are two potential problems with this. First, imaging may be inadequate for diagnostic purposes, or worse, provide fictitious information resulting in false-positive diagnoses. The second, and more recently recognized problem because of unfamiliarity with pediatric body CT techniques, is unnecessary radiation exposure to the individual. This latter point has been emphasized recently and has fundamentally changed the way that radiology personnel view CT in children as well as adults.[6-10]

Because of the increasing impact and potential misuse of MSCT, and because pediatric CT in children is technically challenging,[11] resulting in an unnecessary and excessive amount of radiation exposure,[12] it is critically important that individuals be familiar with a set of practical guidelines before performing pediatric MSCT. In addition, it is helpful to have a basic understanding of the potential risks of CT in this population when comparing the costs and benefits.[13] Finally, since the foundation for applied MSCT in children is a technically sound examination, applications will be addressed only as they illustrate certain technical aspects. Therefore, the following material addresses technical considerations, emphasizing the unique considerations of pediatric CT, and offers general practical guidelines and specific predominantly organ-based strategies, including special applications such as CT angiography. Together with radiation management strategies, successful diagnostic CT examinations will be optimized even for the most challenging pediatric cases.

General Technical Considerations

Of the available imaging modalities, CT offers the most comprehensive assessment of all organ systems. Although MR imaging is superior in many aspects to CT, including evaluation of the central nervous and musculoskeletal systems, information obtained from the lung and bowel is generally inferior to that obtained by CT. This is one reason why CT is used increasingly as a primary imaging option, rather than just as a problem-solving technology. Compared with radiography, ultrasonography, and nuclear medicine, superior anatomical information is obtained through CT. A CT examination is performed in a very consistent fashion, without the operator dependency evident with ultrasonography, and occasionally, MR examina-

tion. Examination times are increasingly faster, in the order of 2 to 10 seconds for entire regions in children. This means that sedation is increasingly infrequent.[14] With the advent of the number of detector rows to, and perhaps exceeding, 64, this should further reduce the need for sedation. This issue of a decreased need for sedation compared with MR imaging is substantial, since "conscious" (now termed *moderate*) sedation requires a great deal of resources and is not without risk. An in-depth discussion of sedation can be found elsewhere.[15] Some routine agents and doses are provided in Table 10-1.

Disadvantages of CT include higher cost compared with sonography and radiography. In addition, intravenous contrast material is often necessary. However, this risk is negligible given the very low severe adverse reaction rate in children.[16] Finally, the amount of radiation that can result from CT examinations can be quite large. This is why familiarity with the radiation risks associated with CT and the pediatric population is so important.

Basically, CT examinations can provide an effective dose of less than 1.0 to nearly 30 mSv.[17] Note that background radiation is about 3.0 mSv per year. Although CT examinations account for the minority (approximately 5%) of all imaging procedures resulting in ionizing radiation,[17] it provides about two thirds of the total amount of medical radiation.[17,18] Therefore, CT is the largest contributor of medical radiation dose. This point is especially important since the use of CT is increasing at a rate of about 10% to 15% per year.[13] The number of CT examinations in children has increased from about 4% to 11%.[18,19] Considering recent data about the number of CT examinations performed in the United States every year, an estimated 7 million examinations are performed on children. These numbers do not reflect the most recent applications of the newest multislice technology, which has the potential for exponential growth in use.

Children are at an increased risk of radiation-induced cancer compared with adults. Organ sensitivity ranges up to 10 times that of adults.[19-21] They also have a longer lifetime in which to manifest radiation-related changes, and a longer lifetime in which to undergo additional CT imaging, with cumulative radiation doses. Finally, an identical exposure to a smaller cross-sectional area in a child, compared with a larger cross-sectional area in an adult, will result in greater energy deposition.[22] For

Table 10-1 Sedative agents for pediatric imaging

Agents	Class	Effect	Dose	Route*	Onset	Duration[†]
Chloral hydrate[‡]	NA	Sedative	50-100 mg/kg, up to 120 mg/kg reported, max single dose 2 g	PO (PR)	20-30 min (rarely up to 60 min)	30-90 min
Sodium pentobarbital	Barbiturate	Sedative	2-3 mg/kg doses titrated q 5-7 min until sedated or max cumulative amount of 8 mg/kg, not to exceed 200 mg	IV (PO, IM)	5-10 min	40-60 min
Fentanyl citrate	Narcotic	Analgesic with sedative properties	1 µg/kg slowly IV q 5-7 min, adult-size patients 25-50 µg per dose, max cumulative dose 4.0 µg/kg	IV	1-2 min	30-60 min for analgesia; sedation may be shorter
Midazolam	Benzodiazepine	Sedative, anxiolytic, amnestic	0.02-0.05 mg/kg IV, titrate using 1/2 original dose (2-4 min) based on effect and oxygen saturation, max bolus dose 1.0 mg	IV (PO)	1-5 min (IV)	20-30 min
Diazepam	Benzodiazepine	Sedative, anxiolytic, amnestic	0.05-0.1 mg/kg IV, max cumulative dose 5.0 mg; 0.2-0.3 mg/kg PO, max cumulative dose 10 mg	IV (PO)	5-15 min (IV)	30-120 min
Methohexital	Barbiturate	Sedative	20 mg/kg in 10% solution	PR	10-15 min	45 min
Morphine	Narcotic	Analgesic with sedative properties	0.1-0.2 mg/kg, max dose 3-4 mg	IV (IM)	3-5 min	Analgesia up to 4 hr; sedation is variable but shorter
Meperidine	Narcotic	Analgesic with sedative properties	1-2 mg/kg, max dose 100 mg	IV (IM)	5-10 min	Analgesia 1-2 hr; sedation is variable but shorter
Naloxone hydrochloride	NA	Narcotic antagonist	0.01-0.1 mg/kg (lower antagonist dose for infant); repeat 2-3 min; titrate to reversal, max dose 2 mg	IV	1-2 min	Max to 20-30 min
Flumazenil	NA	Benzodiazepine antagonist	0.01 mg/kg, max dose (adult) 0.2 mg, max cumulative dose 1 mg	IV	1-3 min; peak effect 6-10 min	Max 60 min but usually <30 min depending on benzodiazepine dose

From American Roentgen Ray Society.[15]
IM, intramuscular; max, maximum; NA, not applicable; PO, per mouth; PR, per rectum.
*Preferred route listed first with alternative route(s) in parentheses.
[†]Duration of sedative effect for imaging purposes. Drowsiness, ataxia, and other effects may have variable durations depending on the agent, dose, and route of administration.
[‡]Thioridazine or hydroxyzine have been reported as adjuncts in children difficult to sedate with chloral hydrate alone.

these reasons, it makes sense that CT protocols, and therefore radiation, are adjusted to suit the pediatric population. However, this has not traditionally been the case. In one investigation, Paterson et al showed that the techniques used for pediatric body imaging were not substantially different than those used for adult imaging (Table 10-2). In particular, tube currents in excess of 200 mA were used routinely for body MSCT even in the smallest children. In addition, often (more than 30% of the time for abdomen helical CT) an examination with up to four phases was performed, increasing the radiation dose in multiples of the number of phases.[12] This investigation (together with two additional articles discussing the potential development of fatal cancer and techniques that were more appropriate for pediatric body CT[20,23]), helped to bring this issue to the attention of medical, industrial, regulatory, and public communities.[6] In the intervening years since these articles have come out, there has been an increasing amount of information regarding contemporary pediatric MSCT, including some evidence that the practice of pediatric CT is now more size-based (Tables 10-3 to 10-5). However, there is still a need for education regarding CT doses, potential risks,[24] and strategies to manage these radiation doses.[4,5]

This chapter's objective is not to provide a detailed discussion of CT risks. However, it is important to realize that this is a highly debated topic.[25-30] Support can be found both for the association of low-level radiation (< 100 to 150 mSv) with the risk of fatal cancer as well as the lack of this association. In general, however, most individuals take the conservative approach to CT in children (as well as adults) and agree that it should be designed to minimize excessive radiation. This is the ALARA (As Low As Reasonably Achievable) principle.

Pediatric Body MSCT Protocols: Practical Approach

The foundation of pediatric MSCT is the adherence to successful techniques. The following material emphasizes these techniques rather than reviews

Table 10-3 Pediatric body helical CT survey of pediatric radiologists (2003)

	Chest	Abdomen
MEAN TUBE CURRENT (MA)		
0-4 yrs	113	125
5-8 yrs	133	146
9-12 yrs	145	161
13-16 yrs	155	175

From American Roentgen Ray Society.[24]

Table 10-2 Survey of helical body CT of 32 neonates, infants, and children

Age group	Body region (No. of scans)	Tube current (mA) Mean	Range	Median	Kilovoltage (kVp) Mean	Range	Median
TUBE CURRENT AND KILOVOLTAGE SETTINGS (2001)							
Group A (0-4 yr)	Chest (5)	184	100-280	170	122	120-130	120
	Abdomen* (5)	220	140-280	200	122	120-130	120
Group B (5-8 yr)	Chest (3)	210	200-220	210	123	120-130	120
	Abdomen (5)	225	200-240	225	125	120-133	120
Group C (9-12 yr)	Chest (6)	229	200-280	223	123	120-130	120
	Abdomen (15)	196	140-240	200	127	120-140	120
Group D (13-16 yr)	Chest (4)	225	160-260	240	125	120-140	120
	Abdomen (15)	204	160-300	180	128	120-140	120
Total		58					
Chest		18	213	100-300	220	123	120-140	120
Abdomen		40	206		200	127		

From American Roentgen Ray Society.[12]
*Abdomen CT includes abdomen or abdomen and pelvis.

Table 10-4 Pediatric body helical CT survey of pediatric padiologists (2003)

mA	Age (yr)			
	0-4	5-8	9-12	13-16
TUBE CURRENT FOR CHEST CT				
<49	3/89 (3%)	0/88 (0%)	0/87 (0%)	0/88 (0%)
50-99	26/89 (29%)	13/88 (15%)	7/87 (8%)	5/88 (6%)
100-149	30/89 (34%)	39/88 (44%)	36/87 (41%)	30/88 (34%)
150-199	7/89 (8%)	7/88 (8%)	14/87 (16%)	16/88 (18%)
>200	3/89 (3%)	9/88 (10%)	10/87 (12%)	15/88 (17%)
Unknown	20/89 (23%)	20/88 (23%)	20/87 (23%)	22/88 (25%)

From American Roentgen Ray Society.[24]

Table 10-5 Pediatric body helical CT survey of pediatric radiologists (2003)

mA	Age (yr)			
	0-4	5-8	9-12	13-16
TUBE CURRENT FOR ABDOMEN CT				
<49	0/88 (0%)	0/87 (0%)	0/88 (0%)	0/87 (0%)
50-99	19/88 (22%)	4/87 (5%)	3/88 (3%)	1/87 (1%)
100-149	32/88 (36%)	39/87 (45%)	25/88 (28%)	17/87 (20%)
150-199	12/88 (14%)	14/87 (16%)	25/88 (28%)	27/87 (31%)
>200	4/88 (5%)	9/87 (10%)	14/88 (16%)	21/87 (24%)
Unknown	21/88 (24%)	21/87 (24%)	21/88 (24%)	21/87 (24%)

From American Roentgen Ray Society.[24]

applications. Applications will be provided only when they illustrate the technical aspects of pediatric CT. The reader is referred to recent publications of more in-depth discussion of clinical applications, as well as some of the debate about CT benefits in certain clinical scenarios.[1,2,13,31]

There are two technical components for performing pediatric CT. The first is patient preparation, and the second is the selection of various technical factors, including contrast media administration and scan parameters such as tube current.

Patient preparation is an important but often overlooked part of the examination. This requires consideration of sedation or anesthesia; intravascular access; the ability to ingest oral contrast media; and interactions with parents or other caregivers, especially with respect to the need for the examination and pain or risks such as radiation exposure. The CT room or suite should be as child friendly as possible. Personnel (including technologists and radiologists) must be able to discuss with family members the indication for the examination, as well

as potential side effects.[25] A lack of attention to these issues can result in nondiagnostic images (e.g., in a poorly sedated child) or dissatisfaction with the service provided.

The second component for successful pediatric MSCT is the choice of technical factors. This can be divided into contrast material administration (both intravenous and oral) and the CT examination parameters. Information obtained from a survey of current pediatric CT practice is important. Ranges of acceptable practice patterns can be determined, and guidelines can be established. This information also provides an idea of the variability of practices in pediatric CT examinations. Various techniques, including CT parameters in a survey of pediatric radiologists for single-slice CT (SSCT), published in 2003, are found in Tables 10-6 to 10-12.[24]

Oral contrast material is routinely used for pediatric abdominal CT, particularly since there is often little fat to separate bowel from adjacent structures (Figure 10-1). There are several types of oral contrast material. We traditionally use an iodinated

Table 10-6 Pediatric body helical CT survey of pediatric radiologists (2003)

ROUTINE USE OF GASTROINTESTINAL CONTRAST MATERIAL	
Esophageal contrast for chest CT	3/89 (3%)
Oral contrast for abdomen CT (non-trauma)	86/92 (93%)
Oral contrast for abdomen CT (trauma)	31/92 (34%)
Rectal contrast for abdomen CT	0/92 (0%)

From American Roentgen Ray Society.[24]

Table 10-7 Pediatric body helical CT survey of pediatric radiologists (2003)

ROUTINE TECHNIQUE OF IV CONTRAST MATERIAL ADMINISTRATION	
Manual (hand) bolus	42/90 (47%)
Power injection with peripheral IV	41/88 (47%)
Power injection with CVL (not PICC)†	14/88 (16%)
Contrast given over fixed time (sec)	33/79 (42%)
Contrast given at specific rate (ml/sec)	28/79 (35%)

From American Roentgen Ray Society.[24]
†Peripherally inserted central venous catheter.

Table 10-8 Pediatric body helical CT survey of pediatric radiologists (2003)

ml/kg	Chest	Abdomen
DOSE OF IV CONTRAST MATERIAL		
1.0	18/90 (20%)	15/89 (17%)
1.5	11/90 (12%)	4/89 (4%)
2.0	52/90 (58%)	62/89 (70%)
2.5	2/90 (2%)	2/89 (2%)
3.0	0/90 (0%)	0/89 (0%)
Unknown	7/90 (8%)	6/89 (7%)

From American Roentgen Ray Society.[24]

Table 10-9 Pediatric body helical CT survey of pediatric padiologists (2003)

ONSET OF DIAGNOSTIC SCANNING WITH RESPECT TO IV CONTRAST ADMINISTRATION: CHEST CT	
During injection	15/87 (17%)
0-10 sec after completion	38/87 (44%)
11-20 sec after completion	22/87 (25%)
21-30 sec after completion	8/87 (9%)
>30 sec after completion	1/87 (1%)
Unknown	3/87 (4%)

From American Roentgen Ray Society.[24]

Table 10-10 Pediatric body helical CT survey of pediatric radiologists (2003)

ONSET OF DIAGNOSTIC SCANNING WITH RESPECT TO IV CONTRAST ADMINISTRATION: ABDOMEN CT	
During injection	9/88 (10%)
0-10 sec after completion	20/88 (23%)
11-20 sec after onset	18/88 (21%)
21-30 sec after onset	24/88 (27%)
>30 sec	14/88 (16%)
Unknown	3/88 (3%)

From American Roentgen Ray Society.[24]

Table 10-11 Pediatric body helical CT survey of pediatric radiologists (2003)

KILOVOLTAGE FOR CHEST CT	
<110	3/90 (3%)
120	59/90 (66%)
130	1/90 (1%)
140	9/90 (10%)
Unknown	18/90 (20%)

From American Roentgen Ray Society.[24]

material mixed with a beverage (Table 10-13). Barium products can also be used. In addition, when it is difficult to get children to drink an unpleasant mixture, the child can drink whatever material he or she wants, such as fruit juice, water, or milk. This will result in better delineation between fluid in the distended lumen and wall and can provide information that high-density luminal contrast may obscure, such as mucosal enhancement.[32] In cases of small bowel obstruction, there is usually

Table 10-12 Pediatric body helical CT survey of pediatric radiologists (2003)	
KILOVOLTAGE FOR ABDOMEN CT	
<110	1/86 (1%)
120	55/86 (64%)
130	5/86 (6%)
140	7/86 (8%)
Unknown	18/86 (21%)

From American Roentgen Ray Society.[24]

Table 10-13 Oral contrast for abdominal and pelvic CT in infants and children*	
Age	**Amount[†] (1.5%-3.0% solution)**
1-6 mo	60-120 ml (2-4 oz)
6-12 mo	120-180 ml (4-6 oz)
1-4 yr	180-270 ml (6-9 oz)
4-8 yr	270-360 ml (9-12 oz)
8-12 yr	360-480 ml (12-16 oz)
12-16 yr	480-600 ml (16-20 oz)
>16 yr	Adult volume

*45-90 minutes before examination.
[†]Can give an additional volume half of original about 15 minutes before examination.

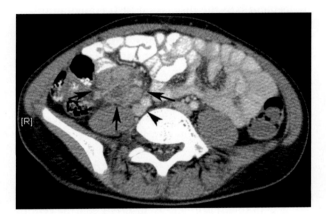

Fig. 10-1 A 10-year-old girl with mesenteric adenitis. Oral and IV contrast-enhanced CT examination shows the inflammatory mass *(arrows)* in the right lower quadrant. This mass is better seen with opacification of adjacent bowel and iliac vessels *(arrowhead)*. Note the lack of intraabdominal fat.

sufficient fluid to delineate the anatomy (Figure 10-2). Administration of oral contrast through a gastric tube should be reserved for only the most critical situations. Rectal contrast is not used routinely. The only exceptions are in cases with the potential for a mass or fluid collection, which is otherwise inseparable from a bowel, particularly in the pelvis.

Intravenous contrast media use can be divided into the following components: type and concentration of contrast material, route of administration, dose of material, rate of administration, injection technique (i.e., power injector versus manual or hand injection), and scan delay (the onset of scanning with respect to the administration of the contrast medium).

In principle, general CT protocols should be essentially based on size (i.e., according to weight). Age-based protocols are an acceptable alternative, although they are not as precise as the size-based

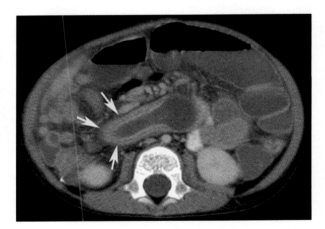

Fig. 10-2 Young, immunocompromised boy. CT was performed to assess for small bowel obstruction. Axial, IV contrast-enhanced CT at the mid-abdominal level shows sufficient delineation of bowel lumen without enteral contrast to demonstrate focal thickening and unobscured mucosal enhancement of a proximal jejunal segment *(arrows)*. Because of the risk of lymphoproliferative disorder, this segment was removed and showed only inflammatory changes.

approach. Protocols should also be adjusted based on the region scanned. For example, tube current can be lower in chest CT, particularly in young children, than in abdomen CT[4,5,23,33-36] (Figure 10-3). In addition, indication-based CT scanning should be built into protocols. For example, when large or high-contrast abnormalities are all that need to be identified, settings that result in slightly lower image quality (i.e., increased image noise) may be appropriate. In situations in which finer detail (e.g., very small abscesses in the liver or small renal

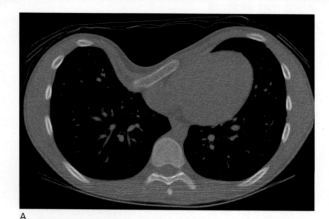

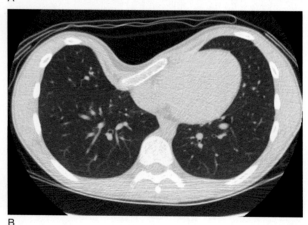

Fig. 10-3 A 17-year-old boy for presurgical evaluation of pectus excavatum deformity. CT examination performed at 120 kVp and 40 mAs displayed in a bone algorithm (**A**) sufficiently demonstrates the deformity. Although there is increased noise, lung detail (**B**) is also sufficient for screening purposes.

lesions) is important, the technique can be adjusted to reduce the amount of image noise.[37]

Low-osmolar contrast media are recommended for pediatric CT[38] because it is more difficult to monitor potentially adverse reactions, particularly in a preverbal or sedated child. In addition, the radiologist and radiology personnel may be unfamiliar with treating contrast allergies or other severe, adverse reactions in young children. In general, iodinated contrast with a concentration of about 300 to 320 mgI/ml is used for pediatric CT. An exception is in some CT angiography in which extremely small test boluses or diagnostic examinations using higher concentration may provide better peak enhancement (see the discussion of CT angiography).

The route of administration is through either peripheral or central venous catheters. Catheter sizes may be quite small in children—as small as 24 gauge. Another unique consideration in children is that the catheter sites may be quite different than those acceptable for adult CT scanning. For example, catheters are often placed in the feet and peripheral locations in the hands. In general, the butterfly-type (fixed metal cannula) is not recommended for pediatric imaging. Angiocatheters provide a safer alternative. Central venous catheters, including subcutaneous infusion ports, are acceptable. Peripherally inserted central venous catheters (PICCs) are not suitable for administration because of their small caliber lumens. The viscous media can also compromise the catheter function. The infant or young child with intraosseous access, reserved for emergency resuscitation (usually for profound shock), is too unstable to be in the CT suite. Although contrast enhancement can be achieved by this route, this access should be replaced by standard vascular catheters before contrast-enhanced CT.

Doses for pediatric scanning range from 1.5 to 2.5 ml/kg (Table 10-14).[39] The dose of contrast

Table 10-14 Pediatric contrast-enhanced abdominal helical CT

Investigator	Injection	Rate	Delay*
RECOMMENDATIONS FOR INITIATION OF DIAGNOSTIC SCANNING			
White	Manual	—	10-20 sec
Luker et al.	Power	1.2 ml/sec	130% of injection duration
Roche et al.	Power	1.7-2.0 ml/kg/min	60-70 sec from onset of contrast injection
Ruess et al.	Power	2.0 ml/sec	10-12 sec
Frush et al.	Manual	0.3-3.5 ml/sec	Mean 29 sec

Citations from summary in Reference 39.
*Delay from end of contrast injection unless stated otherwise.

material for pediatric body MSCT will vary depending on the area to be examined. With the advent of faster scanning, routine contrast amounts are 1.5 ml/kg in neck CT, in chest CT, and for CT angiography. For abdomen scanning, a dose of 2.0 ml/kg is recommended. Weight-based dosing is appropriate, with a limit of 150 ml of contrast.

Administration rates vary. In general, there are two techniques. The first is a fixed rate of administration, anywhere from 1.5 to 5.0 ml/sec. The second technique is to use a fixed duration (or relatively few fixed durations). This technique results in a variable rate of administration, depending on the child's weight. For example, the overall rate of administration for an abdomen CT will be slower in a 15-kg (33-lb) child receiving 30 ml of contrast over a minute (rate of 0.5 ml/sec) than in a 30-kg (66-lb) child receiving 60 ml of contrast over a minute (rate of 1.0 ml/sec). In a recent initial prospective comparison of these two techniques, we have found that either the fixed rate (in this case, 2.0 ml/sec) technique or single duration (60 seconds, with scanning commencing 10 seconds following completion of contrast administration—a 70-second total delay from the onset of administration) provides acceptable enhancement of solid organs (unpublished data). However, we have found that vascular opacification is subjectively better using the faster rate of injection, a principle certainly supported by CT angiographic techniques. In a recent survey of pediatric radiologists, 42% used a fixed duration, and 35% used fixed rates (23% did not know the specific technique) (see Table 10-7).[24]

Recommended contrast administration rates through various sizes of catheters are found in Table 10-15. Power injection should be used whenever possible for administration of contrast in children. Exceptions include situations in which there is inconsistent or no blood return from angiocatheters, or angiocatheters in tenuous locations such as the hand or foot. The use of power injec-

tors with central venous catheters has been addressed. In general, this technique has been found to be successful with complication rates no greater than those associated with manual injection.[40,41] Extravasation detectors are not beneficial for young children, since the amount of the material required to activate the detector may be in excess of the total volume.[42]

One of the most important aspects of IV contrast-enhanced MSCT is the onset of scanning. Proper scanning will optimize enhancement profiles and minimize artifacts (Figure 10-4). This timing of scanning can be through either empirical methods, with delays depending on the administration rate, or through tracking technology. Unlike adult scanning, in which the "scan delay" is routinely determined and usually relative to the initiation of contrast media administration, the onset of scanning in children will vary, depending on several factors. For example, in adult abdomen MSCT, there may be a fixed scan delay from the onset of contrast administration of 65 seconds. This delay in a 10-kg (22-lb) child would be too late for portal venous phase enhancement. In children, the scanning is relative to the *completion* of contrast material. A delay from the completion of contrast administration of about 25 seconds has been shown to provide optimal organ enhancement for general abdomen CT in children.[43,44] See Table 10-14 for a summary of the variation in scan delays for pediatric CT. For neck and chest CT, scanning can commence from 0 to 10 seconds after all contrast has been administered. For CT angiography, the onset of scanning is also critical. Scan delays of 5 to 20 seconds from the onset of contrast administration are used in this case. This is addressed in greater detail later in this chapter.

With bolus tracking, serial iso level slices can be obtained as frequently as every second. With this information, the enhancement of a vessel or organ can be followed (Figure 10-5). This technique can

Table 10-15	Angiocatheter size and suggested rates of administration for pediatric CT angiography

Catheter gauge	Administration rate (ml/sec)
24	1.5
22	2.0
20	3.0-4.0
18	4.0-5.0

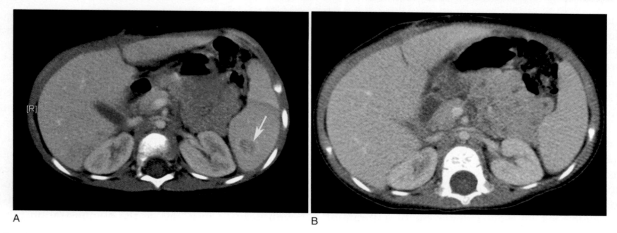

Fig. 10-4 Enhancement artifact caused by early enhancement of the spleen in a young boy with possible lymphoma. **A,** Initial examination was obtained relatively early in contrast enhancement and demonstrates an area of decreased enhancement in the spleen with a more focal low-attenuation center *(arrow)*. **B,** Subsequent evaluation with a reduced dose of contrast (1.0 ml) in a slightly later phase shows a normal spleen. The entire study was normal.

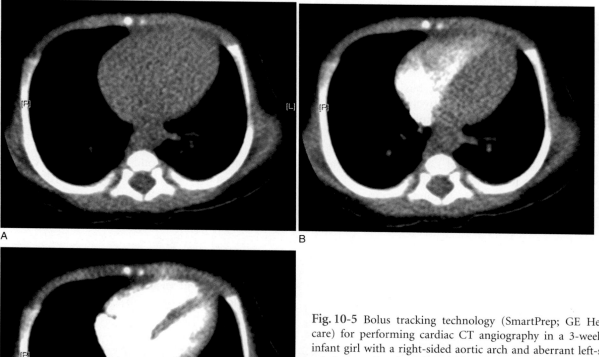

Fig. 10-5 Bolus tracking technology (SmartPrep; GE Healthcare) for performing cardiac CT angiography in a 3-week-old infant girl with a right-sided aortic arch and aberrant left-sided subclavian artery (not shown). Sequential images obtained at 2.0-second intervals through the level of the mid-ventricle before arrival of contrast media (**A**) and during opacification of the right (**B**) and left (**C**) side of the heart. Scanning began after image was obtained in C. For evaluation of the pulmonary arteries, scanning commences once contrast media is seen in the right ventricle (**B**). For aortic or systemic arterial evaluation, scanning commences once contrast is seen in the left ventricle and descending aorta (**C**). Note right-sided descending thoracic aorta *(arrow)*. Borrowed with permission from Springer.[31]

be applied in two settings. First, bolus tracking can be used during the administration of the total volume of contrast, and scanning can commence once the organ or vessel of interest reaches some arbitrarily determined target amount of enhancement.[43] The second method, using a test bolus, has been more successful in adult imaging. However, small test boluses can be used carefully in certain applications in CT angiography of children. These test boluses can be as low as 0.5 ml in neonates.[31]

Another aspect of CT technique consists of the scan parameters that determine the data set acquisition. As mentioned previously, these parameters should be adjusted based on the size of the child, the region scanned, and the scan indication. It is beyond the intent of this chapter to discuss in detail

the various contributions to image quality of various parameters. For a more in-depth discussion, the reader is referred to two excellent reviews.[45,46] However, these parameters will be addressed here briefly to provide some guidance in terms of the effect on image quality for pediatric MSCT. These adjustable parameters include tube current (in milliamperes, or mA), gantry cycle time (seconds), peak kilovoltage (kVp), detector configuration (number of detector rows and detector thickness in mm), and table speed or pitch.

Tube current determines the number of photons, or photon flux. Increasing the tube current increases the number of photons and decreases image noise (or mottle) (Figures 10-6 and 10-7). Tube current has a linear relationship to dose. For example,

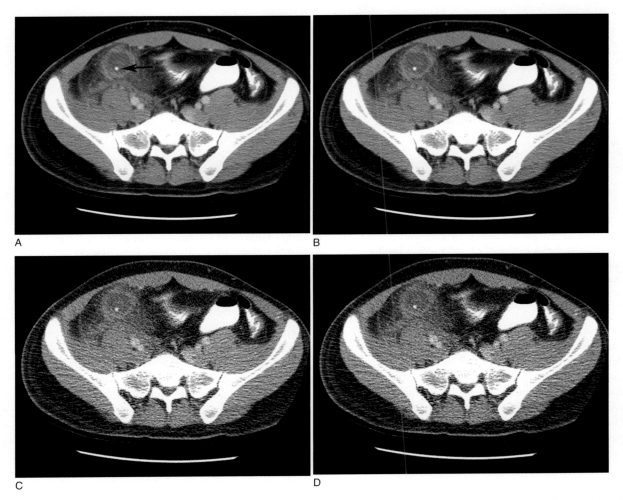

Fig. 10-6 A 28-year old man with complicated appendicitis. Axial, IV contrast-enhanced CT examination in the pelvis performed at 340 mA (**A**) shows a markedly dilated appendix with an appendicolith *(arrow)*. Simulated serial reductions in tube current created by adding noise to the scan data[37] corresponding to 240 mA (**B**), 140 mA (**C**), and 40 mA (**D**) show reduction in image quality. Diagnostic quality is still evident at least as low as 240 mA.

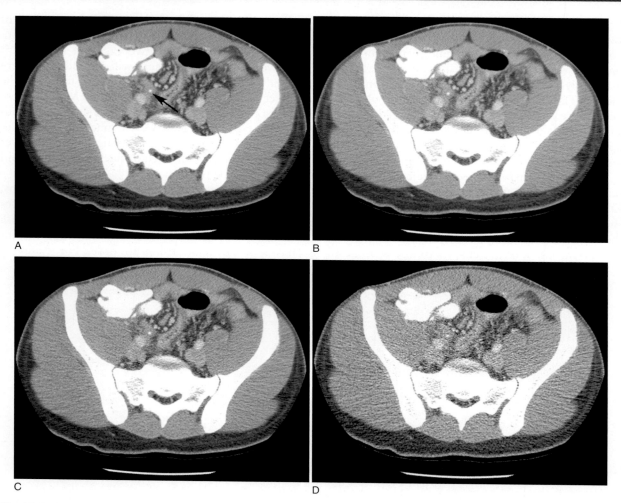

Fig. 10-7 A 20-year-old man with acute appendicitis. Axial, IV contrast-enhanced CT examination in the pelvis performed at 340 mA (**A**) shows a dilated appendix with a small appendicolith *(arrow)*. Simulated serial reductions in tube current created by adding noise to the scan data[37] corresponding to 240 mA (**B**), 140 mA (**C**), and 40 mA (**D**) show reduction in image quality. Diagnostic quality is still evident at least as low as 240 mA but is limited at 40 mA.

doubling the tube current will generally double the radiation dose. Tube current has an exponential relationship to noise, related to the factor change in current. For example, doubling the tube current (a factor of three increase) will decrease noise by a factor of the square root of 2. Likewise, increasing the tube current by a factor of three will decrease noise by a factor of the square root of 3.

Peak kilovoltage contributes to both contrast and noise. With all other parameters constant, decreasing the kilovoltage increases image noise and contrast. The relationship between kVp and radiation dose is nonlinear. For example, decreasing the kVp from 140 to 120 decreases the radiation dose by approximately 35%. In general, there has been

sparse investigation in clinical application of reduced kVp (below 120 to 140) (see Tables 10-11 and 10-12), although recent investigations indicate a growing awareness of the potential benefits in adults. For chest CT, investigators noted an acceptable image quality, with a decrease in dose using as low as 80 kVp.[47] Techniques that have been successful in using relatively reduced kVp can be found in Table 10-16.

Gantry cycle time options are generally 0.4 to 1.0 second. As with tube current, there is a linear relationship between gantry cycle time and radiation dose. Doubling the gantry cycle time (e.g., from 0.5 to 1.0 sec) will approximately double the radiation dose. The combination of gantry cycle time and

Table 10-16   Guidelines for MSCT parameters in children

Weight (lb)	kVp	mAs† SSCT	mAs† MSCT	Slice thickness (mm)	Pitch 4-	Pitch 8-	Pitch 16-	Detector thickness‡ (mm) 4-	Detector thickness‡ (mm) 8-	Detector thickness‡ (mm) 16-	Increment (mm)
CHEST*											
10-19	100-120	40	30	3.75-5	0.75	0.875	0.9375	2.5	1.25	1.25	2.5
20-39	100-120	50	30-40	3.75-5	0.75	0.875	0.9375	2.5	1.25	1.25	2.5
40-59	120	60	40	5	0.75-1.5	1.35	1.375	2.5	1.25	1.25	2.5
60-79	120	70	50	5	1.5	1.35	1.375	2.5	1.25	1.25	2.5
80-99	120	80	60	5	1.5	1.35	1.375	3.75	2.5	1.25	2.5
100-150	120	100-120	70-90	5	1.5	1.35	1.75	3.75	2.5	1.25	2.5
>150	120	120-140	≥110	5	1.5	1.35	1.75	3.75	2.5	1.25	2.5

Weight (lb)	kVp	mAs† SSCT	mAs† MSCT	Slice thickness (mm)	Pitch 4-	Pitch 8-	Pitch 16-	Detector thickness‡ (mm) 4-	Detector thickness‡ (mm) 8-	Detector thickness‡ (mm) 16-	Increment (mm)
ABDOMEN/PELVIS*											
10-19	100-120	60	50	3.75-5	0.75	0.875	0.9375	2.5	1.25	1.25	2.5
20-39	100-120	70	60	3.75-5	0.75	0.875	0.9375	2.5	1.25	1.25	2.5
40-59	120	80	70	5	0.75-1.5	1.35	1.375	2.5	1.25	1.25	2.5
60-79	120	100	80	5	1.5	1.35	1.375	2.5	1.25	1.25	2.5
80-99	120	120	100	5	1.5	1.35	1.375	3.75	2.5	1.25	2.5
100-150	120	140-150	110-120	5	1.5	1.35	1.75	3.75	2.5	1.25	2.5
>150	120	≥170	≥135	5	1.5	1.35	1.75	3.75	2.5	1.25	2.5

*Parameters are based on GE single and multislice scanners.
†Use 0.5 sec gantry time when an option; mA are for 4- and 8-slice MSCT; 16-slice weight-based color-coded mA are loaded on scanner.
‡For anticipated multiplanar reconstructions or 3D rendering, use thinnest detector width (e.g., 0.0625 with 16-slice) at all ages.

Weight (lb)	kVp	mAs† SSCT	mAs† MSCT	Slice thickness (mm)	Pitch 4-	Pitch 8-	Pitch 16-	Detector thickness‡ (mm) 4-	Detector thickness‡ (mm) 8-	Detector thickness‡ (mm) 16-	Increment (mm)
SKELETAL EXAMINATION*											
10-19	80-100	40	30	1.25-2.5	1.5	1.35	1.375	1.25	1.25	0.625	0.5-1.25
20-39	80-100	50	30-40	1.25-2.5	1.5	1.35	1.375	1.25	1.25	0.625	0.5-1.25
40-59	100	60	40	1.25-2.5	1.5	1.35	1.375	1.25	1.25	0.625	0.5-1.25
60-79	100	70	50	1.25-2.5	1.5	1.35	1.375	1.25	1.25	0.625	0.5-1.25
80-99	120	80	60	1.25-2.5	1.5	1.35	1.375	1.25	1.25	0.625	0.5-1.25
≥100	120	100-120	70-90	1.25-2.5	1.5	1.35	1.375	1.25	1.25	0.625	0.5-1.25

*Parameters are based on GE single-slice and multislice scanners. Reconstruct 0.625 data set at 0.5-1.0 mm interval to use for additional planes (e.g., sagittal and coronal). There is no need with submillimeter-thick images for scanning in more than one plane. Protocols generally for finer detail exams such as wrist and ankles. Thicker slices and increase interval for larger regions.
†Consider 80-100 kVp at all ages.

Continued

Table 10-16 Guidelines for MSCT parameters in children—cont'd

| Weight (lb) | kVp | mAs[†] | | Slice thickness (mm) | Pitch | | | Detector thickness[‡] (mm) | | | Increment (mm) |
		SSCT	MSCT		4-	8-	16-	4-	8-	16-	
CT ANGIOGRAPHY											
10-19	80-100	70	60	1.25-2.5	1.5	1.35	1.375	1.25	1.25	0.625	1.0-2.5
20-39	80-100	80	70	1.25-2.5	1.5	1.35	1.375	1.25	1.25	0.625	1.0-2.5
40-59	100	90	80	1.25-2.5	1.5	1.35	1.375	1.25	1.25	0.625	1.0-2.5
60-79	100	120	100	1.25-2.5	1.5	1.35	1.375	1.25	1.25	0.625	1.0-2.5
80-99	120	140	120	1.25-2.5	1.5	1.35	1.375	1.25	1.25	0.625	1.0-2.5
100-149	120	160-180	140-160	1.25-2.5	1.5	1.35	1.375	1.25	1.25	0.625	1.0-2.5
>150	120	≥200	≥170	1.25-2.5	1.5	1.35	1.375	1.25	1.25	0.625	1.0-2.5

*mAs slightly higher than body CT protocols. Use 0.5-second rotation time when an option.
[†]Displayed thickness. For coronal and sagittal reformats, and 3D reconstructions, reconstruct an axial data set at thickness of the detector (e.g., 0.625 for 16-slice scanner) at 0.5-1.0 mm intervals. Multiplanar thickness and interval should be similar to axial. For evaluation of larger structures, especially in larger children (e.g., aorta) the larger detector configuration (2.5 for 8-, and 1.25 for a 16-slice scanner) and a larger reconstructed thickness and interval can be used.
[‡]For larger children (larger vessels), the highest pitch can be used for MSCT.

tube current is mAs. For pediatric scanning, the fastest gantry cycle time is recommended. For example, to obtain a 100 mAs examination, 200 mA at 0.5 second is preferred over 100 mA at 1.0 second. This will reduce periodic motion artifact (e.g., cardiac motion as well as breathing) and will allow one to perform the fastest possible CT examinations, which is beneficial in children with limited breath-holding capabilities (e.g., less than 10 sec).

Detector configuration consists of the number of detector rows as well as detector thickness. Because it is important to perform pediatric CT as fast as possible, one should take advantage of the greatest number of detector rows available. For example, when there is a choice between an 8- or 16-slice mode for helical MSCT examinations, there is no recognized practical benefit obtained by using the 8-slice mode. Although there may be slight trade-offs in terms of slice sensitivity profile (actual reconstructed image thickness) as well as radiation dose, these are minor and do not counterbalance the confusing complexity that comes with increasing the number of selectable parameters or the longer scan time. The thickness of the detectors used will depend, to a large extent, on the application. For multiplanar reformations and 3D reconstructions, the thinnest detector configuration (e.g., 0.625 mm on the General Electric scanner) will provide the

highest quality rendering (Figure 10-8). There is a slight radiation dose penalty because there are more rotations required for the gantry to cover the same z-axis length than if a thicker detector configuration (1.25 mm) is used. This small increase in dose (usually no more than 10%) is acceptable for the improved image quality. However, for general scanning, the detector configuration of 1.25 mm for the 16-slice scanner is acceptable. The larger detector configurations for the 4-slice scanner (e.g., 5 mm) may also be acceptable if thin slices are not necessary for rendering.

There has been scant study of the optimal relationship among table speed, collimation (the concept of pitch), and image quality in pediatric patients. The factor of pitch is becoming less useful when talking about scan protocols. The simplest method is to individually choose the table speed and the total, or effective, collimation (number of detector rows multiplied by detector thickness). This ratio determines pitch. However, earlier work for single-detector CT-based techniques primarily on pitch, and comparison with pitch options for contemporary MSCT techniques has some value. Investigations with single-slice scanners shows that pitches of 1.5 to 2.0 resulted in adequate diagnostic images.[48,49] Based on these findings, pitches of about 1.5 should be the target for MSCT. For patients who approach adult size, higher pitches

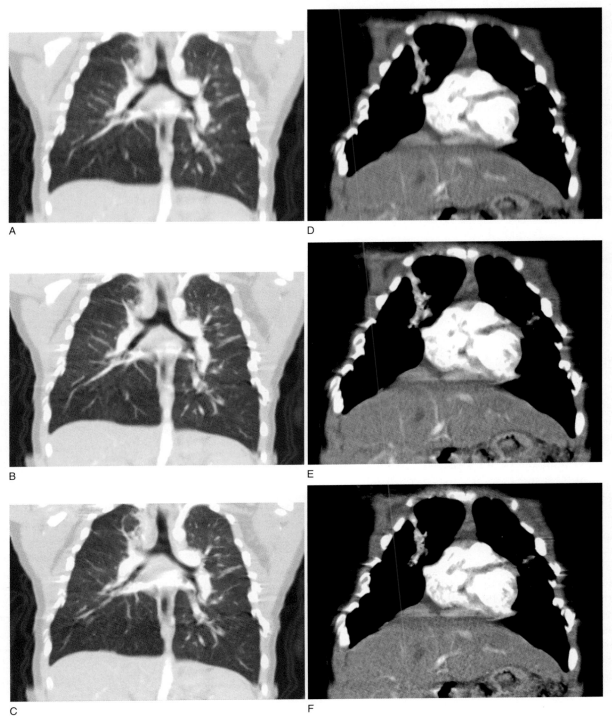

Fig. 10-8 A 15-month-old boy with recurrent right upper lobe atelectasis. IV contrast-enhanced CT was performed to assess for potential mediastinal mass compressing the airway. **A-C,** Lung algorithm coronal reconstructions at nearly identical levels demonstrate the increasing image quality based on 2.5 mm (**A**), 1.25 mm (**B**), and 0.625 (**C**) axial data sets. Each coronal reconstruction was created using a 2.5-mm thickness image at 5-mm intervals. **D-F,** Soft tissue algorithm display of same data set. Note increased detail of hepatic vasculature. Breathing causes artifact, which is seen most clearly at the lateral chest wall, but this does not compromise diagnostic quality. There was no mediastinal abnormality.

(e.g., 1.75 on General Electric scanners) may be performed. For children younger than 3 or 4 years, the helical artifact seen especially at high-contrast interfaces (such as gas-filled bowel and adjacent liver [more common in small children with less intra-abdominal body fat]) has provided annoying artifacts. In this group, pitches at about 1.0 are preferred. Again, for lower-detail assessment, such as follow-up scans, pitches greater than 1.0 may be obtained, even in very young children.

The scan reconstruction interval will depend partly on image review. With electronic review, on picture archive and communications systems (PACS), the image number is less of an issue than with film-based interpretation. As CT technology rapidly evolves to all soft-copy review, thinner intervals with an increased number of images (e.g., intervals at 2.5 mm versus 5.0 mm for hard copy) are appropriate. For rendering, intervals providing overlapping (intervals at about 50%) of slice thickness are preferred.

Specific Pediatric MSCT Techniques

The following section discusses additional unique considerations for region- or organ-based examinations. The general considerations just discussed will apply unless otherwise modified. Regions discussed include the chest and abdomen. Organ systems include abdominal solid organs, the skeletal system, and other applications consisting of airway evaluation and CT angiography.

Special Considerations for Pediatric Chest MSCT

CT is a commonly used modality for chest evaluation and is second only to radiography in terms of frequency of use.[50] MSCT offers important benefits for pediatric chest evaluation.[51] Patient preparation issues for chest CT include trying to minimize respiratory motion. When possible, breath holding should be performed. If this is not possible, quiet breathing usually provides sufficient diagnostic information (see Figure 10-8). Quiet breathing is supported by investigational work in a canine model in which quiet breathing did not qualitatively affect the ability to detect osteosarcoma metastases.[52] For intubated patients, a brief inspiratory (or expiratory, if necessary for diagnostic purposes) hold may be obtained, requiring coordination of scanning with the respiratory support team. Because MSCT is performed so quickly, these scans

can be performed in 2 to 5 seconds with 16-slice technology. Further increasing the number of detector rows will allow even faster coverage in children. The benefits are obvious in cases of limited breath holding or sedated children. Recently, a technique of an induced respiratory pause for CT examinations in a sedated, nonintubated child has been described.[53] In general, tube currents for chest CT can be lower than those for body CT because of decreased attenuation of the photons for the chest. In addition, kilovoltage can be lower in chest CT in young children (see Table 10-11). Applications for pediatric chest CT have recently been reviewed.[1]

Interstitial lung disease evaluation in children is less well understood and classified than in adults. For that reason, there is little investigation of interstitial lung disease and high-resolution techniques in children, compared with that in the adult population. However, dedicated thin section, higher-resolution CT techniques for adults can provide information that is not available from conventional MSCT chest techniques, including the presence of bronchiectasis, interstitial lobular thickening, and other processes such as alveolitis. This technique in adults has been well described. One needs to decide how important this high-resolution information is in pediatric CT. If this level of detail will potentially affect clinical management, it is necessary to determine whether a complete routine chest CT will be necessary. When no additional information will likely result using routine techniques (which is usually the case), axial CT examinations using thin-slice (e.g., 1.25 mm) images obtained every 5.0 mm, and at an mA about 50% greater than routine chest CT will usually be sufficient. This technique reduces the total amount of radiation. A routine helical CT is not required, and radiation is essentially limited to the slice obtained. The high-resolution images provide the same global evaluation of bone and soft tissue as would be provided by the general helical examination. The examination can be obtained prospectively in a lung or standard algorithm. In general, without breath holding, high-resolution chest CT quality is very unsatisfactory, even with 16-slice technology. In this case, only a few satisfactory images are obtained at end inspiration or expiration when chest movement is minimal.

For evaluation of lung parenchyma, intravenous contrast material is not routinely used. For example, intravenous contrast is not routine for evaluation of bronchiectasis, assessment of asymmetry aeration (where possible mediastinal abnormality is not necessary to document), and evaluation of metastatic disease, which does not typically involve the mediastinum (such as Wilms' tumor or osteosarcoma). Unlike in adults, intravenous contrast is otherwise used routinely for pediatric chest CT primarily because the lack of mediastinal fat (Figure 10-9) can make it difficult to separate vascularity from potential small adjacent abnormalities, such as hilar or mediastinal adenopathy. For evaluation of the chest wall, mediastinal, or

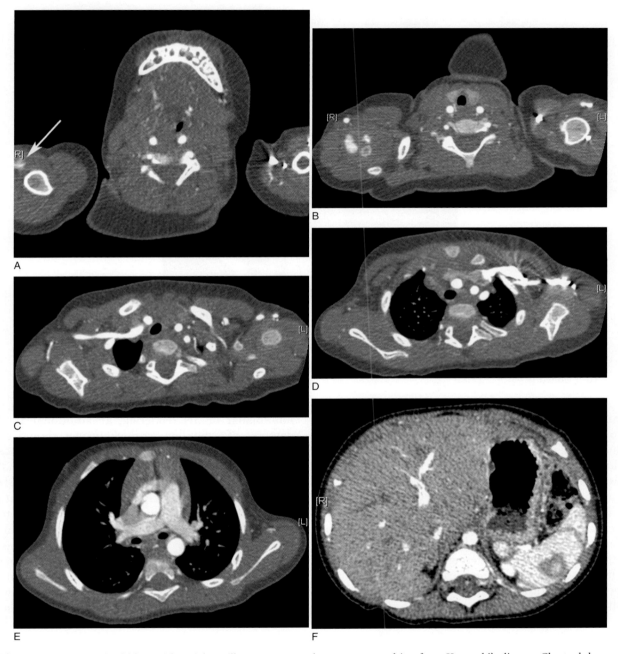

Fig. 10-9 A 14-month-old boy with a right axillary artery pseudoaneurysm resulting from Kawasaki's disease. Chest, abdomen, and pelvis CT angiogram was performed to survey for additional pseudoaneurysms and demonstrates excellent arterial enhancement (1.5 ml/kg IV contrast media) throughout the neck, chest, abdomen, and pelvis (**A-I**). Note slight expansion of axial artery (*arrow*) representing the inferior aspect of the pseudoaneurysm (**A**). Note absence of mediastinal fat (soft tissue in anterior mediastinum is normal thymus). No other pseudoaneurysms were present. Borrowed with permission from Springer.[31]

Continued

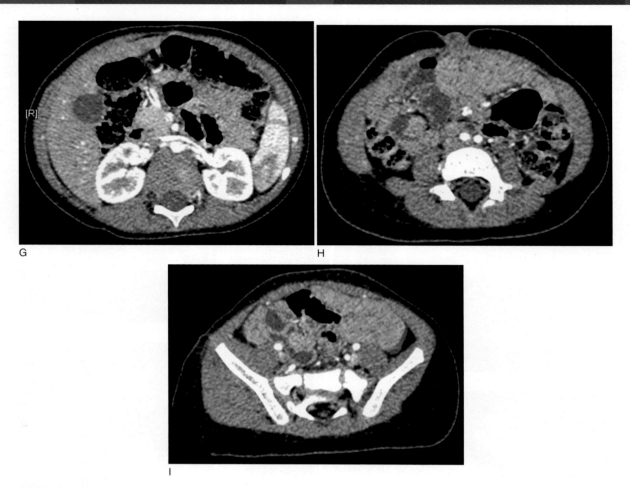

Fig. 10-9 Cont'd

parenchymal masses (especially bronchopulmonary foregut malformations), vascular abnormalities such as rings, and infectious and inflammatory conditions, examinations are most often performed using intravenous contrast media. For pectus excavatum, contrast is not necessary, and the tube current can be reduced from routine techniques by at least 50% (see Figure 10-3). Overlapping slices can be obtained for purposes of multiplanar reconstructions and 3D rendering, if required by the clinical service. Multiphase scanning (e.g., pre- and post-IV contrast media) is rarely necessary and should not be routine.

For airway evaluation, lower tube current (about 30% to 50% reduction from general chest techniques) and kVp (80 to 100) are appropriate. The smallest detector thickness (e.g., 0.625 with 16-slice CT) should be used. Axial image reconstruction can be displayed at 1.5 to 3.75 mm thickness with an interval of about 1.25 to 2.5 mm. For optimal

multiplanar or 3D rendering, an additional axial data set of submillimeter-thick images should be reconstructed at a thickness of 0.5 to 1.0 mm (see Figure 10-8). This will provide improved coronal (or sagittal, if necessary) reconstructions and 3D reformations. This principle of a second axial data set for improved quality rendering is identical to that of CT angiography (discussed later in this chapter). However, the tube current for angiographic evaluation should be higher. The higher tube current therefore should be used when combined assessment of the airway and adjacent arteries is indicated (e.g., in an evaluation of vascular rings and pulmonary artery sling).

Special Considerations for Pediatric Abdomen MSCT

For pediatric abdomen MSCT, multiphase evaluation should be performed only when justifiable. Despite the fact that up to about 30% of abdomen

However, this technique is far less protocol-driven than in adult patients and often requires individualized adjustments in scan technique. For example, since there is a great variation in the size and location of angiocatheters, the ability to provide a predictable onset and level of enhancement is limited. A more in-depth discussion of cardiothoracic CT angiographic techniques has recently been published.[31] Basically, for thoracic cardiovascular CTA, one must have an understanding of the clinical issues that need to be addressed. In addition, one needs to be familiar with the native or postoperative anatomy. For example, the presence of a Glenn (superior vena caval–right pulmonary artery) anastomosis and Fontan (inferior vena cava–left pulmonary artery) anastomosis would mean that the right and left lung would be opacified at different times and different levels depending on whether the administration was through an upper or lower torso vessel.[31] In addition, right-to-left shunts or admixture lesions would increase the chances of an embolic phenomenon into the systemic arterial system with contrast media administration if there is air in the line or syringe (see Figure 10-11).

Generally, 1.5 ml/kg contrast is sufficient for pediatric cardiovascular CT angiography. The thinnest detector configuration, providing the thinnest slice, is preferred. Tube current can be increased by about 30% over general chest or abdomen techniques because of the thinner slice selection. Kilovoltage, even for abdomen CT angiography, can be reduced, in line with that for general chest CT. This is because lower kilovoltage in young children provides increased image contrast. Although the amount of noise is also increased, the contrast-to-noise ratio may improve, considering the relatively greater improvement in image contrast. The rate of administration should be maximized, but even rates between 1.0 and 1.5 ml/sec in infants and young children are acceptable. Empiric delays for CT angiography are between 5 to 20 seconds after the onset of contrast administration. Given this wide range, it is sometimes helpful to use bolus-tracking technology. The tracking can be used during the administration of the contrast dose, with scanning beginning when the desired enhancement of the vessel is achieved. Alternatively, a test bolus may be administered to larger children and teenagers and is similar to that used for adults. In neonates, we have found that the onset of enhancement, particularly of thoracic cardiovascular structures, is often very quick (4 to 6 sec). Because of mandatory hardware delays on some bolus-tracking technology and the delay from the display of the monitoring image from the time the image is actually obtained, there may be an offset of 5 to 7 seconds from the displayed image and actual onset of scanning. In this case, optimal opacification, particularly of the pulmonary arterial system, may be missed. Because of the small volume of contrast for small neonates (i.e., 5.0 ml in a 2.5- to 3.0-kg [5.5- to 7-lb] infant), traditional test bolus amounts of 10 to 15 ml are excessive. A smaller test bolus of 0.5 to 1.0 ml in this population is helpful.[31] Using a higher iodine concentration (370 mg/ml) can provide a better enhancement of these smaller test boluses. To use this small test bolus technique, bolus tracking (using as low as 5 to 10 mAs for the monitoring phase images) is started with images displayed at 1.0-second intervals. When the first tracking image appears, the bolus is administered. The time between the first tracking image and the appearance of the contrast within the right or left ventricle is documented. This is the scan delay, which is used for diagnostic scanning. Further discussion of CT angiographic techniques and underlying principles can be found in the literature.[55]

CONCLUSION

Multislice technology is an extremely valuable modality for a variety of disorders in children. The use of MSCT is expanding. Part of this expansion is due to the unique benefits provided to the pediatric population, mainly faster scanning with thinner slices. The availability of an even greater number of detector rows (e.g., 64) will continue to improve pediatric scanning. However, the pediatric population offers unique challenges for MSCT. These include an increased susceptibility to radiation, an especially important issue when the radiation dose is inappropriately high. Care must be taken to properly balance the scan indications against the potential risks of CT. Once it is determined that a CT is an appropriate examination, the CT technique, including IV contrast administration as well as the individual CT parameters, should be adjusted based on the size of the child, the region (or organ) examined, and scan indication. A familiarity with issues such as radiation dose and special considerations for pediatric techniques will allow appropriate CT examinations to be performed, even in the most difficult and complex cases.

REFERENCES

1. Donnelly LF, Frush DP: Pediatric multidetector body CT, *Radiol Clin North Am* 41:637-655, 2003.
2. Frush DP, Donnelly LF: Helical CT in children: technical considerations and body applications, *Radiology* 209:37-48, 1998.
3. Cohen RA, Frush DP, Donnelly LF: Data acquisition for pediatric CT angiography: problems and solutions, *Pediatr Radiol* 30:813-822, 2000.
4. Frush DP: Pediatric CT: practical approach to diminish radiation dose, *Pediatr Radiol* 32(10):714-717, 2002.
5. Frush DP: Strategies of dose reduction, *Pediatr Radiol* 32:293-297, 2002.
6. Sternberg S: CT scans in children linked to cancer later, *USA Today*, January 22, 2001.
7. Slovis TL: Conference on the ALARA (as low as reasonably achievable) concept in pediatric CT: intelligent dose reduction, *Pediatr Radiol* 32:217-218, 2002.
8. Society for Pediatric Radiology and National Cancer Institute: Radiation and pediatric computed tomography: a guide for health care providers, 2002. www.pedrad.org, www.cancer.gov
9. Rogers LF: Taking care of children: check out the parameters used for helical CT, *Am J Roentgenol* 176:287, 2001.
10. Rogers LF: Low-dose CT: how are we doing? *Am J Roentgenol* 180:203, 2003.
11. Frush DP, Soden B, Frush KS, et al: Improved pediatric multidetector CT using a size-based color-coded format, *Am J Roentgenol* 178:721-726, 2002.
12. Paterson A, Frush DP, Donnelly LF: Helical CT of the body: are settings adjusted for pediatric patients? *Am J Roentgenol* 176:297-301, 2001.
13. Frush DP, Applegate K: Computed tomography and radiation: understanding the issues, *J Am Coll Radiol* 1:113-119, 2004.
14. Pappas JN, Donnelly LF, Frush DP: Marked reduction in the frequency of sedation of children using new multislice helical CT, *Radiology* 215:897-899, 2000.
15. Frush DP, Bisset GS, Hall SC: Pediatric sedation: The practice of safe sleep, *Am J Roentgenol* 167:1381-1387, 1996.
16. Cohen MD, Smith JA: Intravenous use of ionic and nonionic contrast agents in children, *Radiology* 191:793, 1994.
17. UNSCEAR 2000 Medical radiation exposures, annex D. United Nations Scientific Committee on the Effects of Atomic Radiation Report to the General Assembly; New York.
18. Mettler FA, Wiest PW, Locken JA, et al: CT scanning: patterns of use and dose, *J Radiol Prot* 20:353-359, 2000.
19. Brenner DJ: Estimating cancer risks from pediatric CT: going from the qualitative to the quantitative, *Pediatr Radiol* 32:228-231, 2002.
20. Brenner DJ, Elliston CD, Hall EJ, et al: Estimated risks of radiation-induced fatal cancer from pediatric CT, *Am J Roentgenol* 176:289-296, 2001.
21. Pierce DA, Shimizu Y, Preston DL, et al: Studies of the mortality of atomic bomb survivors. Report 12, part 1, Cancer. 1950-1990, *Radiat Res* 146:1-27, 1996.
22. Frush DP: Practical approach to manage radiation exposure. In Carty H, Brunelle F, Stringer D, Kao S: *Pediatric Imaging*, ed 2. Philadelphia: Elsevier Churchill Livingstone, 2005.
23. Donnelly LF, Emery KH, Brody AS, et al: Minimizing radiation dose for pediatric body applications of single-detector helical CT, *Am J Roentgenol* 176:303-306, 2001.
24. Hollingsworth CL, Frush DP, Cross M, et al: Helical CT of the body: a survey of techniques used for pediatric patients, *Am J Roentgenol* 180:401-406, 2003.
25. Lee CI, Haims AH, Monico EP, et al: Diagnostic CT scans: assessment of patient, physician, and radiologist awareness of radiation dose and possible risks, *Radiology* 231:393-398, 2004.
26. Brenner DJ, Doll R, Goodhead DT, et al: Cancer risks attributable to low doses of ionizing radiation: assessing what we really know, Proc *Natl Acad Sci USA* 100:13761-13766, 2003.
27. Cohen BC: Cancer risk from low level radiation, *Am J Roentgenol* 179:1137-1143, 2002.
28. Cameron JR: Longevity is the most appropriate measure of health effects of radiation, *Radiology* 229:14-15, 2003.
29. Wagner LK: The "healthy worker effect": science or prejudice? *Radiology* 229:16-17, 2003.
30. Hall EJ, Brenner DJ: The weight of evidence does not support the suggestion that exposure to low doses of x-rays increases longevity, *Radiology* 229:18-19, 2003.
31. Frush DP, Herlong JR: Pediatric CT angiography, *Pediatr Radiol* 35:11-25, 2005.
32. Donnelly LF: Commentary: oral contrast medium administration for abdominal CT–reevaluating the benefits and disadvantages in the pediatric patient, *Pediatr Radiol* 27:770, 1997.
33. Rogalla P, Stover B, Scheer I, et al: Low-dose spiral CT: applicability to paediatric chest imaging, *Pediatr Radiol* 28:565-569, 1998.
34. Lucaya J, Piqueras J, Garcia-Peña P, et al: Low-dose high-resolution CT of the chest in children and young adults: dose, cooperation, artifact incidence, and image quality, *Am J Roentgenol* 175:985-992, 2000.
35. Ambrosino MM, Genieser NB, Roche KJ, et al: Feasibility of high-resolution, low-dose chest CT in evaluating the pediatric chest, *Pediatr Radiol* 24:6-10, 1994.
36. Ambrosino MM, Roche KJ, Genieser NB, et al: Application of thin-section low-dose chest CT (TSCT) in the management of pediatric AIDS, *Pediatr Radiol* 25:393-400, 1995.
37. Frush DP, Slack CC, Hollingsworth CL, et al: Computer simulated radiation dose reduction for abdominal multidetector CT of pediatric patients, *Am J Roentgenol* 179(5):1107-1113, 2002.
38. Cohen MD, Smith JA: Intravenous use of ionic and nonionic contrast agents in children, *Radiology* 191:793-794, 1994.
39. Frush DP: Pediatric helical CT: techniques and applications, *Worldwide Radiol J* 9:17, 1999.
40. Kaste SC, Young CW: Safe use of power injectors with central and peripheral venous access devices for pediatric CT, *Pediatr Radiol* 26:499, 1996.
41. Herts BR, O'Malley CM, Wirth SL, et al: Power injection of contrast media using central venous catheters: feasibility, safety and efficacy, *Am J Roentgenol* 176:447-453, 2001.
42. Nelson RC, Anderson FA Jr, Birnbaum BA, et al: Contrast media extravasation during dynamic CT: detection with an extravasation detection accessory, *Radiology* 209:837-843, 1998.
43. Frush DP, Spencer EB, Donnelly LF, et al: Optimizing contrast-enhanced abdominal CT in infants and children using bolus tracking, *Am J Roentgenol* 172:1007, 1999.

44. Frush DP, Donnelly LF, Bisset GS: Technical innovation: effect of scan delay on hepatic enhancement for pediatric abdominal multislice helical CT, *Am J Roentgenol* 176: 1559-1561, 2001.

45. McNitt-Gray MF: AAPM/RSNA physics tutorial for residents: topics in CT: radiation dose in CT, *Radiographics* 22:1541-1553, 2002.

46. Rydberg J, Liang Y, Teague SD: Fundamentals of multichannel CT, *Radiol Clin North Am* 41:465-474, 2003.

47. Sigal-Cinqualbre AB, Hennequin R, Abada HT, et al: Low-kilovoltage multi–detector row chest CT in adults: feasibility and effect on image quality and iodine dose, *Radiology* 231:169-174, 2004.

48. Vade A, Demos TC, Olson MC, et al: Evaluation of image quality using 1:1 pitch and 1.5:1 pitch helical CT in children: a comparative study, *Pediatr Radiol* 26:891-893, 1996.

49. Vade A, Olson MC, Vittore CP, et al: Hepatic enhancement analysis in children using Smart Prep monitoring for 2:1 pitch helical scanning, *Pediatr Radiol* 29:689-693, 1999.

50. Frush DP, Donnelly LF, Chotas HG: Contemporary pediatric thoracic imaging, *Am J Roentgenol* 175(3):841-851, 2000.

51. Denecke T, Frush DP, Li J: Eight-channel multidetector CT: unique potential for pediatric chest CT, *J Thorac Imaging* 17:306-309, 2002.

52. Coakley FV, Cohen MD, Johnson MS, et al: Effect of breathing on the detection of in vivo simulated pulmonary nodules by spiral CT, *Clin Radiol* 53:506-509, 1998.

53. Long FR, Castile RG, Brody AS, et al: Lungs in infants and young children: improved thin-section computed tomography with a noninvasive controlled-ventilation technique: initial experience, *Radiology* 212:588-593, 1999.

54. Siegel MS: Multiplanar and three-dimensional multidetector row CT of thoracic vessels and airways in the pediatric population, *Radiology* 229:641-650, 2003.

55. Fleischmann D: Use of high-concentration contrast media in multiple-detector-row CT: principles and rationale, *Eur Radiol* 13 (suppl)5:M14-20, 2003.

Body Computed Tomography Angiography and Contrast Administration Issues

Friedrich Knollmann

INDICATIONS FOR BODY CT ANGIOGRAPHY

Computed tomography (CT) is now used for practically all vascular diseases in which imaging is indicated and has virtually replaced conventional angiography because of its noninvasive properties. The most common applications include aortic disease, such as aortic aneurysms and aortic dissection, atherosclerotic arterial disease of the renal and mesenteric arteries, and presurgical imaging of arteries (e.g., in living renal and hepatic transplant donors). CT angiography (CTA) in trauma patients, patients with hepatic or pancreatic disease, peripheral CTA, cardiac or neurovascular disease, and pulmonary embolism are discussed in their respective chapters.

Upon review of published guidelines available through the National Guideline Clearinghouse (www.guideline.gov), 46 entries could be found for the key word *CT angiography* as of November 2004. These 46 entries concerned cardiac disorders (11 entries), neurovascular disease (7), trauma (5), pulmonary embolism (3), tumor staging (3), chest pain (3), and peripheral artery disease (2). Since evidence-based guidelines depend on the literature review at the time of publication, the most recent technological advances are typically not considered, and clinical practice may significantly deviate from the guidelines as a result. The lack of high-level evidence for the benefits of multislice CT (MSCT) can be illustrated for body applications in the case of aortic dissection. The National Guideline Clearinghouse offers guidelines for the diagnosis and management of aortic dissection issued by the European Society of Cardiology as the most recent guideline in November 2004, which is based on a review of the literature from 2001. In this guideline, CT is described as the most commonly used technique for diagnosing aortic dissection, but limitations are noted in comparison to a greater sensitivity and specificity of MRI (100% versus 90% and 85% for CT). This assessment has its roots in a study that used helical CT technique in only a fraction of cases.[1] In addition, the temporal resolution of the CT methods in this study was much less than what is available today, not to mention the option of EKG gating, which has since been made available.

In the review just discussed, the advances of MSCT are not even mentioned or distinguished from the results of the single detector row method. Therefore, to fully appreciate the potential of MSCT, one has to directly review the latest journal articles in the field. Even there, the diagnostic benefit of MSCT over single-row CT is quite difficult to document, although the method is obviously much better suited for diagnosing aortic dissection than single-row CT. It becomes obvious that evidence-based analyses fail to reveal the expected clinical benefits of MSCT at this time. Such comparative evidence may actually never become available, since manufacturers have started to phase out the development and distribution of single-row detector imagers.

Although there is an apparent lack of evidence, we do not believe that we need formal proof of the obvious improvements offered by MSCT and see little use in trying to prove its benefits by clinical comparisons to former diagnostic standards. With modern 16-row detector scanners, imaging time has been reduced dramatically while gaining z-axis spatial resolution at the same time. The faster examination speed eliminates motion artifact, particularly breathing artifacts, which are unavoidable at scan times of more than 20 seconds. The other advantage of a short exam time is that optimal intraarterial contrast can be maintained throughout the exam.

MSCT protocol options for contrast administration are reviewed in Table 11-1.

Oral Contrast Media

As compared with single row detector CT, few specifics apply for oral contrast media. Three different types of contrast are used, almost exclusively for abdominal imaging: barium-based formulations, iodinated ionic contrast agents, and water-based agents (so-called *negative contrast agents* with water attenuation). For angiographic MSCT applications, it is important to avoid radiopaque oral contrast materials, which obstruct the view of the vasculature in three-dimensional reconstructions. Therefore, we increasingly use hyperosmotic, watery contrast agents for abdominal MSCT applications, in particular for the workup of upper abdominal disease. Others have used plain tap water for this purpose. The advantage of a hyperosmotic watery solution is that the agent is not absorbed by the upper GI tract and thus remains effective over a longer passage through the digestive tract. Pancreatic cancer is one important application in which the use of radiopaque oral contrast agents has been abandoned.

The timing of oral intake is important and depends on where the suspected disease is assumed to be located. For colonic disease, retrograde air insufflation is preferred and allows the reconstruction of virtual colonoscopy images. For the assessment of retroperitoneal lymph nodes, radiopaque contrast is administered orally, ideally at least 1 hour before the scan, with the last 200 ml taken immediately before the patient is placed on the CT couch.

Intravenous Contrast Media

Iodine concentration

In Europe, nonionic IV contrast agents with iodine concentrations of 370 to 400 mg/ml are broadly available, and some authors have argued that such agents are better suited for MSCT applications than lower-concentration agents. The logic behind such recommendations is usually a comparison of two agents given at the same total injection volume. Since the higher concentrated agent involves a greater total amount of iodine in such a comparison, it is not surprising that the higher concentration results in a stronger contrast effect. This result

Table 11-1   Body CTA protocol

Indication	Patient with aortic or arterial disease, protocol is adapted to exact problem
Protocol designed for (scanner type)	LightSpeed 16 Pro
Patient preparation	Informed consent obtained for contrast administration
Oral contrast	—
IV contrast administration	Iomeprol, 400 mg I/ml
Volume/injection rate/delay	1. 90-120 ml / 3.5 ml/sec / bolus tracking 2. Saline chaser 40 ml / 3.5 ml/sec / starts upon completion of contrast injection
Tube settings	
kV	120
mA	320, tube current modulation ("automA, smartmA"), noise index = 12, max = 320 mA, min = 100 mA
Detector configuration	16*1.25 mm
Gantry speed (sec)	0.5
Table speed	17.5 mm/rotation
Reconstructed slice thickness	3.75 mm, no overlap, and 1.25 mm with 0.8 mm increment for 3D processing
Anatomical coverage	Jugular crest–pelvic floor
Reconstruction kernel	Standard
Breath hold	Inspiration
Window settings	900/80

Postprocessing	Depending on exact clinical context, volume rendering for visualization of
	    pathological findings and anatomy
	Other Additional image reconstruction series according to the discretion of
	    the attending radiologist

Typical dose	CTDI = 15 mGy, DLP = 438 mGycm at 70 cm scan length

is not caused by the contrast concentration, however, and can be compensated for by a higher injection rate on the side of the lesser-concentrated agent. Typically, the contrast effectiveness is determined by the iodine delivery rate (IDR), which is the amount of iodine administered within 1 second, and is dependent on both the flow rate of the contrast solution and its iodine concentration.

The maximal flow rate, in turn, depends on the size of the venous cannula, vascular resistance, and independent factors such as contrast viscosity and maximum injection pressure. Since increases in iodine concentration for a given agent result in a markedly elevated viscosity, the IDR does not increase with higher concentrated agents.

In an experimental setting, the highest achievable injection rates for different contrast agents were tested under defined conditions, using a plastic IV line as a mock vein system and commercially available IV cannulae. For this experiment, the injection pressure was limited to 21 bar, and the microprocessor-controlled injection pump discontinued the injection at higher pressure. Injection rates of 4, 5, 6, and 8 ml/sec were tested in four consecutive trials (Figures 11-1 to 11-4).

According to these measurements, the limited injection pressure led to aborted injections at higher flow rates for the higher concentrated agents, and the maximum iodine delivery rate was achieved with less-concentrated agents.[2]

Timing of the Data Acquisition

For arterial CT angiograms, the interindividual variability of the ideal scan start time is a significant

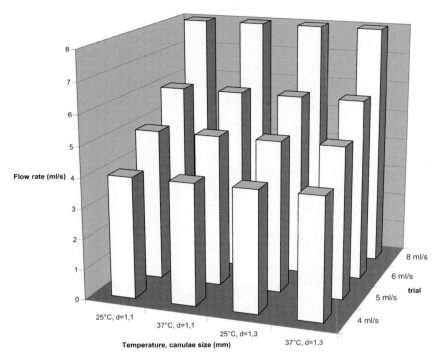

Fig. 11-1 Maximal injection rates achieved for iopromide 300. All injection trials were completed at the designated flow rate.

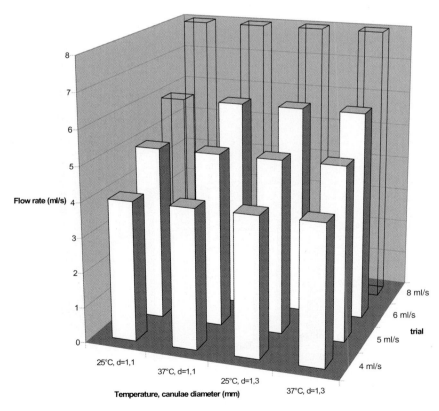

Fig. 11-2 Maximal injection rates achieved for iopromide 370. At higher injection rates, the injection was prematurely stopped because the pressure limits were exceeded *(transparent boxes).*

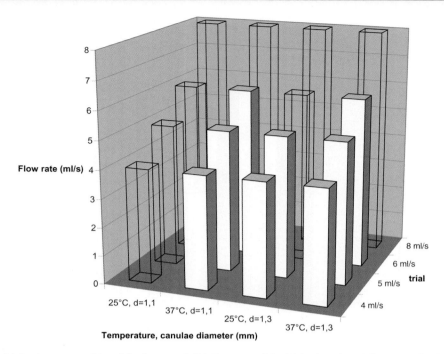

Fig. 11-3 Maximal injection rates achieved for iomeprol 400. Because of the high viscosity of the agent, the injection failed at the smallest cannula size and with the agent at room temperature.

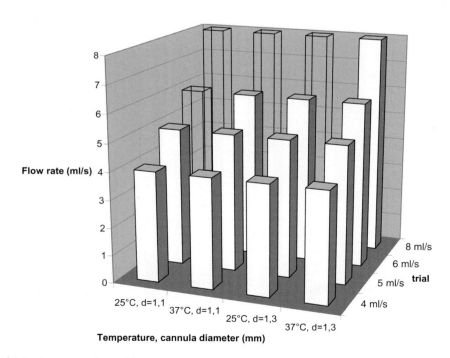

Fig. 11-4 Maximal injection rates achieved for iodixanol 320.

factor. For an individually optimized scan start time, two approaches are possible: injection of a small amount of contrast agent, and repeated scans over a predefined period to determine the time until peak enhancement in the arterial territory. This is then used as the scan delay in a subsequent contrast injection of a larger contrast volume, or a bolus tracking method, which performs repeated scans until significant contrast enhancement is observed in the arterial territory followed by an automated scan initiation (Figure 11-5).

With MSCT, the bolus tracking method is now used for most arterial angiograms, except for applications in which a test injection is performed for perfusion imaging anyway, such as in stroke protocols.

With the bolus tracking method, the onset of contrast enhancement can be individually captured to trigger the diagnostic CTA series. The duration and time course of contrast enhancement, however, are to be determined before the bolus tracking series begins and cannot be adjusted afterward. Obviously, the contrast injection period should not exceed the data acquisition time, since the contrast volume injected after data acquisition would not contribute to image contrast at all. Since the scan duration depends on the anatomical examination volume and table speed, and the time from the injection start to scan start varies, the optimal injection protocol should also vary between individuals. Therefore, it is important to devise scan protocols that result in a sufficiently long duration of contrast effect, which raises the question of how much contrast enhancement is sought (Figure 11-6).

A comparison of intraarterial attenuation with visual estimates of contrast quality indicates a good agreement (Figures 11-7 and 11-8).

One conclusion from the visual assessment of arterial contrast quality is that with an intraluminal attenuation of greater than 280 HU, not 5% of images were rated as less than satisfactory.

The test bolus technique offers the advantage of tailoring not only the onset of data acquisition to the individual contrast effectiveness, but also of adjusting the contrast injection rate and total volume to the individual by using a pharmacokinetic simulation technique (Topfit, G. Fischer, Stuttgart) (Figures 11-9 and 11-10).

With 16-row MSCT, practically all examinations are completed in less than 20 seconds. Thus the amount of contrast agent does not limit image quality. Usually, 200 ml is regarded as the upper limit of permissible contrast volume for an

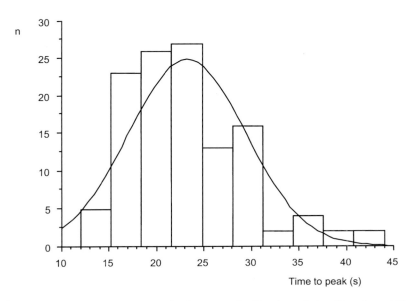

Fig. 11-5 Variability of the time-to-contrast appearance in the aorta of a 20-ml test bolus. Data from 138 patients.

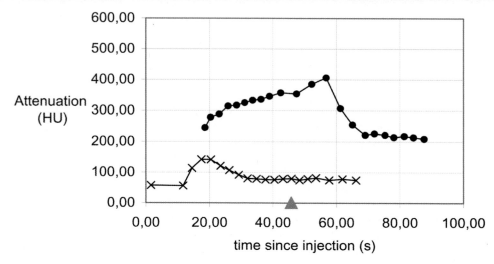

Fig. 11-6 Time course of arterial contrast enhancement following a test bolus (*crossed line*; 40 ml iopromide, 370 mg I/ml) and a diagnostic contrast bolus (*circles*; 150 ml iopromide).

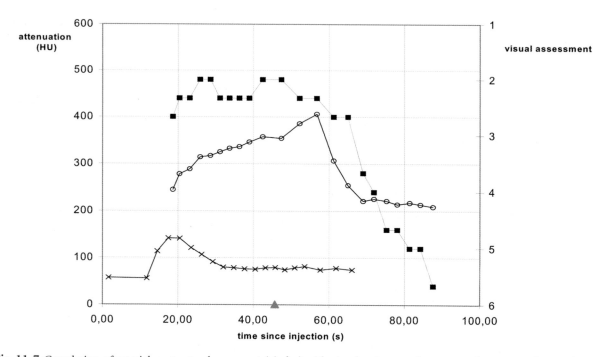

Fig. 11-7 Correlation of arterial contrast enhancement (circles) with visual estimates of contrast enhancement (squares).

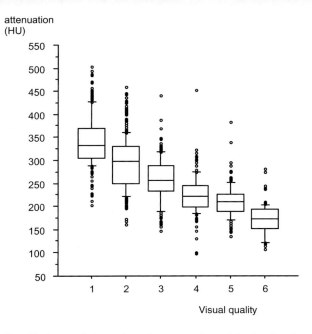

attenuation
(HU)

Visual quality

Fig. 11-8 Correlation of aortic attenuation with visual estimates of contrast enhancement quality from 36 electron beam CT examinations. *1* indicates best image quality; *6* indicates worst image quality.

individual adult patient. With 16-row MSCT, seldom is more than a 100 ml bolus required, which has led to significant contrast agent savings.

Although the individual test bolus technique can be used to tailor an optimal injection protocol to each patient, the approach is too time consuming to be practical at the moment. Because of the short acquisition period in MSCT, dual-phase contrast injections with an early fast injection followed by a slower maintenance injection rate are not necessary to obtain consistently good image quality. It has proved sufficient to empirically select a contrast volume that will safely allow complete contrast enhancement of the arterial system during the typical exam period with a generous "reserve" volume for delayed contrast circulation in some individuals, and then to use a bolus-tracking technique. Also, each contrast volume can be reduced by 20 to 40 ml per injection by using a saline flush with the same flow rate as the initial contrast injection.

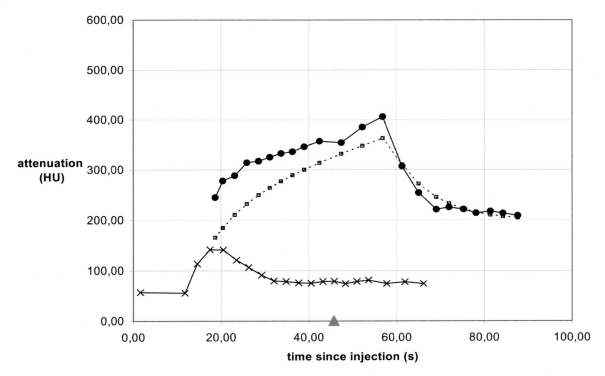

attenuation
(HU)

time since injection (s)

Fig. 11-9 Comparison of predicted attenuation with measured results. Measured aortic attenuation after test bolus injection *(crossed line)*. These data were entered into the pharmacological simulation model. Predicted aortic attenuation for a 150-ml bolus of iopromide, injected at 3.5 ml/sec *(dotted line)*. Measured attenuation following the injection of the same protocol *(solid line)*. The measured aortic attenuation closely follows the predicted attenuation.

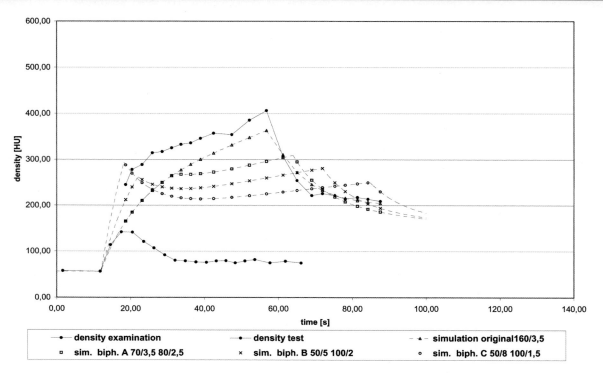

Fig. 11-10 Simulation of the effect of biphasic contrast injection for a 160-ml volume of iopromide, based on a test bolus injection. Contrast protocols are given as volume (ml)/flow rate (ml/sec) for each phase.

AORTIC MSCT

The general MSCT protocol presented at the beginning of this chapter offers a complete diagnosis of the entire aorta, including the supraaortic branches and the iliac arteries. The most important indications include aortic dissection and aortic aneurysms. The clinical setting for diagnosing aortic dissection typically includes patients who present with an episode of acute chest pain, and differential diagnoses include myocardial infarction, pulmonary embolism, and aortic dissection. All three diagnoses can be approached with MSCT, although the differential diagnosis of myocardial infarction is typically addressed by EKG and laboratory tests. Pulmonary embolism is discussed in a separate chapter, and aortic dissection will therefore be the focus of this discussion.

Rationale

In aortic imaging, aortic diameter measurements and an analysis of aortic wall morphology are the primary concerns. In a simplified approach, the normal aortic diameter is no greater than 30 mm, and a diameter of greater than 50 mm is generally considered an indication for intervention. In one recent investigation,[3] it has been shown that surgical repair of abdominal aortic aneurysms does not yield any survival benefit in aneuryms of less than 5.5 cm. However, the measurement of aortic diameters is based on in vivo experience with single detector row CT, and often the diameter of the aorta can be overestimated if the largest axial diameter is measured, since curved sections of the aorta result in axial images that contain an oblique section of the vessel. With high-resolution CT techniques and postprocessing tools that allow reconstructions of the aorta along its longitudinal axis, cross-sections that are truly perpendicular to the aortic axis can be obtained. If no such tools are available, an approximation can be achieved by measuring the shorter axial diameter of the aorta in sections of the aorta that run in an oblique orientation to the axial plane. Even with the sophisticated vessel tracking tools, care needs to be taken to consider intraluminal thrombus, since postprocessing software tools tend to track the contrast–medium-filled lumen of the aorta only. The decision to operate on patients with an aortic aneurysm is based on less-sophisticated image analysis, and the potential benefit of a more accurate analysis remains to be established. This fact can be viewed as the main reason that the more elaborate method has not become the standard of clinical care in most institutions. With the advent of endovascular graft repair of aneurysms, however, the necessity of a more exact preinterventional measurement has made such postprocessing methods necessary, since the endovascular prosthesis must fit perfectly to prevent complications such as an endoleakage. Since the three-dimensional curved reformat procedure is greatly facilitated by almost isotropic voxel size, MSCT has gained an important advantage over MRI in this indication and is now used as the standard of care.

Parameter Choice

Tube voltage of 120 kV has the advantage of a 20% dose savings over 140 kV, while being closer to the ideal voltage for the effectiveness of iodinated contrast agents. Even lower voltages, however, would lead to unacceptable loss of image quality in adults. To adapt tube current to image quality requirements, tube current modulation is now available on many recent scanner types.[4] With the generic autoMA modulation used on GE LightSpeed scanners, tube current is adapted to estimated body attenution, wihch is estimated from a scout scan. If more than a single scout is used, dose modulation uses the last scout scan. Then, the software predicts the tube current that will be necessary to obtain a certain noise level for the first selected reconstruction slice thickness. The latter condition is important, since different initial slice thickness selections would result in very different tube current selections. Empirically, a "noise index" of 12 has been found to consistently yield diagnostic image quality with an initial slice thickness of 3.75 mm. This slice thickness can still be used for film documentation in an environment without complete PACS coverage and without excessive print numbers, while most important image details are documented. Using tube current modulation as a dose-saving method, the upper limit is set at 320 mA to avoid the selected noise level leading to a higher effective radiation dose than with a fixed tube current in obese patients, while the lower limit of 100 mA keeps mediastinal image noise at an acceptable level throughout the examination.

Image Interpretation

Although three-dimensional volume-rendering techniques are excellent tools for visually conferring a diagnosis, a review of axial or reformatted images is still necessary to exclude rupture of an aortic aneurysm (Figure 11-11).

Despite the attractiveness of the volume-rendered images, these renderings do not reveal that the aneurym has ruptured, and if used as the sole source of imaging diagnosis, would thus hide the immediate urgency for surgery (Figures 11-12 to 11-15).

For an assessment of aortic wall morphology, including the diagnosis of aortic dissection, review of the axial images is the preferred mode of diagnosis, since MIP and volume-rendering reconstructions as projection methods obscure the cross-sectional vessel wall anatomy (Figure 11-16, A).

Despite EKG gating, a double contour was detected at the dorsal aspect of the aortic root. Although this was not considered to indicate type A dissection, such motion artifacts can make it impossible to clearly rule out local dissection (Figure 11-16, B-D).

Minor artifacts may remain visible in patients in whom the heart rate often cannot be reduced to an extent that would be deemed ideal for artifact-free cardiac CT (Figure 11-17, A).

Intramural aortic hematoma presents as a thickening of the aortic wall with blood attenuation. Although some recommend a precontrast exam of the entire aorta to rule out such lesions, there is little evidence that such lesions cannot be reliably diagnosed with the contrast-enhanced series in a thin-slice MSCT study alone (Figure 11-17, B).

RENAL ARTERY IMAGING

Renal artery CTA can be considered exemplary for body CTA. A review of the literature reveals 42 citations in the PubMed database of the National Library of Medicine (as of November 2004) for the search term *renal arteries CTA*. However, there are no formal comparisons of MSCT with the

Text continued on p. 216

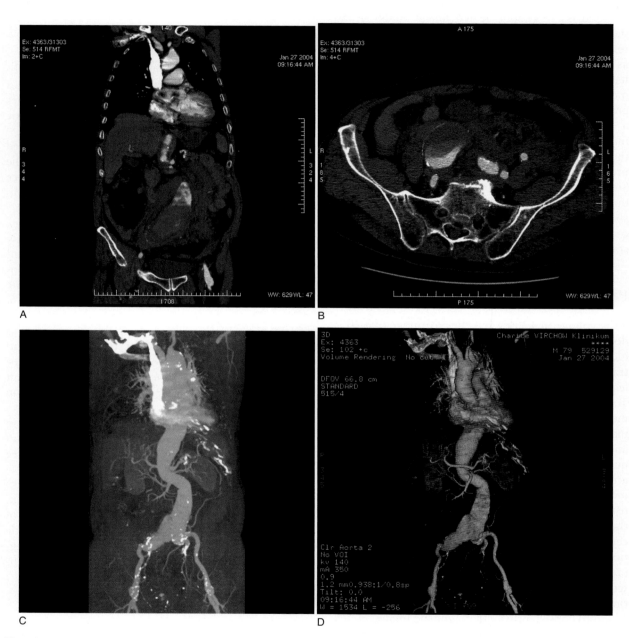

Fig. 11-11 A, Coronal reformat of an aortic series demonstrates periaortic hemorrhage as an indicator of a ruptured aneurysm. **B,** In the axial plane, the extent of intraabdominal hemorrhage is also evident. **C,** Upon 3D postprocessing, the extent of the aneurysm is visualized impressively in an MIP reconstruction after automatic elimination of bony structures (autoBone feature, Advantage Windows workstation, GE Medical Systems). **D,** Volume rendering also impressively depicts aortic anatomy, including the major arterial branches. In this instance, the involvement of the iliac arteries was an important feature for surgical planning.

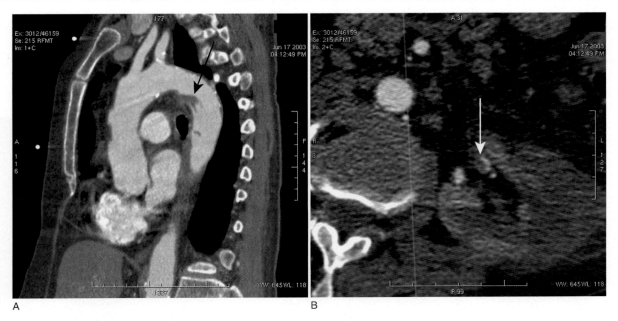

A   B

Fig. 11-12 A, As in Figure 11-11, MIP and volume-rendering techniques would not display intraaortic thrombi *(arrow)*, as in another patient **(B)**. Emboli have caused renal infarction, and an embolus *(arrow)* is detected in a major renal artery branch in the renal hilum.

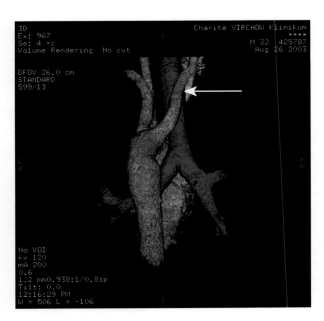

Fig. 11-13 Volume rendering is important in the visualization of anatomical variations, as in this patient with an arteria lusoria *(arrow)*. The arteria lusoria is a right subclavian artery that leaves the aortic arch as the last supraaortic branch and thus forms a sling running dorsal to the esophagus and the trachea *(red)*. In patients requiring surgery, it is important to note and communicate this abnormality. Color-coded volume-rendering reconstructions have found broad acceptance by vascular surgeons.

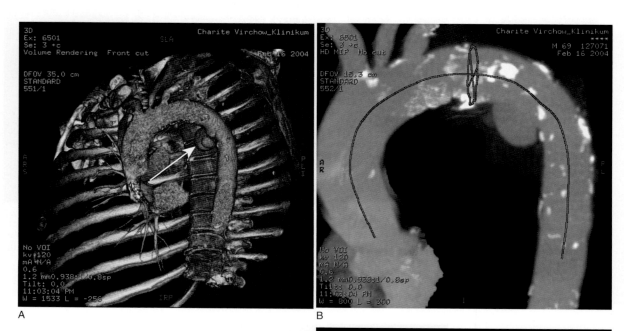

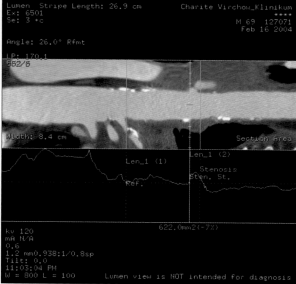

Fig. 11-14 A, For the planning of endovascular procedures, 3D renderings have become essential. In this instance, a ruptured atherosclerotic aneurysm *(arrow)* of the aortic arch needed to be repaired. **B-C,** To determine the length of an endovascular prosthesis, the distance from the aneurysm neck (marked green as "Len_1(2)") to the supraaortic arteries (marked green as "Len_1(1)") had to be determined. This is greatly facilitated by automatic determination of the aortic center line, followed by a curved reformat of the aorta. By using this method, the required length of an endovascular prosthesis of the aortic arch can be determined with great accuracy.

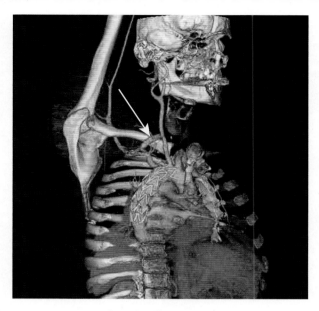

Fig. 11-15 When the subclavian artery ostium is "sacrificed" in favor of the endovascular repair option, it is important to determine the exact location of the left carotid artery to avoid fatal neurovascular complications. In our index case, a carotid-subclavian artery bypass *(arrow)* was used afterward to treat arm ischemia in a patient who was treated by endovascular repair of a type B aortic dissection.

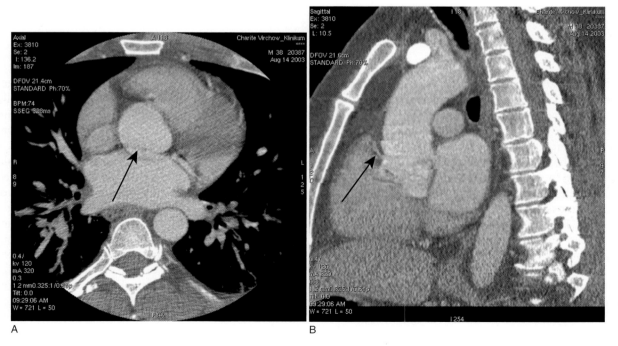

A   B

Fig. 11-16 A, In patients with acute-onset chest pain, motion artifacts *(arrow)* in the aortic root commonly make it difficult to rule out type A aortic dissection in images without EKG gating (or even with EKG gating), if the reconstruction time is not optimized. Thus, to rule out type A dissection, an EKG-gated protocol is recommended, as discussed in Chapter 6. **B,** A hint of motion artifacts *(arrow)* as the cause of the double contour is evident upon coronal reformat reconstruction.

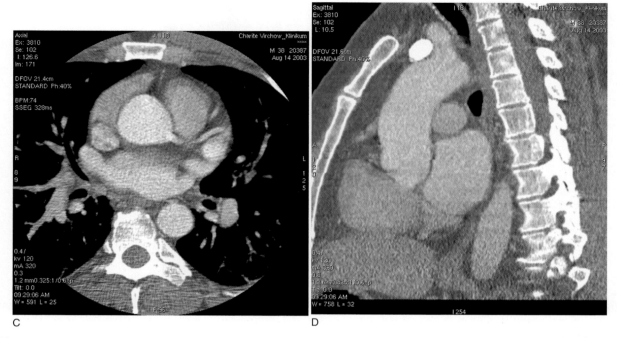

Fig. 11-16 cont'd **C,** Upon reconstruction at an earlier time, 40% of the RR-interval, the double contour disappeared. **D,** Even at that time, however, minor motion artifacts remained visible in the sagittal reformat.

traditional gold standard, CTA, for diagnosing renal artery stenosis, and the only pertinent references for a comparison with conventional angiography concern the evaluation of living renal donors.[5] For detecting accessory renal arteries, MSCT has been found to be equivalent to conventional angiography according to these data. There is evidence, however, that single-row CT is a capable diagnostic method for diagnosing renal artery stenosis.[6-8] Single-slice spiral CT of the renal arteries is limited by a 2- or 3-mm slice thickness, maximal tube load that may limit the scan length, and scan duration. Even so, the test qualities of single-detector row CTA for detecting high-grade renal stenoses have been reported as more than 90%. The formal evidence that MSCT is better than either single-row CTA or conventional angiography remains limited at this time. Formal evidence regarding the use of single-row CTA for the preoperative depiction of renal vasculature and the detection of lumbar veins is incomplete[9] (Figures 11-18 to 11-20).

The color-coded, volume-rendered images convey a more realistic view, which is generally greatly appreciated by the referring clinician and makes explaining a diagnosis to the patient more convincing.

As a rule of thumb, the CT slice thickness should not exceed the diameter of the smallest target vessel, since even with overlapping reconstruction, thicker slices may not be able to effectively depict the target vessel or a stenotic target vessel. Thus, for a complete analysis of accessory renal arteries, 1.25-mm slice thickness is recommended. Accordingly, sub-millimeter slices may add even smaller vascular details, although the clinical impact of the additional detail remains to be investigated.

It may be concluded that despite incomplete formal numbers on the superiority of MSCT angiographic diagnosis over single-row CTA, the benefit of high spatial resolution, fast scan acquisition, and complete anatomical coverage for CTA applications is clinically obvious.

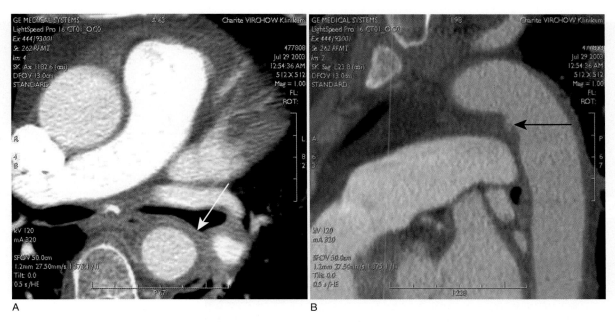

Fig. 11-17 A, Although the diagnosis of frank dissection has its own complications, another important diagnosis is that of an aortic wall hematoma *(arrow),* which is today considered a precursor or equivalent of frank dissection. **B,** Sometimes an atherosclerotic ulceration *(arrow)* can be seen as the cause of aortic wall hematoma. In addition to visualization of dissection or a precursor lesion, MSCT offers a complete diagnosis of ischemic complications. Although dissection of the ascending aorta is an established indication for surgical repair, dissection of the distal aorta can often be treated without surgery, unless ischemic complications make surgical intervention necessary. Such complications include progressive widening of the thoracic aorta, progressive hemorrhagic pleural effusions, renal or mesenteric ischemia, or lower extremity ischemia. Endovascular treatment of such complications is increasingly used, particularly in older patients with a high surgical risk. Endovascular procedures such as aortic stenting and fenestration of the dissection membrane (alone or in combination with stenting of the main aortic branches) is greatly facilitated by a complete aortic CT-angiogram.

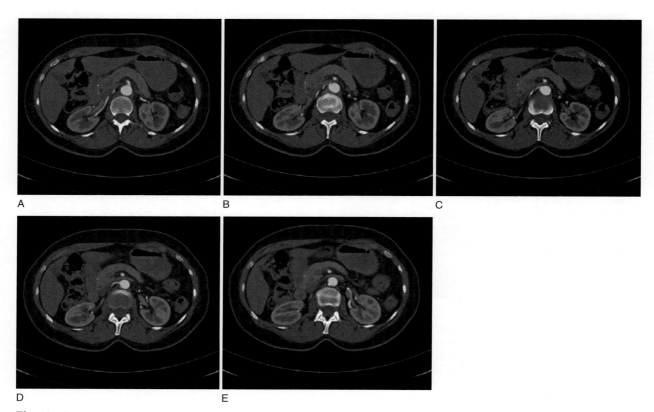

Fig. 11-18 A-E, Simple clinical examples can demonstrate the advantages of MSCT. In a living renal donor, MSCT was performed to determine renal artery anatomy. With a single-slice CT image, the smallest realistic slice thickness for renal artery imaging would amount to 3 mm. Upon review of the 3-mm slices, both renal arteries were nicely depicted, and no abnormality was noted.

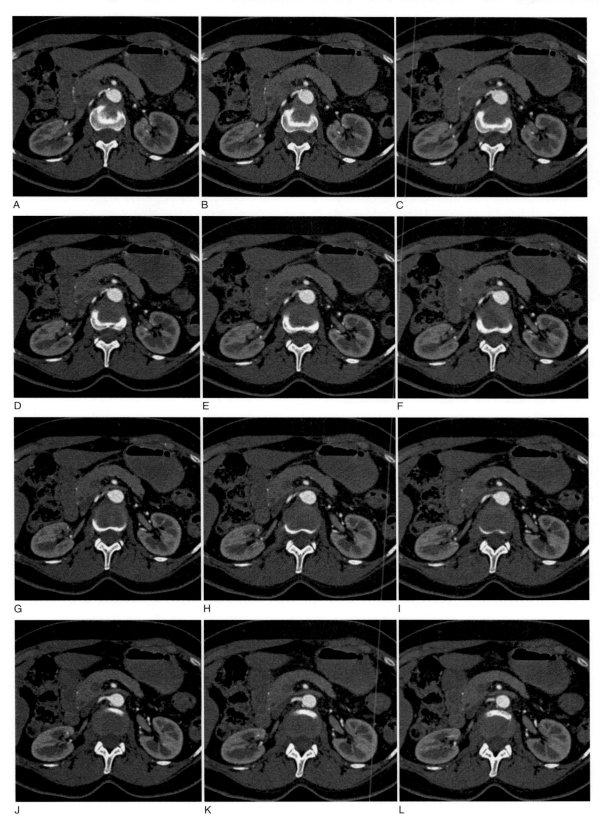

Fig. 11-19 Upon review of the 1.25-mm slices, which were reconstructed from the same helical raw data set using a 50% overlap, second thoughts arose, because the right renal artery seemed to have either two ostia, or was disturbed by respiratory artifact.

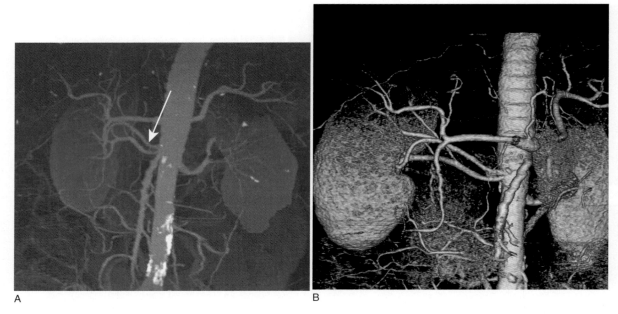

A   B

Fig. 11-20 A, To resolve the dilemma presented in Figure 11-19, a 3D MIP reconstruction of the renal arteries was performed, which clearly documented the presence of an accessory right renal artery *(arrow).* **B,** Volume-rendering reconstruction provides an even more impressive depiction.

REFERENCES

1. Nienaber CA, von Kodolitsch Y, Nicholas V, et al: The diagnosis of thoracic aortic dissection by noninvasive imaging procedures, *N Engl J Med* 328:1–9, 1993.
2. Knollmann F, Schimpf K, Felix R: Iodine delivery rate of different concentrations of iodine-containing contrast agents with rapid injection, *Fortschr Roentgenstr* 176:880–884, 2004.
3. Lederle FA, Wilson SE, et al: Immediate repair compared with surveillance of small abdominal aortic aneurysms, *N Engl J Med* 346:1437–1444, 2002.
4. Kalra MK, Maher MM, Toth TL, et al: Techniques and applications of automatic tube current modulation for CT, *Radiology* 233:649–657, 2004.
5. Kapoor A, Kapoor A, Mahajan G, et al: Multispiral computed tomographic angiography of renal arteries of live potential renal donors: a review of 118 cases, *Transplantation* 77:1535–1539, 2004.
6. Galanski M, Prokop A, Chavan A, et al: Renal artery stenosis: spiral CT angiography, *Radiology* 189:185–192, 1993.
7. Wittenberg G, Kenn W, Tschammler A, et al: Spiral CT angiography of renal arteries: comparison with angiography, *Eur Radiol* 9:546–551, 1999.
8. Kim TS, Chung JW, Park JH, et al: Renal artery evaluation: comparison of spiral CT angiography to intra-arterial DAS, *J Vasc Intervent Radiol* 9:553–559, 1998.
9. Lewis GR, Mulcahy K, Brook NR, et al: A prospective study of the predictive power of spiral computed tomographic angiography for defining renal vascular anatomy before live-donor nephrectomy, *Br J Urology* 94:1077–1081, 2004.

CHAPTER 12.

Musculoskeletal Multislice Computed Tomography

Michael Rieger

MUSCULOSKELETAL IMAGING WITH MULTISLICE CT

Multislice CT (MSCT) was introduced in 1992 with the advent of dual slice scanners. This technology was improved with the implementation of 4-slice scanners in 1998, 8-slice scanners in 2000, and 16-slice scanners in 2002. In 2004, the first 64-slice devices were installed. The technical enhancements that CT devices have experienced over the past years have dramatically improved image quality and clinical applications. MSCT offers the considerable advantage over single-slice CT of larger volume acquisition and a much higher spatial resolution along the longitudinal axis with ultra-thin slices. Scanning can be performed much faster, resulting in improved temporal resolution and reduced motion artifacts. The spectrum of indications has been extended, and the examination algorithm has evolved as a major advantage of MSCT in musculoskeletal imaging.

Postprocessing

In comparison to single-slice CT, MSCT took a fundamental step from a cross-sectional view to a truly three-dimensional (3D) imaging modality that allows arbitrary cut planes as well as excellent displays of the data volume. The base for high-quality 2D and 3D reconstructions is the appropriate image acquisition with appropriate acquisition protocols. Single-slice CT suffered from a disproportion between the resolution in the axial plane, x-axis and y-axis, which is mostly a function of geometry and detector design, and the longitudinal resolution, z-axis, which is a function of the slice thickness. To generate an isotropic volume in cases of nonisotropic volume, raw-data interpolation steps are necessary. This disadvantage has been overcome with the latest generation of MSCT, which allows acquisition of near-isotropic voxel, a prerequisite for depiction of highly detailed 2D and 3D images.[1] To take full advantage of these capabilities, production of multiplanar reformatted (MPR) images has become an integral part of musculoskeletal examinations. Sections in the same image quality as the source data can be obtained in any plane. Positioning of the body part, which should be examined, in the gantry becomes less important because any plane can be reformatted from the acquired volume. This capability simplifies examination, especially of traumatized patients. Imaging data from joints within casts can be reformatted retrospectively into orthogonal planes.[2]

Different 3D rendering techniques have proved valuable in the diagnosis of various pathological findings and for therapy planning in musculoskeletal disorders. For 3D postprocessing, two different algorithms are commonly used. The surface shaded display (SSD) algorithm takes the first voxel encountered along a projection ray that exceeds a user-defined threshold value and defines the position and attenuation value of that voxel as the surface of the object. No additional information along the projection ray contributes to the viewed image. Therefore, SSD images are only capable of demonstrating gross 3D relationships but fail to display lesions hidden beneath the bone surface (Figure 12-1). As a result of this technical disadvantage, some fractures (especially those that are not dislocated) may be underdiagnosed. In addition, SSD also tends to demonstrate stairstep artifacts.

The other 3D rendering technique, volume rendering (VR), makes use of the entire data set and

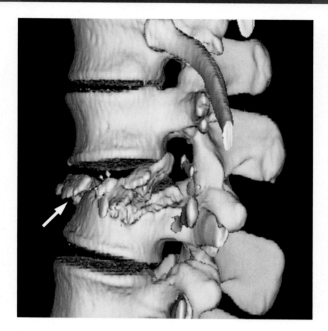

Fig. 12-1 Oblique sagittal surface-rendered image of a traumatized patient. The 3D reconstruction demonstrates a burst fracture of the third lumbar vertebral body. Depiction of the osseous fragments of the cover plate of the vertebral body *(arrow)*. Because of the reconstruction mode used, only the osseous structures are displayed.

thus conveys more information than SSD. In VR, the contributions of each voxel along a line of sight from the viewer's eye through the data set are summarized. This process is repeated many times to determine each pixel value in the displayed image. VR can show multiple internal and overlying features, and the displayed intensity is related to the amount of bone encountered along a line extending through the volume (Figure 12-2). The flexibility of the VR algorithm allows the radiologist to tailor the degree of surface shading and bone opacity to the actual clinical problem. These advantages have made VR superior to SSD for a variety of MSCT applications.[3,4] When performing 3D rendering techniques, it is important to calculate the source data in a standard reconstruction kernel instead of a bone algorithm. This is explained by the much higher image noise of the transverse images when reconstructed with the bone algorithm. As a result of that image noise, certain randomly distributed soft tissue pixels gain equally high attenuation values as bone. They may then appear in the VR images, reducing the image quality and possibly altering the coherence of the displayed structures.[5]

Volume Coverage and Image Quality

Anatomical coverage is the display of structures surrounding the region in which the diagnosis is established. Adequate landmarks must be provided if treatment decisions are to be made from CT scans. For single-slice CT, anatomical coverage can be calculated by multiplying slice width by pitch by exposure time. For example, in a slice width of 1 mm, a pitch of 1, and a 100-second helical acquisition, the coverage would be 100 mm. Most musculoskeletal applications require greater coverage. On the one hand, lengthening the coverage by increasing the slice width or the pitch in single-slice CT will degrade the images and hamper the production of high-quality reformations. On the other hand, because of the collimation of a narrow x-ray fan in a single-slice CT, only a fractional amount of the emitted quanta of the x-ray tube accounts for the image. As a consequence, tube cooling may become a problem for the acquisition of a greater musculoskeletal volume.[6,7] MSCT has overcome these disadvantages of single-slice CT and can image large anatomical volumes because of the simultaneous registration of a multiplicity of sections during each rotation without the drawback of using increased slice width. Simultaneously, this means a more efficient use of the x-ray tube. As a result, state-of-the-art scanners allow nearly unlimited anatomical coverage with ultra-thin submillimeter slices combined with high-speed data acquisition.

UNIVERSAL MUSCULOSKELETAL APPLICATIONS

Skeletal Trauma

Because of the advantages just described, MSCT referrals for examinations of musculoskeletal disorders and pathologies has increased greatly. In cases of musculoskeletal trauma, MSCT has two major roles: to define or exclude a fracture that was equivocal at plain radiography and to determine the extent and the classification of a previously diagnosed or suspected fracture and thus provide guidance for therapy (Table 12-1). MSCT will also

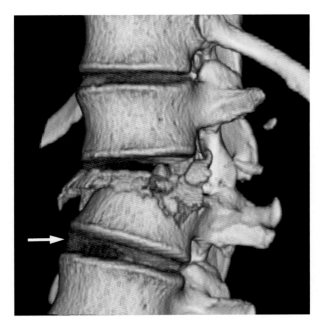

Fig. 12-2 Oblique sagittal volume-rendered image of the same patient shown in Figure 12-1. The volume-rendering reconstruction mode allows depiction not only of the osseous structures of the lumbar spine but also of the intervertebral discs *(arrow).*

Table 12-1	CT Protocol of Skeletal Fractures
Indication	Suspected skeletal fracture
Protocol designed for	LightSpeed 16
Patient preparation	Not required
Scanning plane	Axial
Oral contrast	—
IV contrast	—
Tube settings	
kV	100-140
mAs	60-200
Gantry speed (sec)	0.5-0.8
Table speed (mm/sec)	13.75
Slice thickness (mm)	0.63-1.25
Reconstruction interval (mm)	0.3-0.6
Anatomical coverage	Suspected injured area
Reconstruction kernel	Bone (and standard, if the evaluation of soft tissue and 3D reconstructions are required)
Breath hold	Inspiration only in thoracic skeleton
Postprocessing	2D reconstructions in at least two planes; 3D volume-rendering reconstructions in complex fractures

provide additional information about pathologies in anatomically complex areas such as shoulder girdle, spine, pelvis, and middle face.

For the detection of injury, some skeletal regions are examined primarily by MSCT instead of plain radiography. Examples include severe spinal or pelvic injuries and suspected skeletal fractures in polytraumatized patients. In addition, MSCT can detect soft-tissue abnormalities. The major advantage of VR is its capacity to display multiple tissues and show their relationship to one another. VR programs retain all of the information within the data set and display one or more tissues, depending on the chosen protocol. This technique is helpful in musculoskeletal applications, where it may be particularly important to display the relationship of bone to soft tissue.[3,8]

Infection and Tumor

There are other musculoskeletal applications for MSCT besides trauma, which have only been briefly addressed. An increasing number of examinations are being performed for the evaluation of known or suspected musculoskeletal infection. MSCT with 2D or 3D reconstructions is useful for detecting infections and abscesses, for determining which compartments are involved, and for describing the extent of an infection. In this situation, it is necessary to apply intravenous contrast medium. MSCT is also used to evaluate cortical bone and associated soft-tissue masses in suspected osteomyelitis. The presence of sequester can be verified, and the response to therapy monitored.

MSCT is useful for defining the full extent of primary and metastatic bone tumors. Although MR imaging has become the leading modality for evaluating the extent of bone and soft-tissue neoplasms, CT is nearly as efficacious and remains superior to MR imaging in the detection of cortical destruction and lesion calcification. In comparison to bone scintigraphy, which is an excellent screening study for metastases, MSCT is much more specific.[6]

INTRINSIC TRAUMATIC APPLICATIONS

Skull and Facial Fractures

Facial fractures are a common result of direct trauma (e.g., a traffic accident or a fist fight). The complex anatomy of this region requires detailed imaging free of superposition. Therefore, for characterization and classification of facial fractures, helical CT is considered the standard imaging modality (Table 12-2).

CT in at least two orthogonal planes (axial and coronal) is the standard examination procedure for making a reliable and precise diagnosis for treatment planning.[9,10] Narrow-collimation (0.6 to 1.2 mm) axial acquisition yields a volume that allows the creation of MPR and VR images with very high spatial resolution. Sections can be obtained in any plane. Because of the nearly isotropic viewing, MPR images have approximately the same spatial resolution as the original sections (Figure 12-3). Therefore, the need for direct coronal imaging of facial fractures (as with single-slice CT) is avoided. Dental artifacts, which often degrade direct coronal images, can be evaded with MSCT and MPR.[2] Philipp et al. (2003)[9] examined the use of 0.5-mm slice thickness instead of 1-mm thickness. They found no clear incremental advantage of using the ultra-high resolution because of the decreased signal-to-noise ratio. However, this ultra-high mode improved the delineation of thin osseous lamellae, but these were of no clinical relevance in the study. They suggest the use of 1-mm slices for the scanning of the face and 0.5-mm slices only when findings are inconclusive. When the thin primary source images of the facial skeleton are used and thicker MPRs (e.g., 5 mm) are performed in any plane calculated with a standard reconstruction kernel and an average projection mode, the brain can be examined without a rescan. Therefore, patients suspected of having facial fractures and intracranial hemorrhage can be examined in a "one-stop shop" mode (Figure 12-4). Another advantage modern MSCT holds over single-slice CT is the possibility of calculating high-resolution images of the temporal bone in patients with suspected fracture

Table 12-2	AO classification of facial fractures	
Type A	Undislocated fractures, dislocation of fragments <2 mm
Type B	Dislocated fractures with a dislocation >2 mm
Type C	Multifragmentary, complex fractures with no contact between the two main fragments, which means a dislocation of fragments >5 mm

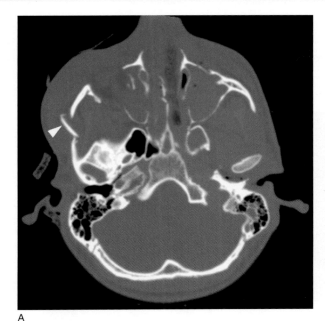

A

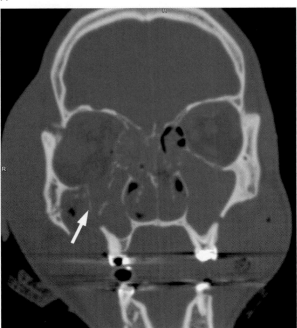

B

Fig. 12-3 Axial source image (A) and coronal reformatted image (B) of facial fractures. The images in two different planes show multiple facial fractures, including the orbital floor *(arrow)* and is depicted in the coronal reformation (B) and the zygomatic arch *(arrowhead)* shown in the axial image (A).

from the acquisition data without rescanning this specific area. The images are reconstructed, if necessary, in two planes in a high-resolution bone window-level setting. Pathologies of the temporal bone and the inner ear can be described in detail.

Spinal Trauma

Radiologists and trauma surgeons are constantly trying to reduce the time it takes to adequately image trauma victims and to simultaneously improve diagnostic quality. Considering the devastating consequences, especially for patients in whom a spine injury has been missed at examination, all individuals who have sustained trauma must be assessed for spinal fractures. Ideally, this should be ruled out within minutes after a patient's admission to the emergency room. In many cases, however, patients who have sustained severe trauma are uncooperative or unstable, and are thus difficult to examine clinically. A rapid but accurate diagnosis of the patient must therefore be performed. The diagnosis must detect the entire extent of the injury, including the characterization and classification of the fracture. It must also indicate whether a fracture is stable (Table 12-3).

Possible spinal cord damage caused by the narrowing of the spinal canal, bone fragments, hematoma, or intervertebral disc material must be detected quickly. When choosing the best imaging algorithm for evaluation of spine fractures, the radiologist is often hampered by time limitations, lack of patient cooperation, and hemodynamic instability or coexistent traumatic lesions.[11,12] Radiological standards are in a constant state of development. At this time, it seems that the issue at hand is not whether radiological imaging should be performed, but rather, what kind. This shift has been accelerated by the advent of helical CT and, in particular, MSCT, with its intrinsic ability to provide reconstructions of the highest quality.[13] As indicated by Imhof and Fuchsjäger (2002),[14] various authors have shown that conventional radiographs miss 23% to 57% of all cervical spine fractures. At best, this may simply lead to a delayed diagnosis. At worst, it could result in disastrous mismanagement of the patient's condition.

Because of these results, many advocate emergency spiral CT as the first imaging method in severe spinal trauma patients or in patients with high or moderate risk. High-risk patients include those with multiple injuries, those with abnormal

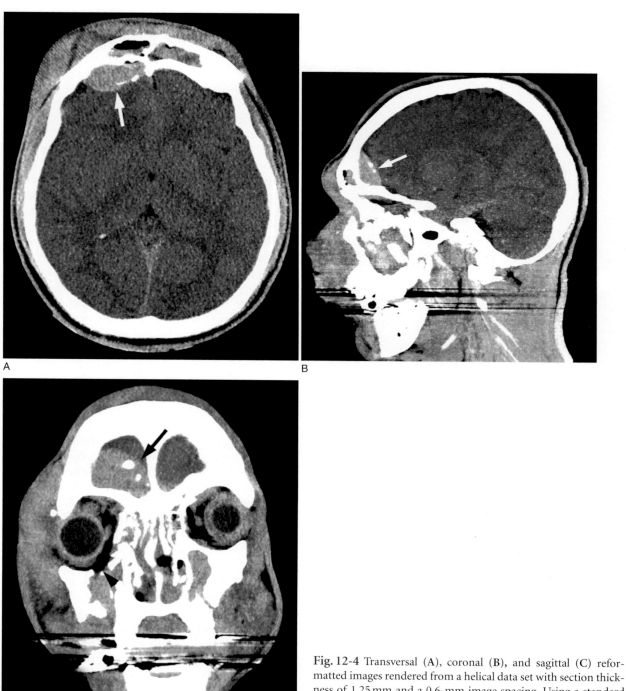

A

B

C

Fig. 12-4 Transversal (**A**), coronal (**B**), and sagittal (**C**) reformatted images rendered from a helical data set with section thickness of 1.25 mm and a 0.6-mm image spacing. Using a standard reconstruction kernel and an average projection mode, intracerebral injuries like this epidural hematoma *(arrows)* can be depicted in different planes as well as facial fractures *(arrowhead)* without needing a new scan.

Table 12-3	Magerl/AO classification of spinal fractures
Type A	Compression fractures A1—Impaction fracture A2—Split fracture A3—Burst fracture
Type B	Distraction fractures B1—Dorsal laceration (predominantly ligamentous) B2—Dorsal laceration (predominantly osseous) B3—Ventral laceration through the intervertebral disc
Type C	Rotatory fractures C1—Type A with rotatory component C2—Type B with rotatory component C3—Rotatory shear fracture

mental status, and those older than 50 years with an injury mechanism, which is very suggestive of severe spinal trauma. This group has an anticipated cervical spine fracture risk of 11.2%. The moderate-risk group, with a fracture risk of 4.2%, includes those patients 50 years or younger with a high-energy mechanism of injury and patients older than 50 years with a moderate-energy mechanism of injury. Only in the low-risk group (with a potential fracture risk of 2.1% in patients 50 years or younger with a moderate-energy mechanism of injury) can conventional radiographs be performed and trusted as the sole modality.[15,16] For the optimal workup of patients with severe spinal trauma, Imhof and Fuchsjäger (2002)[14] concluded that MSCT with reconstructions rules out or confirms bone abnormalities (e.g., fractures, dislocation) with the highest precision. Conventional radiographs are diagnostically insufficient. As many as 57% of cervical spine cases produce false-negative results.[14]

Injuries of the thoracic and lumbar spine can be detected with a high sensitivity and specificity, because these injuries can be depicted without superposition (e.g., by the shoulder or other skeletal structures) and because reconstruction in any plane is possible. When the discrepancy between MSCT and conventional radiography in polytraumatized patients with fractures of the thoracic and lumbar spine was measured, the following results arose: (1) there was no discrepancy between both modalities in 4% of the thoracic and 33% of the lumbar spine; (2) fracture only diagnosed in the CT examination: 33% of the thoracic and 22% of the

lumbar spine; (3) multislice CT gave additional information concerning the extent, the characterization, and the classification in 63% of the thoracic and in 44% of the lumbar spine.[17] Wintermark et al. (2003)[12] examined the quality of MSCT images of the thoracic and lumbar spine in 100 severe trauma patients. CT images were regarded as interpretable in 100% of cases. Motion or misregistration artifacts occurred, but the artifacts did not substantially alter the diagnostic value of MSCT results in any of the cases. Fractures could be easily distinguished from nutrient artery channels and other fracture-mimicking entities. All vertebral levels were visible at MSCT. Performing CT examination without conventional radiography is less time consuming and diminishes the need for patient manipulation and the potential hazards for unstable fractures. Therefore, MSCT can replace conventional radiography and can be the sole modality performed in patients who have sustained severe trauma (Figure 12-5).

MSCT allows evaluation of the intervertebral disc in trauma patients. By performing 2D MPR reconstructions in a sagittal, coronal, and oblique transversal plane parallel to the endplates of the vertebral bodies, MSCT facilitates the imaging of traumatic and degenerative herniated vertebral discs. Soft-tissue evaluation requires calculation of the source images in a standard reconstruction kernel and MPRs in an average mode. Disc-caused stenoses of the spinal canal and the intervertebral foramen, combined with a compression of the nerve roots, can be diagnosed. By using additional volume-rendering reconstructions, a traumatic discoligamentous disruption of the lumbar spine can be detected (Figure 12-6). In addition, MSCT enables the detection of injuries near the spine, such as hematomas.

Pelvic Trauma

Pelvic injuries primarily occur as a result of accidents with high kinetic energy secondary to either a motor vehicle collision or a high-velocity fall. They can result in potentially devastating and fatal consequences. Pelvic injuries are correlated with significant morbidity and a reported mortality between 10% to 29%. This percentage is a result of the complications of pelvic ring disruptions, which, because of the high energy involved, are usually combined with multiple injuries and high injury severity scores (ISS).[18] Pelvic fractures can produce significant

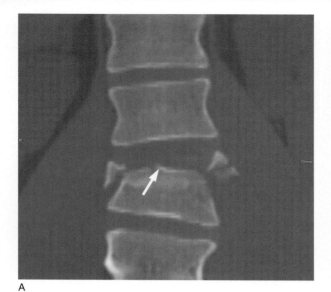

A

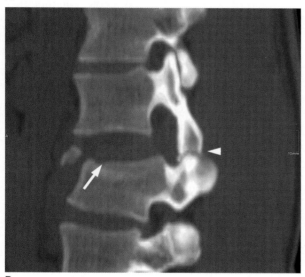

B

Fig. 12-5 Coronal (**A**) and sagittal (**B**) reformatted images of the lumbar spine. The images show a compression fracture of the third vertebral body of the lumbar spine with a segmental extension of the intervertebral space crabwise, indicating an injury of the intervertebral disc *(arrows)*. The extension of the intervertebral space shows indirect an injury of the intervertebral space *(arrowhead)*.

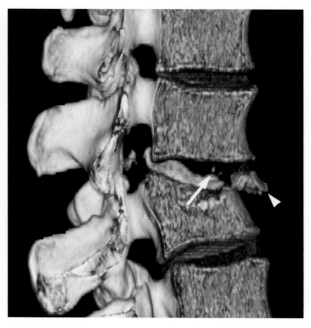

Fig. 12-6 Sagittal surface–rendered CT image with a cut through the center of the lumbar spine of the patient shown in Figure 12-5. VR view shows an impaction fracture of the third lumbar vertebral body combined with a discoligamentous disruption *(arrow)*. A small fragment *(arrowhead)* of the ventral part of the vertebral body is torn off. The second vertebral body shows light ventral shift, indicating a segmental instability.

hemorrhage from iliac arterial branches, the presacral venous plexus, and a large bulk of cancellous bone, especially if posterior structures are disrupted. A study of 1400 patients found a mortality of 5.5% with simple pelvic fractures and 39% for complex pelvic trauma. In patients with pelvic fracture and hemorrhagic shock, which develop in as many as 52% of patients, mortality is approximately 40%. Immediate recognition of a pelvic ring disruption and determination of pelvic stability is a vital component in trauma evaluation during the critical first hour after the injury occurs.[19] Because the clinical examination of severely injured patients is usually limited, it is essential that the radiological diagnostic workup is efficient. Diagnostic demands include rapid availability and feasibility combined with an accurate detection of the extent of the pelvic and accompanying injuries. However, because of the complexity of pelvic fractures and the precise pathological anatomy, characterization and classification (Table 12-4) of the fractures are not easily demonstrated by conventional radiographs, and in many cases details of the fractures are not visible. Plain films miss approximately 30% of pelvic fractures detected by CT. In sacral trauma, conventional radiography missed 29% of sacroiliac diastasis, 57% of acetabular rim fractures, and 34% of vertical shearing fractures. In addition, plain films missed up to 40% of intraarticular

Table 12-4	Tile/AO classification of pelvic fractures
Type A	Stable fractures A1—Ischial fractures A2—Iliac fractures A3—Sacrum coccyx fractures
Type B	Rotationally unstable fractures B1—Open book B2—Lateral compression B3—Combination of open book and lateral compression
Type C	Rotationally and vertically unstable fractures C1—Unilateral vertical unstable C2—Unilateral vertical unstable, opposite rotational unstable C3—Bilateral vertical unstable

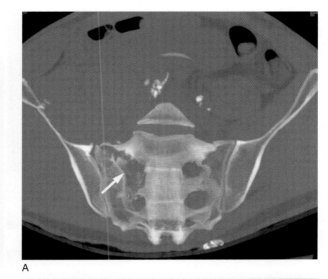

A

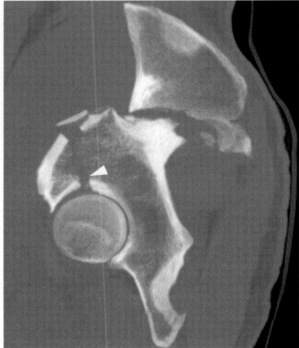

B

fragments and 50% of femoral head fractures visualized with CT.

Because of the limited image volume with thin slices, single-slice CT is inferior to MSCT, which allows for high-resolution source images and for secondary high-quality 2D and 3D reconstructions. This increased performance in comparison to single-slice CT provides more information regarding the extent of fractures and the spatial arrangement of fracture fragments. MSCT has become an outstanding and effective tool for understanding complex fracture patterns, particularly when combined with multiplanar 2D or 3D reconstructions (Figures 12-7 and 12-8). Subtle fractures, especially those orientated in the axial plane, are better seen with MPR or 3D volume-rendered images.[18,20] For simultaneous evaluation of osseous and vascular pathologies, the use of intravenous contrast medium is necessary. Pelvic fractures accompanying hematomas are displayed as hyperdense areas; active bleeding is shown as contrast medium extravasations. Localization and extent of the area will permit an assessment of blood loss. MSCT covering the pelvis with an optimized technique in the arterial phase allows the detection of arterial extravasation, which requires immediate interventional therapy (Figure 12-9). In addition, the volume of extraperitoneal pelvic hemorrhage is also a potentially important marker for the presence of pelvic arterial injury. Blackmore et al. (2003)[21] demonstrate that patients with low pelvic CT

Fig. 12-7 A, Images show fractures of the pelvic ring combined with, **B,** an acetabular fracture. Oblique coronal and sagittal reformatted images of the pelvic in a patient suffering from a severe crush trauma. Images show fractures of the posterior pelvic ring *(arrow)* combined with an acetabular fracture *(arrowhead)*. The right sacral foramina are involved by the fracture. Bony fragments cause stenoses of the foramina. In addition, reformations demonstrate a comminuted fracture of the iliac bone.

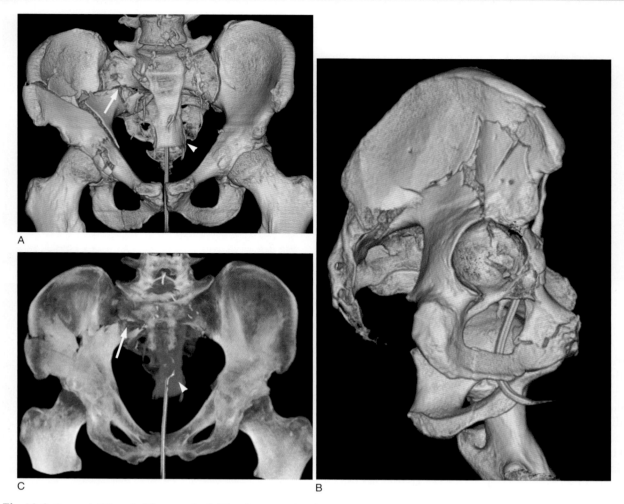

Fig. 12-8 Coronal (**A**) and oblique sagittal (**B**) volume-rendered CT images and 3D MIP reformation (**C**) of a polytraumatized patient with a severe crush trauma to the pelvis (same patient as shown in Figure 12-7). VR (**A, B**) and MIP (**C**) reconstructions depict the extent of the comminuted pelvic fracture involving the dorsal pelvic ring *(arrows)* and the iliac bone—including the anterior articular lip of the acetabulum. In addition, coronal reconstructions (**A, C**) show a fracture of the anterior pelvic ring of the right side without a dislocation. The urinary bladder *(arrowheads)* is partially filled with contrast medium, and a urinary catheter is inserted. Images show a displacement of the bladder, indicating an injury of the neck of the bladder.

hemorrhage volumes (< 200 ml) had only a 5% probability of pelvic arterial injury, whereas subjects with high volumes of pelvic hemorrhage (> 500 ml) had a 45% probability of pelvic arterial injury.

EXTREMITY TRAUMA

The aim of extremity fracture treatment is accurate anatomical repositioning of the fragments, the recovery of the proper angulatory deformity, and early mobilization. The extent of dislocation of

fragments in conventional radiographs is often not detectable and requires further diagnostics for exact characterization and classification, especially in complex fractures involving articular joints. The current AO/ASIF ("Arbeitsgemeinschaft für Osteosythesefragen"/Association for the Study of Internal Fixation; OTA: Ortopedic Trauma Association) classification of fractures of different areas enables very accurate classification (Table 12-5).

Different studies demonstrate that the inter- and intraindividual reproducibility of the AO/ASIF classification on the basis of conventional radiographs resulted in only moderate agreement. For example,

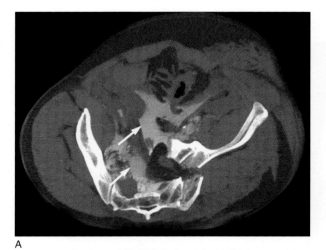

A

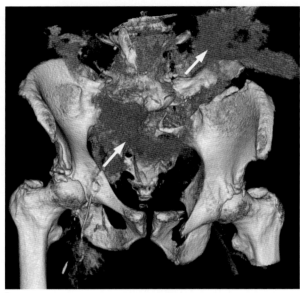

B

Fig. 12-9 Axial source image (**A**) and oblique coronal reformatted volume-rendered image (**B**) of a patient with severe crush trauma to the pelvis. Images show rotationally and vertically unstable fractures of the left side (AO classification type C1) with a distinct dislocation of the left side of the pelvis, associated with a significant, active hemorrhage indicated by a severe contrast medium extravasation (*arrows*), which is red in the volume-rendered image (**B**).

Table 12-5 Classification of fractures

AO CLASSIFICATION OF DIAPHYSEAL FRACTURE, MID-SHAFT FRACTURES

Type A	Simple fractures with cortical disruption for at least 90% of the bone circumference A1—Spiral A2—Oblique A3—Transverse
Type B	Multifragmentary, wedge fracture, always some contact between the two main fragments B1—Torsion wedge B2—Bending wedge B3—Fragmented wedge
Type C	Multifragmentary, complex fractures with no contact between the two main fragments C1—Complex spiral C2—Segmental C3—Complex irregular

AO CLASSIFICATION OF ARTICULAR FRACTURES

Type A	Extraarticular, may be intracapsular, but do not involve the joint surface
Type B	Part of the articular surface involved, the remainder being still connected to the diaphysis
Type C	Complete articular fracture with the articular surface disrupted and completely separated from the diaphysis

different investigators identically classified only 38% of proximal humerus fractures. Similar results were found in studies involving distal radius and distal tibia fractures. Therefore, it does not seem reasonable to classify complex intraarticular fractures with only conventional radiographs. However, axial CT can also be challenging when one attempts to interpret regions of complex anatomy, such as the ankle and hindfoot. For example, the precise localization of the articular facets of the subtalar joints may be difficult to appreciate on routine axial scans. High-resolution reconstructions created from the CT data provide an additional perspective that can improve depiction of the subtalar joint anatomy. MSCT is extremely sensitive in the detection of fractures, and source images together with rendered reconstructions can display the spatial relationship of fracture fragments in complex anatomical regions. Removal of plaster casts and splints is just as unnecessary as hazardous positioning maneuvers (Figure 12-10). This provides a considerable advantage for the attending physician deciding on whether to use conservative or surgical treatment. Complementary CT examination of intraarticular distal tibia fractures caused a change in surgical treatment in 64% of patients; in 82% of the cases, CT provided additional information concerning fracture characterization and classification.

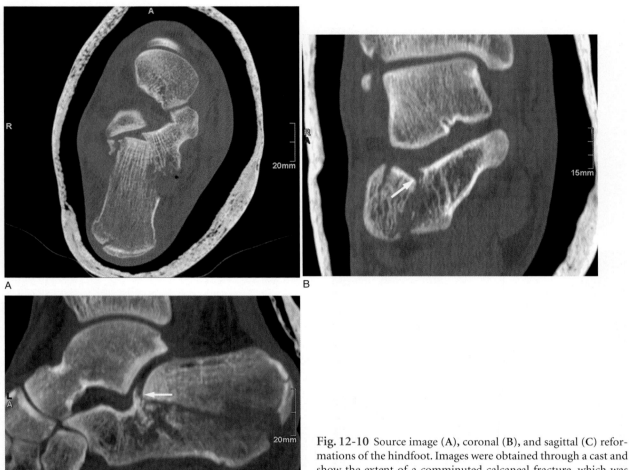

Fig. 12-10 Source image (A), coronal (B), and sagittal (C) reformations of the hindfoot. Images were obtained through a cast and show the extent of a comminuted calcaneal fracture, which was the result of a jump from a significant height. The orientation of the fracture fragments is clearly depicted on these views, and the intraarticular nature of the fracture *(arrows)* is demonstrated.

The speed of MSCT in comparison to single-slice technique is advantageous in situations in which the patient may have difficulty lying still. This is particularly important in areas such as the sternoclavicular joint or shoulder girdle, because the patient must remain motionless.[22,23]

3D reconstructions enable radiologists to highlight and display the individual osseous and soft-tissue components of complex anatomy. With volume rendering, for example, it is possible to demonstrate both the tendons and bones of the hands, the ankle, and the hindfoot, because the tendons in these areas are surrounded by fat and have an attenuation of approximately 90 HU, which is intermediate between the attenuation of bone and muscle[8] (Figure 12-11).

In patients with traumatic extremity injuries, particularly those with suspected vascular involvement, MSCT has been advocated as an alternative noninvasive diagnostic tool for imaging both osseous and vascular pathologies. Single-slice CT angiography has been recognized as a fast, noninvasive, and feasible tool that allows 3D assessment of the vasculature and of vascular pathologies. For this reason it is used to diagnose acute vascular injuries and to evaluate arterial runoff in the proximal extremity after trauma.[24] Because of its advantages over single-slice CT, MSCT has the potential to further improve the diagnostic workup of traumatic arterial injuries. Single-slice CT angiography of large volumes calls for a relatively large collimation (i.e., 3 to 5 mm),

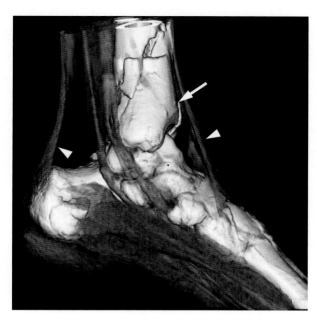

Fig. 12-11 Volume-rendered MSCT image of the ankle and hindfoot in a patient who sustained an acute twisting injury. VR image depicts a pilon fracture of the distal tibia *(arrow)* and demonstrates both the tendons *(arrowheads)* and bones of the ankle and the hindfoot. This is possible because the tendons are surrounded by fat.

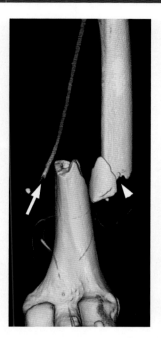

Fig. 12-12 Volume-rendered MSCT angiogram in a 27-year-old man with blunt trauma to the left upper leg. VR view shows an abrupt contrast material stop with irregular edge at the distal segment of superficial femoral artery, which is laterally deviated, indicating arterial rupture *(arrow)*. Image also shows a severely dislocated fracture of the femur shaft *(arrowhead)* at the level of arterial interruption. During surgery, the superficial femoral artery was found disconnected at fracture level.

which affects spatial resolution along the z-axis and image quality of 3D reconstructions. On the contrary, MSCT angiography of the entire extremity can be performed with 1.25-mm collimation and high pitch in a relatively short acquisition time. On the one hand, this yields an improved spatial resolution along the z-axis and therefore enhanced visualization of small arteries. On the other hand, it considerably reduces the amount of contrast medium required and also reduces motion artifacts (Figures 12-12 and 12-13). In the emergency room setting, MSCT imaging permits immediate evaluation of the involved extremity concerning osseous and vascular pathologies as well as rapid examination of other body regions that may be injured (Table 12-6).

After stabilization of life-threatening conditions, polytraumatized patients require a fast, reliable, and comprehensive diagnostic workup so that a therapy plan can be chosen. The most common error in the first phase after a patient is admitted is a delayed and insufficient diagnostic workup, which impairs the prognosis. The polytrauma patient has thus greatly benefited from the introduction of

MSCT, whose speed permits a whole body evaluation within a few seconds in very thin slices (1.25 mm) during the application of one bolus of intravenous contrast medium. Using these source images, transverse, sagittal, and coronal reformations (e.g., 5 mm) can be performed for diagnosing injuries of the brain, neck, thorax, abdomen, and pelvis—as well as thin-slap reformations of the skeletal system in any plane. In fact, there is no longer any need for other diagnostic modalities when evaluating injuries in polytraumatized patients (Figure 12-14). Whole body CT starts with an examination of the head without contrast medium to detect intracerebral hematomas, contusions, and traumatic subarachnoidal bleedings. To display soft tissue, a standard algorithm and an average reconstruction mode is used. The same source images can be used for thin-slap reconstructions in any plane, calculated in a maximum intensity projection mode, for detecting facial fractures.

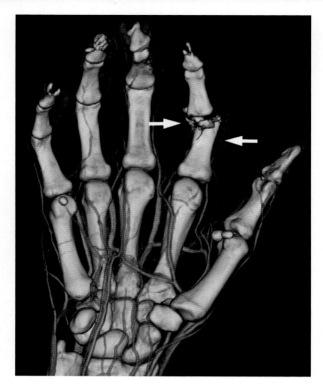

Fig. 12-13 Volume-rendered MDCT angiogram in a 19-year-old man with blunt trauma to the right hand. VR view shows occlusion of the ulnar and radial proper palmar digital arteries of the forefinger *(arrows)*. Image also shows a subcapital fracture of the proximal phalanx. Surgery confirmed the presence of both occlusions that were attributed to disconnection of the ulnar arteries and dissection of the radial digital arteries.

Table 12-6	CT Protocol for Whole-Body CT
Indication	Polytraumatized patients
Protocol designed for	LightSpeed 16
Patient preparation	Not required
Scanning plane	Axial
Oral contrast	—
IV contrast	2 × body weight
Flow	3 ml/sec
Tube settings	
kV	120-140
mAs	120-200
Gantry speed (sec)	0.4
Table speed (mm/sec)	27.5
Slice thickness (mm)	1.25
Reconstruction interval (mm)	0.6-1.0
Anatomical coverage	Whole body
Reconstruction kernel	Standard
Breath hold	—
Postprocessing	2D reconstructions in at least two planes; 3D volume-rendering reconstructions in complex fractures

For the neck and body stem examination, the patient's arms should be elevated. If this is not possible, the arms should be placed very close to the body so that they are inside the largest display field of view (DFOV) to avoid artifacts. The DFOV should be adapted to the size of the anatomical region. The scan begins at the skull base with a DFOV adapted to the neck down to the third thoracic vertebra with a short overlap and an adjusted DVOF down to the proximal femur during an intravenous contrast medium bolus. The time lapse of the contrast application must be adapted so that the data of the neck and thorax are acquired in an arterial phase to recognize potential arterial injuries like dissections and aneurysms. To detect potential injuries, the data of the abdomen and pelvis must be scanned in the parenchymal phase for optimal attenuation of the parenchymal organs. The same data can be used for high-resolution reconstructions of the skeletal system. The implementation of the Innsbruck Emergency Algorithm (Figure 12-15) not only accelerated radiological diagnostics but also improved radiological quality.[17]

VIRTUAL 3D PLANNING OF CORRECTIVE OSTEOTOMY

By providing virtual perspectives that simulate the anatomical and pathological reality in a patient and by allowing interactive control on rendering parameters, computer-assisted, 3D reconstruction of imaging data sets has enabled the creation of a virtual reality environment. This assists in the determination of diagnosis and preoperative planning. High-resolution, 3D reconstruction of MSCT data of the skeletal system (e.g., a malunited forearm), planned for a corrective osteotomy and transferred

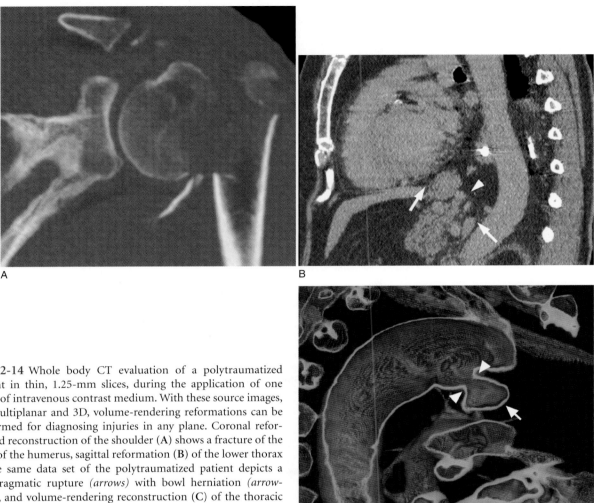

Fig. 12-14 Whole body CT evaluation of a polytraumatized patient in thin, 1.25-mm slices, during the application of one bolus of intravenous contrast medium. With these source images, 2D multiplanar and 3D, volume-rendering reformations can be performed for diagnosing injuries in any plane. Coronal reformatted reconstruction of the shoulder (**A**) shows a fracture of the neck of the humerus, sagittal reformation (**B**) of the lower thorax of the same data set of the polytraumatized patient depicts a diaphragmatic rupture *(arrows)* with bowl herniation *(arrowhead)*, and volume-rendering reconstruction (**C**) of the thoracic aorta performed with a cut demonstrates a traumatic thoracic aneurysm of the aorta *(arrow)* and the neck of the aneurysm *(arrowheads)*.

in a suitable CAD software, may assist the surgeon in making crucial decisions by providing a preoperative perceptibility of the individual operation territory and recognition of possible limitations. In addition, it may also offer objective details concerning the appropriate position of the distal radius fragment and determination of the form and size of required bone graft.

Virtual operation planning of malunited distal radius fractures comprises two main procedures: carrying out the virtual osteotomy of the radius and predicting the final position of the distal radius fragment after osteotomy. The first procedure is initiated by segmentation of the bony structures of the forearm and wrist of both upper extremities and by creation of a 3D, surface-rendered model using thin multislice source data (Figure 12-16). The latter is then imported into a virtual modeling system, which enables a natural interaction with the digital 3D model via haptic feedback. With this software, the virtual osteotomy is performed (Figure 12-17). The second procedure of operation planning is dedicated to transferring the virtual result of reposition in the operation theater either digitally to a navigation system or by producing a repositioning device that, when placed in the osteotomy gap during surgical operation, would restore the original position of the distal

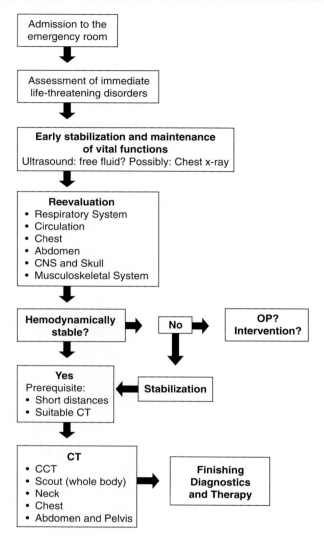

Fig. 12-15 Innsbruck Emergency Algorithm.

articular fragment. For this purpose, the surface-rendered models of the right and left wrists are transferred to an image fusion program. After being appropriately mirrored, the ulna and the proximal radius of the involved forearm are digitally fused with those of the healthy forearm that were used as a reference. To simulate its original position, the distal articular radius fragment is then fused with the contralateral side, resulting in the creation of a wedge-shaped gap in the osteotomy region (Figure 12-18). In cases of producing a template, the virtual wedge-shaped gap at the osteotomy site is computed, and a 3D model that resembles the gap is then created (Figure 12-19). According to the form and size of the gap's model, a synthetic template of stereolithography material is manufactured, which is firmly placed intraoperatively between the proximal and the distal radius to assist in reproducing the original location of the distal fragment. After placement of the osteosynthesis, the repositioning device is then replaced with a bone graft.[25]

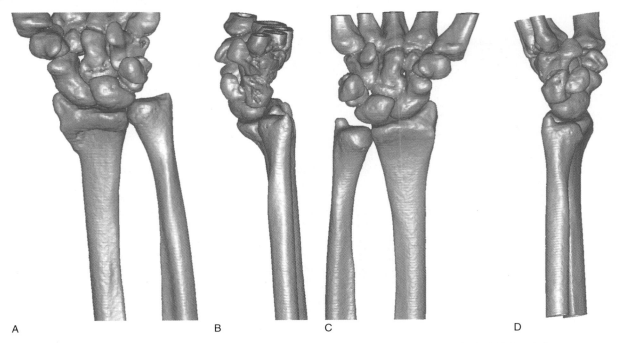

Fig. 12-16 Coronal and sagittal surface-rendered CT images of healthy *(right)* (**C, D**) and involved *(left)* (**A, B**) forearm, as reconstructed by the segmentation program. Left images show malunited distal radius fracture, ulnar positive variance, and subluxation of distal radioulnar joint.

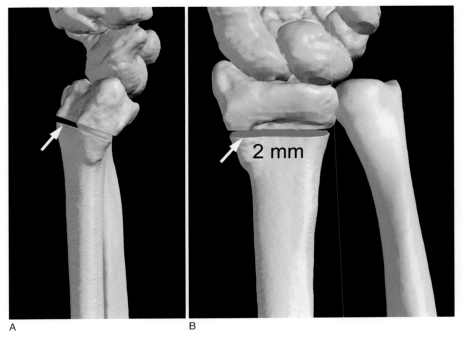

Fig. 12-17 Coronal (**A**) and sagittal (**B**) surface-rendered CT images of involved forearm, as reconstructed by virtual osteotomy program, showing a level of previously performed osteotomy of the distal radius *(arrows)*.

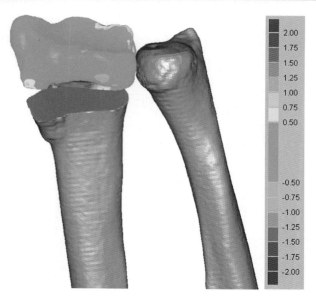

2.00	
1.75	
1.50	
1.25	
1.00	
0.75	
0.50	
-0.50	
-0.75	
-1.00	
-1.25	
-1.50	
-1.75	
-2.00	

Fig. 12-18 Coronal surface-rendered color-coded CT image of both forearms, as reconstructed by the image fusion program, showing fused ulnae and proximal radius fragments as well as the fused distal radius fragments of both sides. The image depicts the automatic repositioning of distal radius fragments and resulting wedge-shaped gap at the osteotomy site. Color-coding of distal radius fragments reveals that fusion error of the majority of distal radius fragments was within +0.5 mm as indicated by the color-coded scale *(right)*.

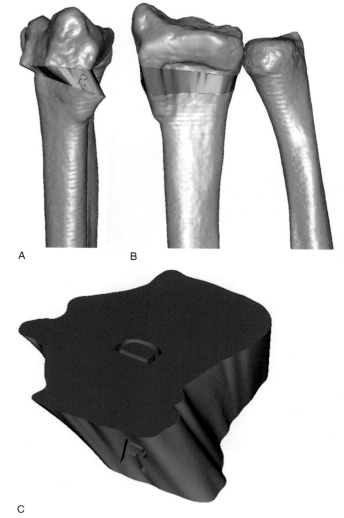

Fig. 12-19 3D virtual model of wedge-shaped osteotomy gap *(right)* and sagittal (**A**) and coronal (**B**) surface-rendered CT image of involved forearm *(left/middle)*, demonstrating final results of virtual osteotomy with wedge-shaped disc in situ.

REFERENCES

1. Philipp MO, Kubin K, Mang T, et al: Three-dimensional volume rendering of multidetector-row CT data: applicable for emergency radiology, *Eur J Radiol* 48(1):33–38, 2003.
2. Rydberg J, Buckwalter KA, Caldemeyer KS, et al: Multisection CT: scanning techniques and clinical applications, *Radiographics* 20(6):1787–1806, 2000.
3. Pretorius ES, Fishman EK: Volume-rendered three-dimensional spiral CT: musculoskeletal applications, *Radiographics* 19(5):1143–1160, 1999.
4. Kuszyk BS, Heath, DG, Bliss DF: Skeletal 3-D CT: Advantages of volume rendering over surface rendering, *Skeletal Radiol* 25(3):207–214, 1996.
5. Alkadhi H, Wildermuth S, Marincek B, et al: Accuracy and time efficiency for the detection of thoracic cage fractures: volume rendering compared with transverse computed tomography images, *J Comput Assist Tomogr* 28(3):378–385, 2004.
6. Buckwalter KA, Rydberg J, Kopecky KK, et al: Musculoskeletal imaging with multislice CT, *Am J Roentgenol* 176(4):979–986 2001.
7. Ohnesorge B, Flohr T, Schaller S, et al: The technical bases and uses of multi-slice CT, *Radiology* 39(11):923–931, 1999.
8. Choplin RH, Buckwalter KA, Rydberg J, et al: CT with 3D rendering of the tendons of the foot and ankle: technique, normal anatomy, and disease, *Radiographics* 24(2):343–356, 2004.
9. Philipp MO, Funovics MA, Mann FA, et al: Four-channel multidetector CT in facial fractures: do we need 2 .003 0.5 mm collimation? *Am J Roentgenol* 180(6):1707–1713, 2003.
10. Rosenthal E, Quint DJ, Johns M, et al: Diagnostic maxillofacial coronal images reformatted from helically acquired thin-section axial CT data, *Am J Roentgenol* 175(4):1177–1181, 2000.
11. Daffner RH: Helical CT of the cervical spine for trauma patients: a time study, *Am J Roentgenol* 177(3):677–679, 2001.
12. Wintermark M, Mouhsine E, Theumann N, et al: Thoracolumbar spine fractures in patients who have sustained severe trauma: depiction with multi-detector row CT, *Radiology* 227(3):681–689, 2003.
13. Berlin L: CT versus radiography for initial evaluation of cervical spine trauma: what is the standard of care? *Am J Roentgenol* 180(4):911–915, 2003.
14. Imhof H, Fuchsjäger M: Traumatic injuries: imaging of spinal injuries, *Eur Radiol* 12(6):1262–1272, 2002.
15. Blackmore CC, Ramsey SD, Mann FA, et al: Cervical spine screening with CT in trauma patients: a cost-effectiveness analysis, *Radiology* 212(1):117–125, 1999.
16. Blackmore CC, Emerson SS, Mann FA, et al: Cervical spine imaging in patients with trauma: determination of fracture risk to optimize use, *Radiology* 211(3):759–765, 1999.
17. Rieger M, Sparr H, Esterhammer R, et al: Modern CT diagnosis of acute thoracic and abdominal trauma, *Radiology* 42(7):556–563, 2002.
18. Wedegartner U, Gatzka C, Rueger JM, et al: Multislice CT (MSCT) in the detection and classification of pelvic and acetabular fractures, *Rofo Fortschr Geb Rontgenstr Neuen Bildgeb Verfahr* 175(1):105–111, 2003.
19. Stambaugh LE, Blackmore CC: Pelvic ring disruptions in emergency radiology, *Eur J Radiol* 48(1):71–87, 2003.
20. Falchi M, Rollandi GA: CT of pelvic fractures, *Eur J Radiol* 50(1):96–105, 2004.
21. Blackmore CC, Jurkovich GJ, Linnau KF, et al: Assessment of volume of hemorrhage and outcome from pelvic fracture, *Arch Surg* 138(5):504–508, 2003.
22. Burkhardt M, Gansslen A, Uder M, et al: New possibilities in fracture visualization by means of CT: reconstructions, 3D plannings–difficult joint fractures–modern management–improved visualization and operative planning in joint fractures, *Zentralbl Chir* 128(1):34–39, 2003.
23. Novelline RA, Rhea JT, Rao PM, et al: Helical CT in emergency radiology, *Radiology* 213(2):321–339, 1999.
24. Soto, JA, Munera F, Morales C, et al: Focal arterial injuries of the proximal extremities: helical CT arteriography as the initial method of diagnosis, *Radiology* 218(1):188–194, 2001.
25. Rieger M, Gabl M, Gruber H, et al: CT virtual reality in the preoperative workup of malunited distal radius fractures: preliminary results, *Eur Radiol* 14–25, 2004.

13.

Multislice Computed Tomography of the Genitourinary System

Benjamin M. Yeh

CT is a primary modality for evaluation of the urinary tract, and to a lesser extent for evaluation of the genital tract. In particular, CT is used for detailed evaluation of renal parenchyma and morphology. The development of multislice CT (MSCT) allows higher z-axis resolution and faster image acquisition than previously possible, and combined with PACS, greater diagnostic evaluation of the ureters and vessels and improved visualization of renal processes. CT remains a less than optimal tool for evaluation of genital disease, but it is useful in first-line evaluation of lower abdominal and pelvic pain as well as evaluation of tumor extent for presurgical planning. Knowledge of the capabilities and limitations of MSCT allows the radiologist to use MSCT appropriately and for the greatest possible patient care.

The aim of this chapter is to review the MSCT strategies for genitourinary imaging and to provide evidence-based guidelines for the performance and interpretation of these studies.

TERMINOLOGY FOR MULTIPHASE MSCT OF THE KIDNEY

Phases of Enhancement

Contrast enhancement of the kidneys is unlike that of other abdominopelvic organs due to the compartmentalized structure and physiology of the kidneys. Knowledge of this is crucial for the evaluation of renal disease. The kidneys are highly vascular organs and receive 25% of the resting cardiac output. Approximately 90% of renal blood flow goes to the renal cortex. After administration of a bolus of intravenous contrast material, opacification of the renal arteries and renal cortex is typically seen nearly simultaneously with enhancement of the abdominal aorta. Opacified blood flows rapidly into the low-resistance glomeruli of the renal cortex, and then almost as rapidly, it flows back out into the renal veins. The renal veins and portions of the suprarenal inferior vena cava are opacified even during the typical "early arterial" phase of contrast enhancement when other abdominal organs show minimal, if any, parenchymal enhancement. In contrast, slower-flowing blood supplies the renal tubules of the renal medulla, which is supplied by the tubular vascular network. Therefore, the medullary pyramids enhance much more slowly than the renal cortex. The medulla is clearly distinguished from the cortex during early phases of enhancement (*corticomedullary phase*). The enhancement of the cortical and medullary vascular networks eventually demonstrates similar enhancement during the later phases of contrast enhancement, called the *nephrographic phase*. Because of filtration and concentration of intravenous contrast material, the renal collecting system opacifies intensely with contrast as time passes. This latter phase is called the *excretory phase* of contrast enhancement and may persist in normal individuals more than 24 hours after contrast administration. The phases of contrast are summarized in Table 13-1, and examples are shown in Figure 13-1.

1. Early arterial (or arteriographic) phase. Typically acquired after a scan delay of 20 seconds. This early phase of contrast enhancement allows for optimal arterial evaluation and may be acquired after a fixed scan delay or after an individualized delay determined by a test bolus or by bolus-tracking software.
2. Late arterial (or corticomedullary) phase. Typically acquired after a scan delay of 45 seconds. The renal cortex is well enhanced. Hypervascular lesions, such as many renal cell carcinomas,

Table 13-1 Indications for acquisition of nonenhanced and multiphase postcontrast images

Phase	Indications
Nonenhanced	Nephrolithiasis Diagnosis of hemorrhage Diagnosis of angiomyolipoma Baseline for confirmation of subsequent enhancement
Early arterial (arteriographic) 20-second delay	CT arteriogram for arterial anatomy
Late arterial (corticomedullary) 45-second delay	Detection of hypervascular tumors Evaluation of normal renal veins
Nephrographic 90 to 200-second delay	Detection of parenchymal masses Evaluation of venous thrombosis
Excretory More than 200-second delay	Evaluation of renal collection system

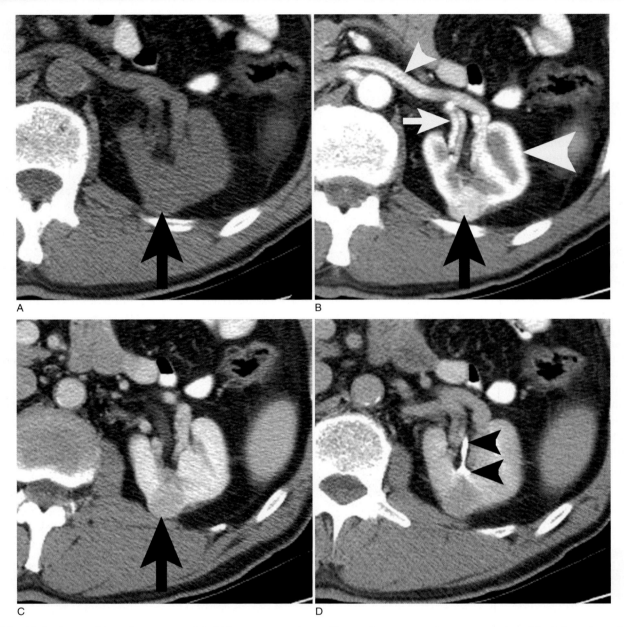

Fig. 13-1 Phases of CT enhancement of the kidney. **A,** Nonenhanced image shows a posterior contour bulge of the kidney *(arrow)*. **B,** Corticomedullary phase demonstrates enhancement of the renal cortex *(large arrowhead)* but not of the medulla. The renal vein *(small arrowhead)* and renal artery *(small arrow)* are both opacified. A renal cell carcinoma *(large arrow)* is noted posteriorly. **C,** Nephrographic phase. Uniform enhancement of the renal parenchyma is seen. The renal cell carcinoma is again visualized posteriorly *(arrow)*. **D,** Delayed phase shows excreted contrast in the renal collecting system *(arrow)*.

may be most conspicuous during this phase of contrast.[1,2] The medulla is poorly enhanced during this phase of contrast.

3. Nephrographic phase. Typically acquired after a scan delay of 90 to 200 seconds. The renal cortex and medulla exhibit a similar degree of contrast enhancement. The relatively uniform renal parenchymal enhancement allows maximum sensitivity for parenchymal lesion detection.[1,2]

4. Excretory phase. The scan delay for optimally imaging the collecting system is variable and may range from 3 to 15 minutes, or longer. These

images help in the detection of urothelial lesions and filling defects in the renal collecting system.

Streamlining the MSCT Evaluation of the Kidneys

As just described, the kidneys may be imaged and re-imaged during different phases of contrast enhancement to emphasize different aspects of renal pathology. However, repeated CT imaging increases the radiation dose delivered to the patient, decreases the life of the CT x-ray tube, increases data storage demands, and increases the number of images that a radiologist must interpret for a particular examination. A study of 31 renal tumors (16 renal cell carcinomas and 15 cysts) demonstrated that although the specificity of both the nephrographic and corticomedullary phases were 100% for determination of malignancy, the nephrographic phase was more sensitive for renal cancers (16 of 16 versus 11 of 16 cancers detected).[1] Another study of 417 renal lesions showed that nephrographic phase evaluation was more sensitive than corticomedullary phase evaluation for lesion detection (389 versus 259 lesions detected) and that the addition of the corticomedullary phase to the nephrographic phase images did not result in an increased number of tumors identified. In particular, lesions in the medulla were more frequently identified by nephrographic phase imaging (111 lesions detected) than by corticomedullary phase imaging (25 lesions detected).[2] In light of such findings, the corticomedullary phase may not contribute significantly to the detection of renal cell carcinoma and may be reasonably excluded from routine CT screening of the kidneys.

The excretory phase of contrast does not require the acquisition of an extra set of images of the urinary tract. To reduce the patient radiation dose and the number of images for the radiologist, the excretory phase of contrast can be combined with other phases of contrast. This can be done by splitting the contrast bolus so that a small bolus of intravenous contrast (40 ml) is given to opacify the collecting system 4 minutes or more before administration of a larger contrast bolus (80 to 110 ml).[3] The resultant CT images have uniform enhancement of the renal parenchyma as well as opacification of the collecting system. A typical CT protocol for such imaging is shown in Table 13-2.

CT Evaluation of Hematuria

Several studies before the introduction of MSCT have shown that 17% to 22% of patients who present with hematuria will have urinary disease requiring treatment, and approximately 1% to 3% of patients will be diagnosed with a urological malignancy (Table 13-3).[4-6] In these studies, the prevalence of significant urologic disease varied with the patient population and depended on whether hematuria was gross or microscopic. Subsequent studies have shown a high sensitivity of CT for urinary stones as well as other urological pathology, but specific outcome data regarding the impact of MSCT for evaluation of hematuria remain sparse.[7,8]

Table 13-2 Split bolus CT urogram

Step	Description
1. Nonenhanced	Nonenhanced CT of the kidneys through the pelvis
2. Mini bolus	Pre-bolus 40 ml intravenous contrast; wait 4 minutes
3. Parenchymal bolus	Bolus 110 ml intravenous contrast; wait 100 seconds
4. Combined nephrographic and excretory phase	Thin-section CT through the abdomen and pelvis

Table 13-3 Prevalence of significant urological disease in patients with hematuria*[4-6]

Author	Number of patients	Significant urological disease	Malignancy
Murakami et al[5]	1034	22%	2.3%
Ritchie et al[6]	76	17%	2.6%
Thompson[4]	85	22%	1.2%

*Significant disease includes pyelonephritis, nephrourolithiasis, renal parenchymal disease, vascular thrombosis, and vascular malformations.

NONENHANCED CT

Renal Stone Disease

Nonenhanced CT is much more sensitive for renal and ureteral calculi than intravenous urography. Furthermore, nonenhanced CT is useful for identifying causes of flank pain other than nephrolithiasis, such as aortic aneurysm, perirenal abscess, and bony fractures. In a prospective trial of 93 patients referred for clinically suspected renal colic, a change in the treatment plan was made in 57 patients (61%) based on findings at nonenhanced CT.[9]

Detection of Stones

CT is the most sensitive cross-sectional modality for direct visualization of renal and ureteral calculi. The sensitivity of helical CT for depicting a renal or ureteral stone is 94% to 98%, whereas that of ultrasonography is approximately 20%, and intravenous urogram is 52% to 59%.[10-13] The vividness of direct stone visualization at CT is affected by several factors, including CT technique and stone composition. In general, calcified stones are more conspicuous and of higher CT attenuation than noncalcified stones, such as uric acid, struvite, and cystine stones.[14] Use of higher kilovolt (kV) settings (120 and 140 kV) and higher tube current (mA) allows visualization of smaller diameter stones than lower kilovolt and tube current settings,[14] likely caused by decreased noise. Also, use of thinner slice thickness improves visualization of small stones (Figure 13-2), particularly for poorly calcified stones such as pure uric acid, struvite, and cystine stones.[15]

Secondary signs of ureteral obstruction are useful for determining whether calcified focus is a ureteral stone. In particular, hydroureter is a useful sign because this occurs in 70% of patients with ureteral stones, and hydronephrosis and perinephric fat stranding occurs in 50% and 49%, respectively.[16] In addition, the obstructed kidney may be swollen and demonstrate slightly lower CT attenuation (5 to 10 HU lower) than the contralateral kidney in up to 87% of cases.[16] Another less-reliable sign of ureteral obstruction is decreased CT attenuation of the tips of the medullary pyramids near the calyces. It should be noted that absence of hydroureteronephrosis does not imply absence of ureteral obstruction; early ureteral obstruction

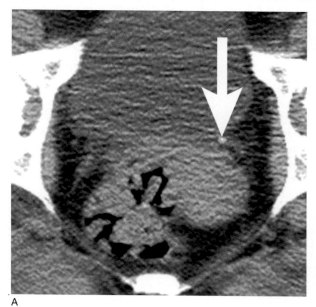

A

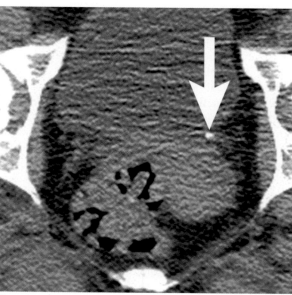

B

Fig. 13-2 CT slice thickness and stone visualization. **A**, 5-mm slice thickness CT image shows a small stone at the ureterovesical junction *(arrow)*. **B**, 2.5-mm slice thickness CT image shows the same *(arrow)* stone more vividly despite increased image noise. However, CT scans obtained at thinner slice thickness may increase radiation dose.

may not have resulted in dilation of the ureter by the time of CT examination. Also, in children, perinephric fat stranding has been shown to be a relatively infrequent finding in ureteral stone obstruction, occurring in only 1 of 20 patients examined in one study.[17]

Differentiation of Stones from Phleboliths

A problem with nonenhanced CT is that stones, particularly in the pelvis near the ureterovesical junction, must be differentiated from phleboliths. Although phleboliths commonly demonstrate a radiolucent center at plain film radiography, this sign was not useful at CT for distinguishing phleboliths from ureteral stones. In a clinical study of 50 patients with 120 phleboliths, only 1% of phleboliths showed a definite radiolucent center at CT, whereas 34% of the same phleboliths showed a radiolucent center at plain film radiography.[18] A similar study of 150 phleboliths showed central lucency in 95 phleboliths at plain film radiography but in none at CT.[19] In a separate study of CT in 442 patients, of whom 136 had ureteral calculi, it was found that a thin rim of soft tissue surrounding a calcification (the "soft tissue rim sign") (Figure 13-3) was seen in 105 of 136 ureteral calculi (sensitivity 77%) and in 20 of 259 phleboliths (8%, specificity 92%).[20] In a different study of 65 patients, the soft tissue rim sign was shown to be a specific but usually superfluous sign of an intraureteric stone since at least three other signs of ureteral obstruction were seen in 64 of the 65

patients (98.5%) with ureteral stones.[21] The converse sign, the "comet tail sign," (Figure 13-4) in which a thin linear soft tissue structure is seen leading up to a calculus without an associated rim of soft tissue around the calculus, is often described as a characteristic of a phlebolith rather than a ureteral stone. However, the comet tail sign is neither sensitive nor specific for phleboliths, and, when observed in patients with ureteral obstruction, was shown to actually represent a ureteral calculus in 50% to 67% of cases.[21] Use of a computer work station or PACS, which allows dynamic scrolling of axial CT images as well as 3D reformations, is also useful for defining the path of a ureter and determining whether a calcification is within or external to a ureter. In the rare case when a CT examination is equivocal for location of a calcification, intravenous contrast material may be administered to opacify the renal collecting system, allowing more vivid depiction of the ureter relative to the calcification.

Radiation Dose

A disadvantage of CT relative to other imaging modalities for renal stone evaluation is the relatively high radiation dose delivered to the patient. Using

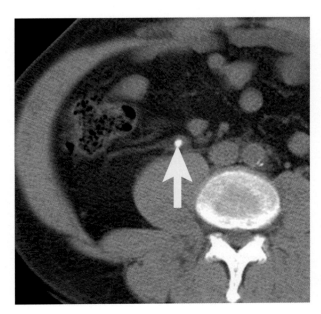

Fig. 13-3 Soft tissue rim sign. A ureteral stone *(arrow)* is surrounded by a thin layer of soft tissue density. Although the finding of the soft tissue rim sign is suggestive of a ureteral stone, this sign is only seen in 77% of ureteral stones and may be seen in up to 8% of phleboliths.[20]

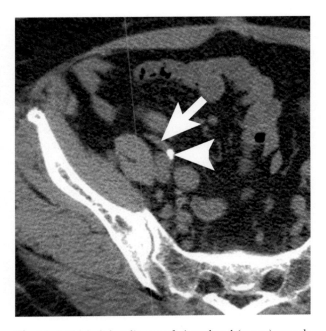

Fig. 13-4 Phlebolith. A linear soft tissue band *(arrow)* extends to a punctate calcification *(arrowhead)*, a finding known as the *comet tail sign.* This finding suggests the calcification is a phlebolith rather than a ureteral stone.

a standard abdominal CT technique of 120 kV and 240 mA, the radiation dose is estimated to be three times that of three-film intravenous urography.[22] Several modifications of CT technique, including higher pitch, lower tube current (mA), and lower kilovoltage, can decrease radiation dose, but each adjustment will decrease image quality. Fortunately, since renal stones are generally high-attenuation structures, a decrease in image quality may not result in a significant decrease in CT accuracy for stone detection. A CT phantom experiment with 37 calcium oxalate stones (ranging from 2 to 8 mm scanned at 120 kV and tube current ranging from 20 to 170 mA) showed 100% sensitivity for stone detection and was noted down to 80 mA.[23] In a separate experiment, in which patients weighing less than 91 kg (200 lb) were scanned once with a mean tube current of 160 mA and again with identical imaging parameters (except for a reduced tube current of 100 mA), the accuracy for stone detection was not significantly decreased with the lower tube current. In this experiment, radiation dose was decreased by 25% for multidetector row and 42% for single-detector row CT.[24] Other evaluations of low-radiation dose CT for detection of nephrolithiasis were performed with clinical findings and follow-up as the reference standard for the presence of stones. One such study demonstrated sensitivities of 90% to 95% for ureterolithiasis at MSCT when patients were scanned with 120 kV and 30 mA, complemented by additional scans at 60 or 120 mA as needed when excessive image noise was noted.[25] A separate study compared a CT pitch of 3.0 to a pitch of 1.5 and showed no significant decrease in CT sensitivity for renal stone detection.[26] It should be noted, however, that combinations of such decreased current and increased pitch have not been studied and would likely result in unacceptably poor image quality.

Prognosis of Ureterolithiasis

The size and location of ureteral stones are predictive of whether the ureteral stones will pass with conservative medical management or whether surgical intervention will be required. At CT, a stone 4 mm or smaller in axial diameter will have a greater than 75% likelihood of passing with conservative management, whereas stones 9 mm or larger are less than 50% likely to pass without invasive intervention. Similarly, stones identified in the mid-ureter or more distally have a greater than 60% likelihood of passing without the need for invasive intervention, whereas more proximal stones are less than 50% likely to pass without intervention.[10]

INTRAVENOUS CONTRAST-ENHANCED MSCT

Nephrotoxicity of Intravenous Contrast Material

Intravenous contrast-enhanced CT allows highly detailed evaluation of the urinary tract. A limitation is the potential nephrotoxicity of iodinated contrast material, which is a particular concern in patients with urological disease, since such patients may have decreased functional renal reserve.

Renal toxicity caused by iodinated contrast materials is called *contrast-induced nephropathy* and is defined by a greater than 25% rise in serum creatinine or an absolute increase from baseline creatinine by more than 0.5 mg/dl. In most cases, the rise in serum creatinine normalizes within 2 weeks, but acute renal failure that requires dialysis will occur in fewer than 1% of patients. Half of these patients will require dialysis for the rest of their lives. In general, contrast-induced nephropathy is associated with a higher rate of in-hospital complications and mortality.

The most important risk factor for development of contrast-induced nephropathy is poor baseline renal function, but other risk factors include diabetes, hypertension, history of renal disease (in particular, recent worsening of renal dysfunction), congestive heart failure, and dehydration at the time of intravenous contrast administration. Patients receiving nephrotoxic drugs may also be at higher risk for renal injury.

There are three basic concepts in the prevention of contrast induced nephropathy:
1. Hydration
2. Type and quantity of administered contrast material
3. Pharmacotherapy before and after contrast administration

Patients at higher risk for contrast-induced nephropathy may be hydrated vigorously before and after administration of iodinated contrast material. In addition, the radiologist may choose to administer a lower dose of contrast or use an isoosmolar contrast agent. Isoosmolar contrast agents, although generally more expensive than the more commonly used hyperosmolar agents, have been shown in some trials to decrease the rate and severity of renal injury,[27] possibly by decreasing the osmotic load on the kidneys and thereby decreasing the energy expenditure of the collecting tubules and preventing microvascular ischemia. Other measures to prevent or lessen the renal risk in these patients is administration of antioxidants such as *N*-acetylcysteine before and after contrast administration[28,29] or administration of intravenous sodium bicarbonate before contrast administration.[30] However, the usefulness of such medical therapy remains controversial.

Distinction of Benign from Malignant Masses

The main radiological goal after the initial detection of a renal mass is characterization of whether the mass is benign or malignant. General guidelines for approaching such masses are as follows:

1. Solid (enhancing) tumors in the kidney that do not contain macroscopic fat must be considered malignant until proven otherwise.
2. A solid renal mass that contains macroscopic fat is almost certainly an angiomyolipoma.

This is a simple distinction in the great majority of cases. Macroscopic fat is considered to have CT attenuation of less than −20 HU, regardless of whether intravenous contrast material was delivered and suggests the mass is an angiomyolipoma (Figure 13-5). Nonenhanced thin-section CT is generally more sensitive for the detection of subtle

macroscopic fat than thick-section–enhanced CT. Pitfalls to avoid include fat that is at the extreme periphery of a renal lesion, because such fat deposits can rarely represent perirenal fat that has been trapped between lobules of tumor.[31] Rare cases of renal cell carcinoma with such an appearance of macroscopic fat have been published.[32] Another pitfall to avoid is that of a fatty mass abutting, but not definitely arising from, the kidney. Such a lesion may represent a fatty malignancy, such as a retroperitoneal liposarcoma (Figure 13-6). Although the finding of macroscopic fat is highly suggestive of angiomyolipoma, 4.5% of angiomyolipomas have minimal fat (nonmacroscopic) at CT, and differentiation of an angiomyolipoma with minimal fat from renal cell carcinoma is difficult. A study of 19 angiomyolipomas with minimal fat and 62 renal cell carcinomas at CT showed that angiomyolipomas tend to have a lower peak enhancement than renal cell carcinoma and also tend to have more homogeneous and prolonged enhancement. However, these features were not definitive for distinguishing the two entities.[33] In particular, papillary and chromophobic subtypes of renal cell carcinomas also tend to have homogeneous and lower peak enhancement[34] and may be misconstrued as angiomyolipomas by such criteria.

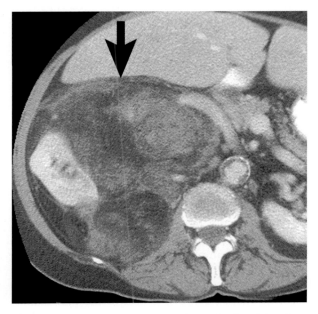

Fig. 13-6 Large fatty masses *(arrow)* not clearly arising from the kidney may be due to retroperitoneal liposarcoma. Differentiation of retroperitoneal liposarcoma from angiomyolipomas may be difficult.

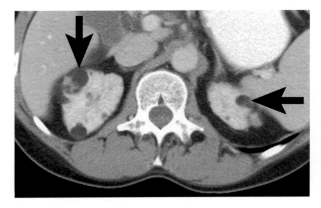

Fig. 13-5 Angiomyelolipoma. Macroscopic fat *(arrows)* in these renal masses strongly suggests angiomyelolipoma.

Renal Tumor Enhancement and Pseudoenhancement

A crucial distinction for characterization of renal masses at CT is whether such masses are solid or cystic. For such an evaluation, comparison of contrast-enhanced images with nonenhanced images is helpful to determine if enhancement occurs with administration of intravenous contrast. Frequently, dense lesions with CT attenuations up to 100 HU may be shown on nonenhanced CT images to be of the same CT attenuation, proving them to be merely hemorrhagic cysts rather than enhancing solid tumors. In general, an increase in CT attenuation of 10 HU or more indicates that a lesion is solid rather than cystic.

However, the finding of increased CT attenuation at contrast-enhanced CT images compared with nonenhanced CT images is not a reliable indicator that a lesion is solid. One reason is partial volume averaging. If voxels representing a cystic lesion include portions of normal enhancing renal parenchyma, then those voxels will demonstrate enhancement caused by partial volume averaging. A study of helical CT of 48 sonographically proven renal cysts demonstrated that significantly more cysts exhibited pseudoenhancement when the slice thickness was more than half the diameter of the cyst, particularly during the nephrographic phase of contrast enhancement.[35] The ideal slice thickness for evaluation of a renal mass should be one third or less of the z-axis diameter of the renal mass, and the region of interest should be drawn carefully on the center slice to stay well within the borders of the mass.

Unfortunately, even with careful assessment, contrast-enhanced MSCT may give a false finding of increased CT attenuation because of a phenomenon called *pseudoenhancement*. Pseudoenhancement refers to the CT finding of false increase by more then 10 HU in CT attenuation of a structure simply because the surrounding tissue has increased attenuation (Figure 13-7). This phenomenon has been well documented in phantom experiments. A study of renal cyst phantom inserts in an anthropomorphic phantom showed pseudoenhancement of greater than 10 HU in 33% of renal cyst phantoms that were 0.7 to 1.5 cm in diameter when CT slice thickness was 50% or less of the cyst diameter. The range of pseudoenhancement was 10.3 to 28 HU and was higher and more common when the background renal CT density was 240 HU rather than 140 HU.[36] In this study, no appreciable pseudoenhancement was noted when cysts were entirely exophytic.[36] Two different studies compared pseudoenhancement between MSCT and single-detector row CT in renal cyst phantoms suspended in baths of diluted iodinated contrast material. One study used 0.5- and 1.5-cm fluid-density rods, and the other used 8- to 28-mm water-filled spheres as phantoms. Both studies found pseudoenhancement was more prominent when the background renal CT attenuation was higher and when MSCT rather than single-detector helical CT was used, regardless of pitch.[37,38]

Solid Renal Masses

Once a renal mass is determined to be solid, the etiology of the mass can be further assessed. The differential diagnosis of a solid renal mass includes renal cell carcinoma (more than 90% of cases), angiomyolipoma with minimal fat, and oncocytoma. Less commonly, a non-fatty solid renal mass will result from transitional cell carcinoma, lymphoma, and metastasis.

Oncocytomas are rare benign tumors of the kidney that classically demonstrate a central stellate scar and a "spoke wheel" appearance of vessels on angiography.[39] Resection is both diagnostic and curative. Transitional cell carcinoma may appear in the calyces and mimic a renal parenchymal mass. In such cases, transitional cell carcinoma tends to be more centrally located in the kidney and may appear as a polypoid-filling defect in the renal collecting system or as an infiltrating mass and may be associated with circumferential wall thickening or calyceal dilatation.[40,41]

Renal lymphoma may have myriad appearances. The prevalence of renal involvement in lymphoma is 30% to 60% at autopsy, but it is only seen in 3% to 8% of patients at CT. Primary renal lymphoma is rare. At CT, renal lymphoma may appear as multiple small, homogeneous-appearing hypoattenuating enhancing masses (Figure 13-8) or may be associated with diffuse infiltration or perinephric encasement. In rare cases, lymphoma may present as a single homogeneous mass. In the vast majority of cases, renal lymphoma is associated with lymphadenopathy.[42]

Metastases to the kidneys are also uncommonly seen at CT but are more common at autopsy, where a prevalence of 2% to 20% has been noted. The most common primary cancers to metastasize to the kidneys are lung, breast, gastric, pancreatic, colon,

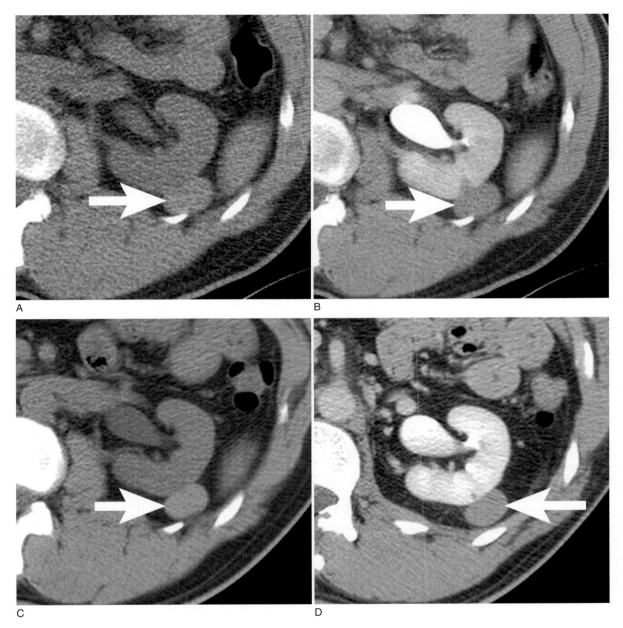

Fig. 13-7 Pseudoenhancement of renal cyst. The following example of a cyst proven at ultrasound illustrates the problem of pseudoenhancement, a phenomenon in which a nonvascularized mass appears to enhance by more than 10 HU when adjacent structures enhance intensely. This may cause the reader to diagnose a solid renal tumor at CT when the lesion is actually a cyst and occurs more commonly when adjacent renal parenchyma enhances intensely and when multidetector row (rather than single-detector row) CT is used. **A,** Single-detector row CT obtained without intravenous contrast demonstrates a slightly high-attenuation exophytic renal mass *(arrow)*. **B,** Administration of intravenous contrast material showed increase of CT attenuation by only 4 HU while the adjacent renal parenchyma enhanced by 180 HU. **C,** The same lesion is imaged 5 years later with a 16-slice multidetector row CT scanner without intravenous contrast. The cyst has decreased slightly in size. **D,** After administration of intravenous contrast, the adjacent renal parenchyma enhanced by 280 HU. The CT attenuation of the cyst increased by 24 HU over that of the nonenhanced CT.

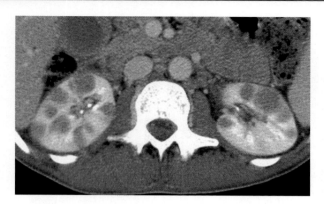

Fig. 13-8 Renal lymphoma. Multiple minimally enhancing intrarenal masses are seen in the kidneys bilaterally.

and melanoma. A study of 27 patients with metastases to the kidneys showed that the masses were small and multifocal in 10 patients, perinephric in 6 patients, and unifocal in 11 patients. Three of the patients (12%) had metastases only in the kidneys.[43]

Cystic Masses

Renal cystic lesions must be approached in a different manner than solid lesions at MSCT. Renal cysts are common and have a prevalence of 20% by age 40 and 33% after age 60. Although most renal cysts remain small and clinically silent, a minority enlarge and may result in abdominal, flank, or pelvic pain.[44] Aspiration alone may temporarily relieve pain, but renal cysts frequently recur with continuation or resurgence of symptoms. Surgical resection, decortication, or ablation may definitively relieve symptoms.[45,46] Occasionally a cyst may represent a cystic renal cell carcinoma or other malignancy, and such lesions must be differentiated from benign cystic disease.

Increasing structural complexity of renal cystic masses has been shown to correlate with increasing likelihood of malignancy. The assessment of renal cysts in this manner is popularly known as the *Bosniak classification,*[47] a set of criteria that was assembled in 1986 and that has been subsequently validated by independent groups[48,49] (Figures 13-9 and 13-10). This list of criteria, with modifications, is summarized in Table 13-4. Some concern has been raised regarding this classification because of a few reports of Bosniak Type II cysts that were later found to be malignant.[48,50] However, in these studies the focus of malignancy was microscopic, or the CT images were not published. A subsequent study of

42 moderately complex cysts (i.e., Bosniak Type IIF) followed for 2 years or longer showed that two were malignant at follow-up, but neither was found to be locally advanced.[44] This study led to the conclusion that moderately complex renal cysts can be followed safely and reassessed for change without undue concern that the cystic masses will become frankly invasive tumors in the interim.

Incidental High-Density Renal Masses

The number of cases of renal cell carcinoma has continued to rise in most populations, possibly because of the increased incidental detection of renal cell carcinoma at imaging for unrelated indications, and possibly because of environmental exposures.[51] As many as 61% of renal cell carcinomas are now detected at imaging obtained for unrelated reasons.[52] Such incidental high-density renal masses are commonly identified at routine CT obtained with a single phase of contrast during the portal venous phase. This presents a diagnostic dilemma for the radiologist because it is difficult to ask all patients with incidental renal masses to return for additional imaging. Although definitive determination of whether a mildly to moderately high attenuation renal mass is solid or cystic is difficult on a single-phase CT scan, stratification of malignancy risk can be made. A study of 57 solid renal cell carcinomas and 37 high-density benign renal cysts at portal venous phase CT showed that a CT attenuation greater than 70 HU or moderate to marked internal heterogeneity was suggestive of renal cell carcinoma.[53] In this study, the sensitivity for renal cell carcinoma by these criteria was 91% (52/57) for each of two readers, with a specificity of 92% (34/37) for reader 1 and 84% (31/37) for reader 2.[53]

Small Renal Lesions

Small renal cell carcinomas tend to grow slowly. At autopsy, renal tumors are identified in 1.5% of the population at gross inspection and more than 22% when the kidneys are examined with 2-mm sectioning.[54] However, renal cell carcinoma is a clinical diagnosis in only 0.03% to 0.3% of patients.[55] Unfortunately, not all small renal cell carcinomas are low grade. At least one radiological study showed that renal cell carcinomas identified when small in size (<3 cm in diameter) may actually be of higher grade and higher local stage than renal cell

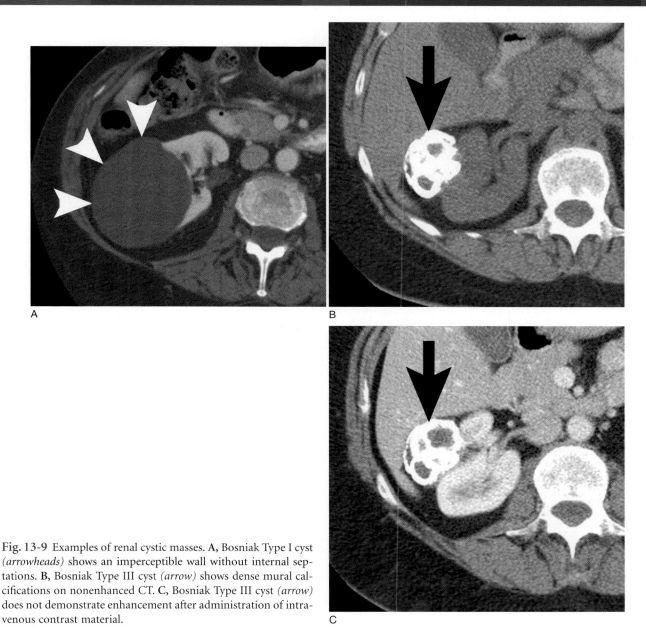

Fig. 13-9 Examples of renal cystic masses. **A,** Bosniak Type I cyst *(arrowheads)* shows an imperceptible wall without internal septations. **B,** Bosniak Type III cyst *(arrow)* shows dense mural calcifications on nonenhanced CT. **C,** Bosniak Type III cyst *(arrow)* does not demonstrate enhancement after administration of intravenous contrast material.

carcinomas identified when larger in size (>3 cm in diameter).[56]

The treatment of renal cell carcinoma is evolving. In many cases of incidentally noted renal tumor, the etiology of the renal tumor is uncertain, and therefore short-term conservative management may be preferred. In addition, surgery may be postponed if the patient refuses or is a poor surgical candidate. In such cases, what is the natural history of renal cell carcinoma? A study of 56 patients with renal cell carcinoma showed that doubling time is extremely variable (mean 610 days, range less than 60 days to more than 6 years), and there is no significant correlation between initial tumor size and doubling time.[57] Another study of 37 patients with renal cell carcinoma showed the mean diameter growth to be 0.36 cm/year (range 0 to 1.1 cm/year).[58] A study focusing on 13 cases of initially asymptomatic small renal cell carcinoma showed a mean growth of 1.32 cm^3/year.[59] In this series, the two patients with fast-growing tumors had symptoms attributable to tumor growth, but no metastases

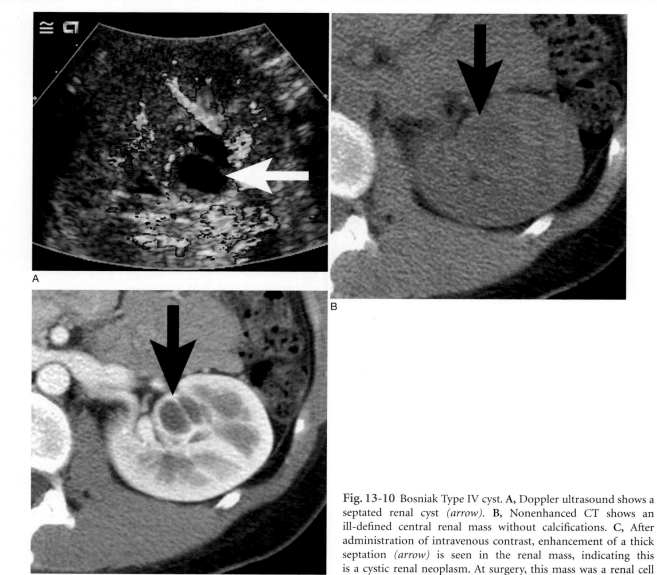

Fig. 13-10 Bosniak Type IV cyst. **A,** Doppler ultrasound shows a septated renal cyst *(arrow)*. **B,** Nonenhanced CT shows an ill-defined central renal mass without calcifications. **C,** After administration of intravenous contrast, enhancement of a thick septation *(arrow)* is seen in the renal mass, indicating this is a cystic renal neoplasm. At surgery, this mass was a renal cell carcinoma.

were later found.[59] Similarly, Birnbaum et al. (1990)[60] showed that in a series of 11 patients with renal cell carcinoma, the mean diameter growth was 0.5 cm/year (range 0.1 to 1.6 cm/year). Based on these reports, close monitoring with reassessment at a later date may be a viable option for patients in whom surgery is not an attractive option.

Preoperative Evaluation of the Kidneys

Advances in renal imaging have been paralleled by advances in surgical and interventional treatment for renal tumors. Laparoscopic nephrectomy is becoming increasingly common for both malignant and benign renal disease. Knowledge of the presence, size, and location of accessory renal arteries and veins is an important factor for preventing surgical complications. A precaval right renal artery (an artery coursing anterior to the inferior vena cava) is of particular concern for laparoscopic nephrectomy since dissection along the anteromedial aspect of the inferior vena cava is often performed with limited direct visualization.[61]

Table 13-4 Malignancy of renal cystic lesion by Bosniak category[44,47,49]

Category	Description	CT features	Approximate likelihood of malignancy
I	Benign simple cyst	Ovoid unilocular lesion Thin/imperceptible wall Sharp parenchymal interface Uniform fluid density (±20 HU)	~0%
II	Benign, high-density cyst Benign, mildly complex cyst	Thin septa Fine curvilinear calcification	~0%
IIF	Moderately complex cyst that requires short-term imaging follow-up	Multiple septa Findings between those of II and III	~5%
III	Possibly malignant complex cyst	Thick or irregular wall or septa Irregular thick calcifications Nonenhancing nodules	~50%
IV	Malignant complex cyst	Irregular enhancing thick wall or septae Enhancing or large nodules	>90%

For treatment of renal tumors, an alternative to radical nephrectomy is partial, or nephron-sparing, nephrectomy. Initially, nephron-sparing surgery was reserved for patients with borderline renal function, a solitary kidney, or a high risk of future renal resection, such as patients with von Hippel–Lindau syndrome or tuberous sclerosis. However, recent studies have shown a similar low risk (0% to 3%) of local recurrence for partial nephrectomy as for radical nephrectomy for treatment of solitary small peripheral renal tumors less than 4 cm in diameter,[62,63] and the indications for nephron-sparing surgery continue to expand. Presurgical evaluation for partial (nephron-sparing) surgery demands accurate assessment of tumor relationship to vessels and the renal collecting system.[64,65] Initial surgical reports focused on resection only of small peripheral renal tumors, but more recent reports suggest that partial nephrectomy may be a reasonable option in patients with centrally located and larger tumors.[66,67]

CT Urography

Evaluation of the renal collecting system is traditionally obtained by plain film conventional intravenous urography, which allows high in-plane resolution as well as relatively lower patient radiation doses. Since the radiation dose of several abdominopelvic plain films is lower than that of CT, multiple images of the renal collecting system may be obtained, which allows a higher likelihood of imaging all segments of the ureters in an opacified state. However, the renal parenchyma is poorly evaluated by conventional intravenous urography. To help this latter deficiency, a CT scan of the abdomen may be performed immediately after the conventional urogram to evaluate the renal parenchyma.[68] Conversely, a contrast-enhanced renal CT may be obtained, followed by plain film evaluation of the collecting system.[69] Although such approaches combine the strength of CT and plain film imaging, logistical coordination of such studies is cumbersome and not always possible.

More recently, several groups have proposed full evaluation of the renal parenchyma and upper tract renal collecting system (renal calices to the distal ureters) by MSCT alone without use of plain film radiography[3,70] (Figure 13-11). In general, this requires thin-section CT imaging through the ureters after excretion of intravenous contrast material. These images can be viewed by scrolling on a PACS system or may be reformatted into coronal urographic images. During evaluation of opacified ureters at CT, one must adjust for the high intensity of excreted contrast material that frequently prevents evaluation for small filling defects in the renal collecting system when images are viewed on soft tissue windows. Dynamic adjustment of window

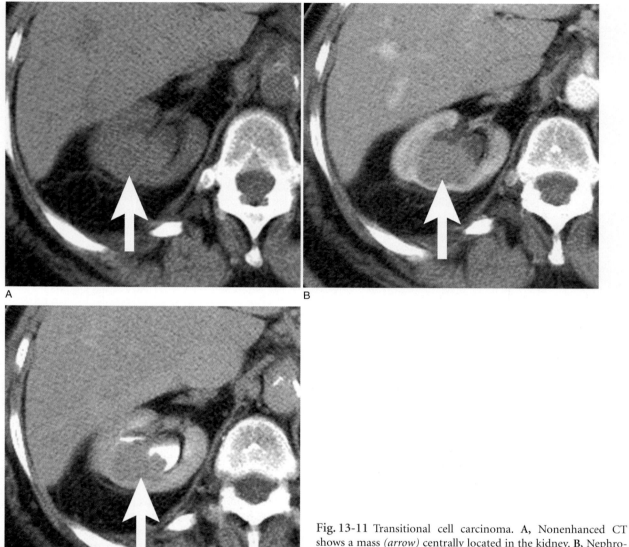

Fig. 13-11 Transitional cell carcinoma. A, Nonenhanced CT shows a mass *(arrow)* centrally located in the kidney. B, Nephrographic phase CT images show the mass *(arrow)* abuts the renal collecting system. C, Delayed-phase CT images show frondlike areas of the mass *(arrow)* extending into the opacified renal collecting system.

and level settings on a work station or use of bone windows will facilitate detection of such lesions (Figure 13-12).

Because of ureteral peristalsis and occasional variable renal excretion of contrast material, portions of the ureteral lumen are frequently not opacified with contrast material at the time of the CT scan (Figure 13-13). Similar to intravenous urography, several techniques have been developed for improving distention of the upper tract collecting system at the time of CT urography. One approach

is to simply scan the patient many times, either on a routine basis[70] or as needed, to improve the likelihood that all segments of the ureters will be opacified with contrast. Alternatively, compression may be placed on the abdomen[3,70,71] over the sacral promontory to prevent urine flow into the distal ureters, thereby improving upper ureteral distention. Imaging of the lower ureters can then be obtained when the compression is released. A third method is to hydrate the patient immediately before the CT scan with either 250 ml or more of intra-

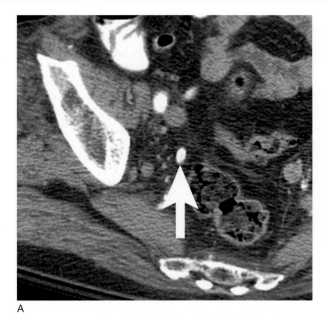

A

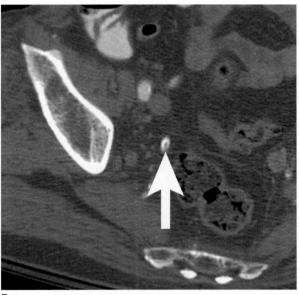

B

Fig. 13-12 Use of bone windows to evaluate the ureters. **A,** CT examination obtained during the delayed phase of contrast shows excreted contrast in the right ureter *(arrow)*, but intraureteral detail cannot be assessed. **B,** When the same image is viewed with bone windows, a filling defect *(arrow)* is revealed. This focus was proved to be transitional cell carcinoma at ureteroscopy.

venous fluid[72] or with water by mouth.[3] A fourth approach is to intravenously administer a diuretic, such as furosemide, immediately before the CT scan.[73] Each of these methods has been shown to improve ureteral opacification or distention with

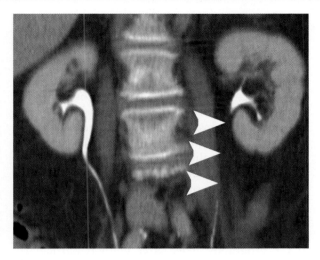

Fig. 13-13 CT urogram demonstrates poor opacification of a short segment of the proximal left ureter *(arrowheads)*.

contrast material, and they may also be used in various combinations.

The question remains, however, whether such efforts to attain distention of the ureters is of diagnostic importance. There appears to be a widely held perception that complete opacification of the ureters is a crucial endpoint of conventional intravenous urography, and this endpoint has been transferred to CT urography. The source of this belief is unclear. In an important but little known study, no upper tract malignancies were identified in 187 retrograde pyelograms performed purely because of underfilling of the upper tracts on intravenous urograms.[74] It would appear that upper tract malignancies manifest on imaging as filling defects or obstruction and do not manifest as underfilling of the ureter. The obsession with complete ureteral opacification may be misguided.

An alternative to re-imaging the patient with cross-sectional CT during the excretory phase of contrast is the use of an "enhanced" CT scout view for ureteral evaluation. This approach has been proposed as a means to decrease the patient radiation dose. If an enhanced scout is used, a low tube kilovoltage of 80 kV and a higher tube current is recommended to maximize the vividness of the excreted contrast material.[75] Preliminary reports of this technique show a similar sensitivity for urinary collecting system pathology as for plain film images.[75] It must be noted that these promising findings are not yet backed by a large body of evidence and need to be independently corroborated by other groups before widespread acceptance.

Another question is whether CT urography can replace intravenous urography for the detection of upper tract urothelial malignancy. One of the traditional reasons for obtaining conventional intravenous urography is to assess the upper tract urothelium. Early studies of CT urography are promising, but it remains to be seen whether the higher contrast resolution and volumetric acquisition of CT urography lends it sufficient sensitivity for upper tract malignancy to replace the higher in-plane spatial resolution and multiple upper tract image acquisitions of conventional urography. Also, it remains to be shown whether the added benefit and convenience of the urographic phase of CT outweighs the associated higher cost and radiation dose of CT urography. This latter point is particularly important, since neither conventional intravenous nor CT urography is sufficiently sensitive to exclude bladder cancer. For bladder cancer, cystoscopy remains a crucial component of the workup in patients with hematuria because the large majority of renal collecting system malignancies occur in the bladder. An estimated 60,000 new cases of bladder cancer will have been diagnosed in 2006, and fewer than 2500 new cases of ureteral cancer will have been found.[76] Unfortunately, this is another area of study with insufficient data, and only small preliminary studies have been published.

CT Cystogram

CT cystography is commonly performed to detect bladder leak, usually after trauma,[77] after surgery, or as a complication of malignancy.[78] CT cystography is less commonly performed to primarily evaluate for bladder malignancy.[79] CT cystography is straightforward and involves an initial nonenhanced CT scan of the pelvis with careful assessment for calcifications, fat stranding, and surgical clips. Subsequently, at least 350 ml of dilute iodinated contrast material (50 mg iodine/ml) is instilled by gravity into the bladder through an indwelling urethral or a suprapubic catheter, according to patient tolerance. Alternatively, the bladder may be filled passively with excreted contrast material if the patient does not void for 30 minutes or longer after intravenous contrast material is given. The pelvis is rescanned once when the bladder is full and once after the contrast material is drained out of the bladder (Figure 13-14). Adequate distention of the bladder with contrast and post-drainage images are important for the detection of subtle bladder tears.

In small series of up to 10 patients, CT cystography has shown a 100% sensitivity for detecting bladder tears,[80,81] but no large series has been reported comparing CT with conventional cystography.[77] If the examination is performed for malignancy, thinner section images (3 mm or thinner) and slightly less concentrated contrast material is administered through the cystostomy catheter to distend the bladder.

REPRODUCTIVE TRACT

Adnexa

Although ultrasound is the modality of choice for first-line evaluation of the female pelvis, MRI and CT may be useful for problem solving and for evaluation of certain disease entities. In the emergency room setting, CT is often the first imaging examination obtained because of its availability in many centers. When identified, adnexal masses must be differentiated from masses of nongynecologic origin and from exophytic uterine masses. Aside from the determination that a mass is in the "adnexal region," the reader can suggest that a mass is of ovarian origin if the ovarian vein can be traced from the inferior vena cava or left renal vein into the pelvic mass. This "ovarian vascular pedicle" sign was shown in one study of 108 ovarian masses and 23 subserosal uterine leiomyomas to be present in 99 of 108 (92% sensitivity) ovarian masses, but was also seen in 3 of 23 subserosal uterine leiomyomas (87% specificity).[82]

An entity with characteristic findings at CT is the mature teratoma, or dermoid cyst, which almost invariably demonstrates a component of macroscopic fat (Figure 13-15). In rare cases, macroscopic fat in an adnexal mass can represent other pathology, such as a tubal lipoma,[83] and rarely is a lesion with macroscopic fat frankly malignant. In a series of 517 mature cystic teratomas, 10.8% were bilateral, 3.5% had torsed, and only 1 (0.17%) was found to have malignant transformation at histopathology.[84] Dermoid cysts themselves are unlikely to undergo malignant transformation, but one report of 141 dermoid cysts showed that associated benign or low-grade malignant epithelial ovarian neoplasms may be present in up to 11.3% of cases.[85] Such "collision tumors" (coexistence of two histologically distinct tumors without histolog-

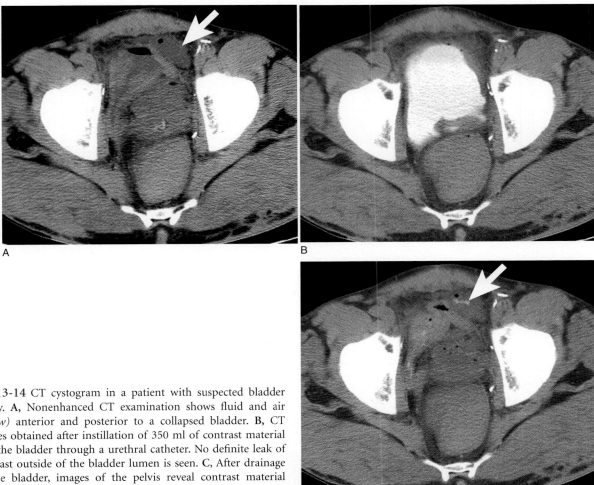

Fig. 13-14 CT cystogram in a patient with suspected bladder injury. **A,** Nonenhanced CT examination shows fluid and air *(arrow)* anterior and posterior to a collapsed bladder. **B,** CT images obtained after instillation of 350 ml of contrast material into the bladder through a urethral catheter. No definite leak of contrast outside of the bladder lumen is seen. **C,** After drainage of the bladder, images of the pelvis reveal contrast material *(arrow)* in a collection of fluid anterior to the bladder, confirming the presence of a bladder leak.

ical admixture) may be suggested if an associated prominent solid component or multiloculated cystic component containing nonfatty fluid is seen at CT.[86]

In the acute setting, physiological adnexal masses should be differentiated from processes requiring immediate intervention. In particular, corpus luteum cysts present as irregular adnexal masses typically less than 3 cm in diameter with a thick hyperdense or vascularized crenulated wall[87] (Figure 13-16) and should not be confused with a periappendiceal abscess. Corpus luteum cysts may cause pelvic pain and present with a small amount of hemoperitoneum and are up to 4.8 cm in diameter.[88]

Once obviously benign etiologies for an ovarian mass are excluded, malignancy must be considered. Features that suggest malignancy include the pres-

ence of solid components of the ovarian mass itself,[89] or the presence of ascites, lymphadenopathy, omental cake, or peritoneal implants (Figure 13-17). Large cystic unilocular or septated adnexal masses without such findings are likely benign cystadenomas (Figure 13-18). A prospective multi-institution study of 280 women suspected to have ovarian cancer at ultrasonography was performed in which each woman underwent further evaluation by CT, MRI, and Doppler ultrasonography. In this study, all three imaging modalities showed similar high accuracy (area under the receiver operating characteristic curves $Az = 0.91$ for each modality) for determining the presence of malignancy, but MRI showed higher accuracy ($Az = 0.91$) for assessment of the ovaries than CT ($Az = 0.85$), which in turn showed insignificantly higher accuracy for

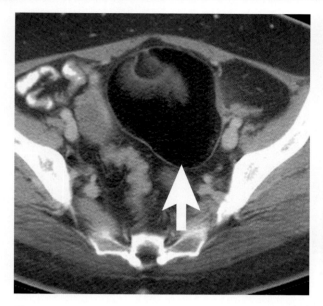

Fig. 13-15 Dermoid. Fat density *(arrow)* in an adnexal mass strongly suggests dermoid.

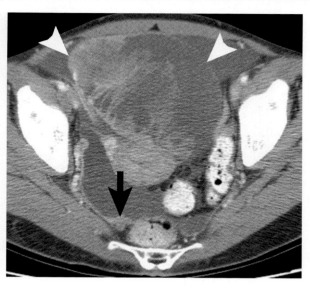

Fig. 13-17 Malignant ovarian mass. Solid and cystic adnexal masses *(arrowheads)* with free fluid and peritoneal implants *(arrow)* suggest a malignancy. Adnexal masses must be differentiated from pedunculated uterine masses.

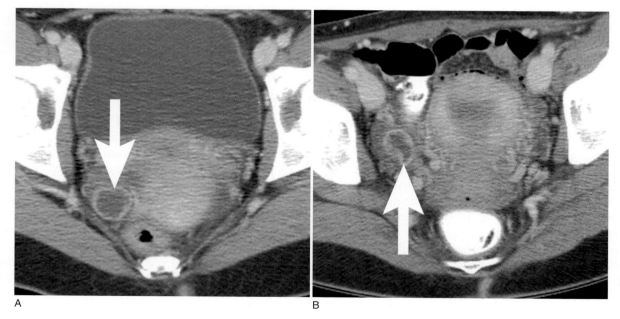

Fig. 13-16 A-B, Examples of corpus luteal cysts. A fluid attenuation structure usually less than 3 cm in diameter with enhancing and crenulated walls is suggestive of a physiological corpus luteal cyst *(arrows)*. Such cysts may be associated with a small amount of intraperitoneal blood and may cause pelvic pain.

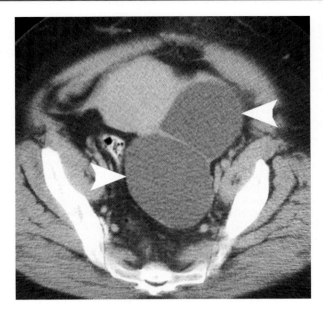

Fig. 13-18 Benign ovarian neoplasm. A unilocular or multilocular adnexal mass *(arrowheads)* without associated free intraperitoneal fluid, lymphadenopathy, or peritoneal implants suggests a benign rather than malignant ovarian neoplasm.

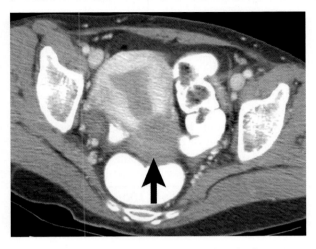

Fig. 13-19 Pseudotumor of the cervix. Delayed enhancement of the cervix *(arrow)* relative to the uterus is normal and should not be mistaken for a cervical mass.

assessment of the ovaries than Doppler ultrasonography (Az = 0.78).[90] This is not to suggest that CT is better than ultrasonography for characterizing ovarian neoplasm but that Doppler ultrasonography may not be a robust method for determining malignancy since it is operator dependent.

At the time of initial presentation, 71% of patients with ovarian carcinoma have peritoneal implants.[91] Although definitive staging of peritoneal implants is obtained at surgery with peritoneal washing,[92] CT shows excellent patient sensitivity (85% to 93%) for detection of peritoneal implants, with area under the receiver operating characteristic curves ranging from 0.89 to 0.93.[93] The CT sensitivity for lesions less than 1 cm in diameter is only 25% to 50%,[93] but a survey of gynecological oncologists showed that 61% of respondents considered debulking down to 1-cm residuals or smaller to be optimal, and an additional 12% considered 1.5- to 2.0-cm residual tumor implants to be optimal.[94] Earlier studies showed that tumor debulking below a threshold of 2-cm residuals offered survival benefit.[95,96]

After initial resection, CT may also be useful for determining disease extent and outlining further management. In particular, the finding of hydronephrosis decreases the likelihood of resectability by 19.4-fold, and pelvic sidewall invasion decreases the likelihood of resectability by 35.6-fold.[97]

Uterus

In general, MSCT is not a robust imaging modality to screen for uterine anomalies or the presence of uterine cancer, nor to evaluate for depth of spread of uterine cancer. The uterine myometrial layers are not well delineated at CT, and the plane of section is frequently not optimal for evaluation of the uterine myometrial layers. In one study of 25 patients with endometrial carcinoma, CT performed poorly compared with MRI. CT demonstrated a sensitivity of 83% and a specificity of 42% for detection of deep myometrial invasion (whereas MRI demonstrated a sensitivity of 92% and a specificity of 90%), and a sensitivity of 25% for detection of cervical involvement (MR showed a sensitivity of 86% and a specificity of 97%).[98] Furthermore, the transverse plane of section is usually not optimal for determination of uterine cancer invasion into the bladder or sigmoid colon. Once uterine malignancy is determined by other means, however, CT may be useful for evaluating distant spread or tumor recurrence.

When evaluating the uterus at contrast-enhanced CT, the reader should be aware that the cervix typically enhances with intravenous contrast later than the uterine corpus. This differential enhancement should not be misinterpreted as cervical cancer or a cervical mass (Figure 13-19).

CT

As for the female reproductive tract, CT also remains of limited value for primary evaluation of the male reproductive tract. CT may be useful for delineation of the extent of abscess formation or for fistulae. If a patient is known to have a malignancy, CT may be useful for evaluating the development of or progression of distant metastases.

CONCLUSION

Knowledge of the advantages and limitations of MSCT contributes to the appropriate use of CT in evaluation of the genitourinary tract. MSCT offers rapid and thorough evaluation of urolithiasis and anatomical evaluation of renal parenchymal disease. Preliminary reports regarding the usefulness of CT urography are promising, and the role of MSCT for evaluation of urothelial lesions continues to evolve. MSCT is useful for the evaluation of the distant spread of tumor, which may occur with genitourinary malignancies.

REFERENCES

1. Birnbaum BA, Jacobs JE, Ramchandani P: Multiphasic renal CT: comparison of renal mass enhancement during the corticomedullary and nephrographic phases, *Radiology* 200:753-758, 1996.
2. Cohan RH, Sherman LS, Korobkin M, et al: Renal masses: assessment of corticomedullary-phase and nephrographic-phase CT scans, *Radiology* 196:445-451, 1995.
3. Chow LC, Sommer FG: Multidetector CT urography with abdominal compression and three-dimensional reconstruction, *Am J Roentgenol* 177:849-855, 2001.
4. Thompson IM: The evaluation of microscopic hematuria: a population-based study, *J Urol* 138:1189-1190, 1987.
5. Murakami S, Igarashi T, Hara S, et al: Strategies for asymptomatic microscopic hematuria: a prospective study of 1,034 patients, *J Urol* 144:99-101, 1990.
6. Ritchie CD, Bevan EA, Collier SJ: Importance of occult haematuria found at screening, *Br Med J (Clin Res Ed)* 292:681-683, 1986.
7. Grossfeld GD, Litwin MS, Wolf JS, Jr., et al: Evaluation of asymptomatic microscopic hematuria in adults: the American Urological Association best practice policy—part II: patient evaluation, cytology, voided markers, imaging, cystoscopy, nephrology evaluation, and follow-up, *Urology* 57:604-610, 2001.
8. Grossfeld GD, Litwin MS, Wolf JS, et al: Evaluation of asymptomatic microscopic hematuria in adults: the American Urological Association best practice policy—part I: definition, detection, prevalence, and etiology, *Urology* 57:599-603, 2001.
9. Abramson S, Walders N, Applegate KE, et al: Impact in the emergency department of unenhanced CT on diagnostic confidence and therapeutic efficacy in patients with suspected renal colic: a prospective survey. 2000 ARRS President's Award. American Roentgen Ray Society, *Am J Roentgenol* 175:1689-1695, 2000.
10. Coll DM, Varanelli MJ, Smith RC: Relationship of spontaneous passage of ureteral calculi to stone size and location as revealed by unenhanced helical CT, *Am J Roentgenol* 178:101-103, 2002.
11. Fielding JR, Silverman SG, Samuel S, et al: Unenhanced helical CT of ureteral stones: a replacement for excretory urography in planning treatment, *Am J Roentgenol* 171:1051-1053, 1998.
12. Sourtzis S, Thibeau JF, Damry N, et al: Radiologic investigation of renal colic: unenhanced helical CT compared with excretory urography, *Am J Roentgenol* 172:1491-1494, 1999.
13. Smith RC, Verga M, McCarthy S, et al: Diagnosis of acute flank pain: value of unenhanced helical CT, *Am J Roentgenol* 166:97-101, 1996.
14. Tublin ME, Murphy ME, Delong DM, et al: Conspicuity of renal calculi at unenhanced CT: effects of calculus composition and size and CT technique, *Radiology* 225:91-96, 2002.
15. Saw KC, McAteer JA, Monga AG, et al: Helical CT of urinary calculi: effect of stone composition, stone size, and scan collimation, *Am J Roentgenol* 175:329-332, 2000.
16. Yaqoob J, Usman MU, Bari V, et al: Unenhanced helical CT of ureterolithiasis: incidence of secondary urinary tract findings, *J Pak Med Assoc* 54:2-5, 2004.
17. Smergel E, Greenberg SB, Crisci KL, et al: CT urograms in pediatric patients with ureteral calculi: do adult criteria work? *Pediatr Radiol* 31:720-723, 2001.
18. Traubici J, Neitlich JD, Smith RC: Distinguishing pelvic phleboliths from distal ureteral stones on routine unenhanced helical CT: is there a radiolucent center? *Am J Roentgenol* 172:13-17, 1999.
19. Kim JC: Central lucency of pelvic phleboliths: comparison of radiographs and noncontrast helical CT, *Clin Imaging* 25:122-125, 2001.
20. Heneghan JP, Dalrymple NC, Verga M, et al: Soft-tissue "rim" sign in the diagnosis of ureteral calculi with use of unenhanced helical CT, *Radiology* 202:709-711, 1997.
21. Guest AR, Cohan RH, Korobkin M, et al: Assessment of the clinical utility of the rim and comet-tail signs in differentiating ureteral stones from phleboliths, *Am J Roentgenol* 177:1285-1291, 2001.
22. Denton ER, Mackenzie A, Greenwell T, et al: Unenhanced helical CT for renal colic—is the radiation dose justifiable? *Clin Radiol* 54:444-447, 1999.
23. Spielmann AL, Heneghan JP, Lee LJ, et al: Decreasing the radiation dose for renal stone CT: a feasibility study of single- and multidetector CT, *Am J Roentgenol* 178:1058-1062, 2002.
24. Heneghan JP, McGuire KA, Leder RA, et al: Helical CT for nephrolithiasis and ureterolithiasis: comparison of conventional and reduced radiation-dose techniques, *Radiology* 229:575-580, 2003.
25. Tack D, Sourtzis S, Delpierre I, et al: Low-dose unenhanced multidetector CT of patients with suspected renal colic, *Am J Roentgenol* 180:305-311, 2003.

26. Diel J, Perlmutter S, Venkataramanan N, et al: Unenhanced helical CT using increased pitch for suspected renal colic: an effective technique for radiation dose reduction? *J Comput Assist Tomogr* 24:795-801, 2000.

27. Aspelin P, Aubry P, Fransson SG, et al: Nephrotoxic effects in high-risk patients undergoing angiography, *N Engl J Med* 348:491-499, 2003.

28. Kay J, Chow WH, Chan TM, et al: Acetylcysteine for prevention of acute deterioration of renal function following elective coronary angiography and intervention: a randomized controlled trial, *JAMA* 289:553-558, 2003.

29. Tepel M, van der Giet M, Schwarzfeld C, et al: Prevention of radiographic-contrast-agent-induced reductions in renal function by acetylcysteine, *N Engl J Med* 343:180-184, 2000.

30. Merten GJ, Burgess WP, Gray LV, et al: Prevention of contrast-induced nephropathy with sodium bicarbonate: a randomized controlled trial, *JAMA* 291:2328-2334, 2004.

31. Helenon O, Merran S, Paraf F, et al: Unusual fat-containing tumors of the kidney: a diagnostic dilemma, *Radiographics* 17:129-144, 1997.

32. Hammadeh MY, Thomas K, Philp T, et al: Renal cell carcinoma containing fat mimicking angiomyolipoma: demonstration with CT scan and histopathology, *Eur Radiol* 8:228-229, 1998.

33. Kim JK, Park SY, Shon JH, et al: Angiomyolipoma with minimal fat: differentiation from renal cell carcinoma at biphasic helical CT, *Radiology* 230:677-684, 2004.

34. Kim JK, Kim TK, Ahn HJ, et al: Differentiation of subtypes of renal cell carcinoma on helical CT scans, *Am J Roentgenol* 178:1499-1506, 2002.

35. Bae KT, Heiken JP, Siegel CL, et al: Renal cysts: is attenuation artifactually increased on contrast-enhanced CT images? *Radiology* 216:792-796, 2000.

36. Birnbaum BA, Maki DD, Chakraborty DP, et al: Renal cyst pseudoenhancement: evaluation with an anthropomorphic body CT phantom, *Radiology* 225:83-90, 2002.

37. Abdulla C, Kalra MK, Saini S, et al: Pseudoenhancement of simulated renal cysts in a phantom using different multidetector CT scanners, *Am J Roentgenol* 179:1473-1476, 2002.

38. Heneghan JP, Spielmann AL, Sheafor DH, et al: Pseudoenhancement of simple renal cysts: a comparison of single and multidetector helical CT, *J Comput Assist Tomogr* 26:90-94, 2002.

39. Newhouse JH, Wagner BJ: Renal oncocytomas, *Abdom Imaging* 23:249-255, 1998.

40. Urban BA, Buckley J, Soyer P, et al: CT appearance of transitional cell carcinoma of the renal pelvis: Part 2. Advanced-stage disease, *Am J Roentgenol* 169:163-168, 1997.

41. Urban BA, Buckley J, Soyer P, et al: CT appearance of transitional cell carcinoma of the renal pelvis: Part 1. Early-stage disease, *Am J Roentgenol* 169:157-161, 1997.

42. Urban BA, Fishman EK: Renal lymphoma: CT patterns with emphasis on helical CT, *Radiographics* 20:197-212, 2000.

43. Choyke PL, White EM, Zeman RK, et al: Renal metastases: clinicopathologic and radiologic correlation, *Radiology* 162:359-363, 1987.

44. Israel GM, Bosniak MA: Follow-up CT of moderately complex cystic lesions of the kidney (Bosniak category IIF), *Am J Roentgenol* 181:627-633, 2003.

45. Lifson BJ, Teichman JM, Hulbert JC: Role and long-term results of laparoscopic decortication in solitary cystic and autosomal dominant polycystic kidney disease, *J Urol* 159:702-705; discussion 705-706, 1998.

46. Stoller ML, Irby PB, III, Osman M, et al: Laparoscopic marsupialization of a simple renal cyst, *J Urol* 150:1486-1488, 1993.

47. Bosniak MA: The current radiological approach to renal cysts, *Radiology* 158:1-10, 1986.

48. Koga S, Nishikido M, Inuzuka S, et al: An evaluation of Bosniak's radiological classification of cystic renal masses, *BJU Int* 86:607-609, 2000.

49. Davidson AJ, Hartman DS, Choyke PL, et al: Radiologic assessment of renal masses: implications for patient care, *Radiology* 202:297-305, 1997.

50. Hartman DS, Weatherby E, III, Laskin WB, et al: Cystic renal cell carcinoma: CT findings simulating a benign hyperdense cyst, *Am J Roentgenol* 159:1235-1237, 1992.

51. Lindblad P: Epidemiology of renal cell carcinoma, *Scand J Surg* 93:88-96, 2004.

52. Jayson M, Sanders H: Increased incidence of serendipitously discovered renal cell carcinoma, *Urology* 51:203-205, 1998.

53. Suh M, Coakley FV, Qayyum A, et al: Distinction of renal cell carcinomas from high-attenuation renal cysts at portal venous phase contrast-enhanced CT, *Radiology* 228:330-334, 2003.

54. Stanley RJ: Inherent dangers in radiologic screening, *Am J Roentgenol* 177:989-992, 2001.

55. Feldman AR, Kessler L, Myers MH, et al: The prevalence of cancer. Estimates based on the Connecticut Tumor Registry, *N Engl J Med* 315:1394-1397, 1986.

56. Hsu RM, Chan DY, Siegelman SS: Small renal cell carcinomas: correlation of size with tumor stage, nuclear grade, and histologic subtype, *Am J Roentgenol* 182:551-557, 2004.

57. Ozono S, Miyao N, Igarashi T, et al: Tumor doubling time of renal cell carcinoma measured by CT: collaboration of Japanese Society of Renal Cancer, *Jpn J Clin Oncol* 34:82-85, 2004.

58. Bosniak MA, Birnbaum BA, Krinsky GA, et al: Small renal parenchymal neoplasms: further observations on growth, *Radiology* 197:589-597, 1995.

59. Rendon RA, Stanietzky N, Panzarella T, et al: The natural history of small renal masses, *J Urol* 164:1143-1147, 2000.

60. Birnbaum BA, Bosniak MA, Megibow AJ, et al: Observations on the growth of renal neoplasms, *Radiology* 176:695-701, 1990.

61. Yeh BM, Coakley FV, Meng MV, et al: Precaval right renal arteries: prevalence and morphologic associations at spiral CT, *Radiology* 230:429-433, 2004.

62. Licht MR, Novick AC: Nephron sparing surgery for renal cell carcinoma, *J Urol* 149:1-7, 1993.

63. Butler BP, Novick AC, Miller DP, et al: Management of small unilateral renal cell carcinomas: radical versus nephron-sparing surgery, *Urology* 45:34-40; discussion 40-31, 1995.

64. Coll DM, Uzzo RG, Herts BR, et al: 3-dimensional volume rendered computerized tomography for preoperative evaluation and intraoperative treatment of patients undergoing nephron sparing surgery, *J Urol* 161:1097-1102, 1999.

65. Coll DM, Herts BR, Davros WJ, et al: Preoperative use of 3D volume rendering to demonstrate renal tumors and renal anatomy, *Radiographics* 20:431-438, 2000.

66. Novick AC: Nephron-sparing surgery for renal cell carcinoma, *Annu Rev Med* 53:393-407, 2002.

67. Hafez KS, Novick AC, Butler BP: Management of small solitary unilateral renal cell carcinomas: impact of central versus peripheral tumor location, *J Urol* 159:1156-1160, 1998.

68. Perlman ES, Rosenfield AT, Wexler JS, et al: CT urography in the evaluation of urinary tract disease, *J Comput Assist Tomogr* 20:620-626, 1996.

69. McCollough CH, Daly TR, King BF, Jr., et al: An auxiliary CT tabletop for radiography at the time of CT, *J Comput Assist Tomogr* 25:876-880, 2001.

70. Caoili EM, Cohan RH, Korobkin M, et al: Urinary tract abnormalities: initial experience with multi-detector row CT urography, *Radiology* 222:353-360, 2002.

71. Heneghan JP, Kim DH, Leder RA, et al: Compression CT urography: a comparison with IVU in the opacification of the collecting system and ureters, *J Comput Assist Tomogr* 25:343-347, 2001.

72. McTavish JD, Jinzaki M, Zou KH, et al: Multi-detector row CT urography: comparison of strategies for depicting the normal urinary collecting system, *Radiology* 225:783-790, 2002.

73. Nolte-Ernsting CC, Wildberger JE, Borchers H, et al: Multi-slice CT urography after diuretic injection: initial results, *Rofo* 173:176-180, 2001.

74. Corrie D, Thompson IM: The value of retrograde pyelography for fractionally visualized upper tracts on excretory urography in the evaluation of hematuria, *J Urol* 138:554-556, 1987.

75. Kawashima A, Glockner JF, King BF, Jr, et al: CT urography and MR urography, *Radiol Clin North Am* 41:945-961, 2003.

76. www.seer.cancer.gov. In: National Cancer Institute, 2004.

77. Vaccaro JP, Brody JM: CT cystography in the evaluation of major bladder trauma, *Radiographics* 20:1373-1381, 2000.

78. Titton RL, Gervais DA, Hahn PF, et al: Urine leaks and urinomas: diagnosis and imaging-guided intervention, *Radiographics* 23:1133-1147, 2003.

79. Beer A, Saar B, Rummeny EJ: Tumors of the urinary bladder: technique, current use, and perspectives of MR and CT cystography, *Abdom Imaging* 28:868-876, 2003.

80. Mee SL, McAninch JW, Federle MP: Computerized tomography in bladder rupture: diagnostic limitations, *J Urol* 137:207-209, 1987.

81. Lis LE, Cohen AJ: CT cystography in the evaluation of bladder trauma, *J Comput Assist Tomogr* 14:386-389, 1990.

82. Lee JH, Jeong YK, Park JK, et al: "Ovarian vascular pedicle" sign revealing organ of origin of a pelvic mass lesion on helical CT, *Am J Roentgenol* 181:131-137, 2003.

83. Baeyens K, Fennessy F, Bleday R, et al: CT features of a tubal lipoma associated with an ipsilateral dermoid cyst (20046b), *Eur Radiol* 14:1720-1722, 2004.

84. Comerci JT, Jr., Licciardi F, Bergh PA, et al: Mature cystic teratoma: a clinicopathologic evaluation of 517 cases and review of the literature, *Obstet Gynecol* 84:22-28, 1994.

85. Okada S, Ohaki Y, Ogura J, et al: Computed tomography and magnetic resonance imaging findings in cases of dermoid cyst coexisting with surface epithelial tumors in the same ovary, *J Comput Assist Tomogr* 28:169-173, 2004.

86. Kim SH, Kim YJ, Park BK, et al: Collision tumors of the ovary associated with teratoma: clues to the correct preoperative diagnosis, *J Comput Assist Tomogr* 23:929-933, 1999.

87. Borders RJ, Breiman RS, Yeh BM, et al: Computed tomography of corpus luteal cysts, *J Comput Assist Tomogr* 28:340-342, 2004.

88. Choi HJ, Kim SH, Kim HC, et al: Ruptured corpus luteal cyst: CT findings, *Korean J Radiol* 4:42-45, 2003.

89. Wagner BJ, Buck JL, Seidman JD, et al: From the archives of the AFIP. Ovarian epithelial neoplasms: radiologic-pathologic correlation, *Radiographics* 14:1351-1374; quiz 1375-1356, 1994.

90. Kurtz AB, Tsimikas JV, Tempany CM, et al: Diagnosis and staging of ovarian cancer: comparative values of Doppler and conventional US, CT, and MR imaging correlated with surgery and histopathologic analysis-report of the Radiology Diagnostic Oncology Group, *Radiology* 212:19-27, 1999.

91. Buy JN, Moss AA, Ghossain MA, et al: Peritoneal implants from ovarian tumors: CT findings, *Radiology* 169:691-694, 1988.

92. van Lankveld MA, Peeters PH, van Eijkeren MA, et al: The value of abdominal CT scans in decision-making during chemotherapy in ovarian cancer, *Med Oncol* 21:41-48, 2004.

93. Coakley FV, Choi PH, Gougoutas CA, et al: Peritoneal metastases: detection with spiral CT in patients with ovarian cancer, *Radiology* 223:495-499, 2002.

94. Eisenkop SM, Spirtos NM: What are the current surgical objectives, strategies, and technical capabilities of gynecologic oncologists treating advanced epithelial ovarian cancer? *Gynecol Oncol* 82:489-497, 2001.

95. Hoskins WJ, McGuire WP, Brady MF, et al: The effect of diameter of largest residual disease on survival after primary cytoreductive surgery in patients with suboptimal residual epithelial ovarian carcinoma, *Am J Obstet Gynecol* 170:974-979; discussion 979-980, 1994.

96. Hunter RW, Alexander ND, Soutter WP: Meta-analysis of surgery in advanced ovarian carcinoma: is maximum cytoreductive surgery an independent determinant of prognosis? *Am J Obstet Gynecol* 166:504-511, 1992.

97. Funt SA, Hricak H, Abu-Rustum N, et al: Role of CT in the management of recurrent ovarian cancer, *Am J Roentgenol* 182:393-398, 2004.

98. Hardesty LA, Sumkin JH, Hakim C, et al: The ability of helical CT to preoperatively stage endometrial carcinoma, *Am J Roentgenol* 176:603-606, 2001.

14.

Peripheral Computed Tomography Angiography

Lionel Meyer-Bisch
Valérie Laurent
Denis Regent

Digital subtraction angiography (DSA) is often considered the standard for peripheral artery disease. Despite its excellent spatial resolution, it is a time-consuming and invasive technique that requires direct arterial puncture. Initially, spiral CT allowed vascular studies, providing a new 3D approach to lesions, whereas DSA and other projection techniques can sometimes overlook less than 360-degree lumen narrowing. Even though conventional CT angiography is well suited for imaging of the head, neck, aorta, and iliac or renal arteries, limited longitudinal coverage makes clinical exploration of inflow and runoff vessels impossible.[1-4] With the introduction of multidetector row systems, acquisition time and z-axis coverage are no longer a problem. MSCT (4-, 8-, or 16-detector rows) provides 3D data sets with a single spiral, ranging from the diaphragm to the ankle and a scanning time suited to a single contrast media infusion.[5-12] Furthermore, a lower dosage of iodinated agent is required with CT angiography than for DSA.

TECHNIQUE

Acquisition

Collimation

The choice of collimation should be considered according to the generation of MSCT; 16-detector row CTs allow millimetric collimation, whereas 4-detector row CTs are limited to 2.5- or 3-mm slices. Even though postprocessed image quality depends mostly on slice thickness, sufficient longitudinal spatial resolution is obtained with 2.5- or 3-mm slices, considering that the aorta and most lower limb vessels run along the z-axis. However, iliac arteries, which are oblique in the three planes, as well as proximal anterior tibial arteries, are better depicted with reformatted images made from millimetric slices. Accordingly, deep femoral artery branches and collateral vascularization are best visualized with later-generation systems (Figure 14-1).

Scanning Duration

The patient is placed in a supine position with the lower limbs immobilized with adhesive tape or dedicated wedges. A scout view is used, and the acquisition is programmed from the diaphragm to the ankle. Tube rotation speed and table feed must allow an acquisition time of less than 50 seconds to avoid venous opacification. Because MSCT permits subsecond tube rotation speed, only the heat capacity may be a limitation. Furthermore, one must take into account that too short an acquisition time (<35 to 40 seconds) may result in a lack of distal vessel opacification.

Infusion

MSCT angiography requires an automatic power injection device and a high rate of infusion, generally 3 to 4 ml/sec. Constant-rate infusion protocol provides arterial enhancement from the supraceliac region to the ankle. Bolus tracking is used to start the acquisition according to the hemodynamic status of the patient. An ROI is placed in the aortic lumen at the celiac trunk level. If a threshold is selected, the acquisition will start automatically. Usual time delay is about 25 to 30 seconds. A 2 ml/kg dose of iodinated contrast media (300 to 350 mg/ml) is injected via an 18- to 20-gauge intra-

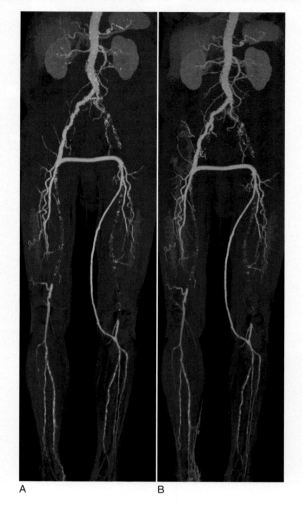

Fig. 14-1 MIP angiograms created from 2.5-mm slices (**A**) and 1.25-mm slices (**B**) in a patient with left iliac occlusion treated by femoral bypass and right superficial femoral occlusion. Collateral vascularization is slightly better depicted with 1.25-mm slices.

venous catheter placed in an antecubital vein. An isoosmolar contrast agent (iodixanol) may be used if toxicity must be reduced. Some authors propose different injection protocols to improve the uniformity of the enhancement and/or to reduce the total dose of contrast media, such as biphasic infusion or additional saline flush.[13,14] Usual contrast volumes remain between 100 and 160 ml (Figure 14-2).

Reconstruction

Raw data are reconstructed using a smooth filter with a 50% to 70% overlapped increment.[15] A 512

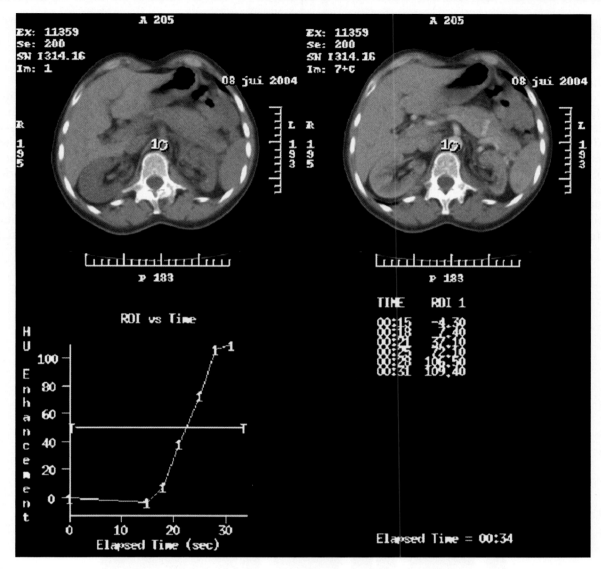

Fig. 14-2 A test bolus or bolus tracking is required for optimum arterial enhancement. The ROI is placed in the aorta at the celiac trunk level.

× 512 matrix and a 40- to 50-cm FOV allow millimetric or better spatial resolution in the x-y plane Reconstruction FOV must be optimized to include peripheral areas at the abdominal level and to improve spatial resolution at the calf level caused by the small diameter of runoff vessels. In these conditions, a 4-detector row CT generates about 900 images (2.5 mm/1.25 mm or 3 mm/1.5 mm), whereas a 16-detector row system produces about 1400 images (1.25 mm/0.8 mm). In addition to the capacities of the imaging system, work stations must be able to process huge amounts of data,

which sometimes prevents the use of a thinner collimation.

Postprocessing

Complete data sets cannot be properly reviewed by clinicians who do not have access to powerful work stations. This step is crucial for image transmission. Furthermore, reviewing axial images alone may result in some misinterpretation because of nonlongitudinal disposition of iliac arteries. Since clinicians are accustomed to conventional angiography, producing pseudoangiographic images of the aorta and lower limb vessels is important.

Volume Rendering

Volume-rendering technique (VRT) shows structures of similar density coded with different colors and opacities. It can easily and rapidly provide an overview of the vessels and the bone structures. Oblique and posterior views around the z-axis are required for a complete analysis of all arterial segments. Wall calcifications are well depicted, but their opacity could hide stenosis. It should also be noted that the apparent vessel section depends on

VRT parameters and needs to be confirmed with other reformatted views (Figure 14-3).

Maximum Intensity Projection

Maximum intensity projection (MIP) is well suited to provide angiographic representations of the data. The main difficulty is in removing the bone structures, which are superimposed on the vessels when the whole volume is projected. With no dedicated software available on the workstation, basic postprocessing tools such as thresholding and subtracting or cutting tools help to remove bones step by step. All of the data should not be processed simultaneously because vessel diameters and enhance-

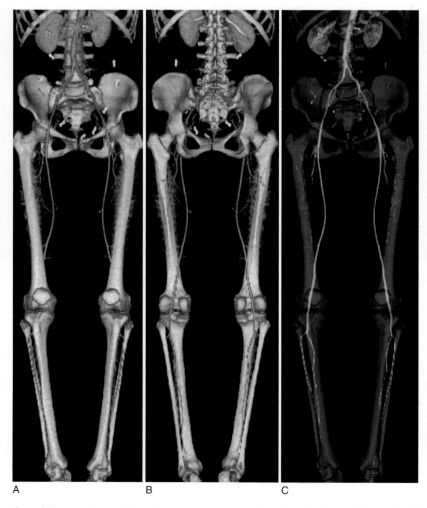

A　　　　　　　　　B　　　　　　　　　C

Fig. 14-3 VRT is fast, but oblique and posterior views are required to show the whole arterial tree (**A, B**). The opacity of bone structures can be reduced to highlight the vessels (**C**).

ment levels are different between inflow and runoff vessels (Figure 14-4).

Automated Analysis

Advanced software provides reformatted longitudinal views of vessels. The operator has to define several points in the vessel lumen along the arterial tree. The software automatically creates a trace between these points that runs along the center of the lumen. Branches may be taken into consideration, and the software can go through occlusions if indicated. The views created cannot provide an overview of the whole arterial tree as MIP views do, but their main advantage is in providing strict axial or orthogonal views of the arteries, which allows more accurate measurements.

Multiplanar Volume Reformation

Multiplanar volume reformation (MPVR) views may be created along oblique planes and therefore also provide strict axial or orthogonal lumen views. It is worth completing MIP views with MPVR analysis to better study stenosis, particularly when calcified, and to unfold the iliac axes.[16] However, MPVR should not be the only postprocessing modality, since it will not provide an angiography-like overview.

Choice of Postprocessing Method

Because some clinicians are not accustomed to reviewing radiological exams on work stations, if CTA is to gain widespread acceptance, it must provide images at least as informative as conventional angiography. Thus angiography-like MIP views are most often used. With such images, patients can be easily informed about their pathology and therapeutic options. Vascular surgeons are provided with a quick overview of the arterial tree, and the comparison of pre- and post-procedure exams is made easier. Since MSCT data sets code for a real 3D volume, it is interesting to project the data volume with MIP algorithm on several planes around the z-axis to highlight anterior or posterior lesions. MPVR views should be created to grade significant stenosis and study iliac arteries, or to provide information about aneurysm sizing. If dedicated software is available, diameter or surface measures of pathologic arterial segments are easily obtained.

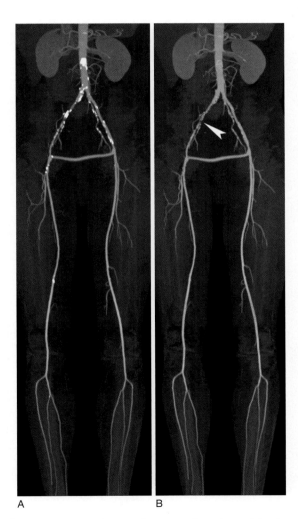

A   B

Fig. 14-4 MIP algorithm allows pseudoangiographic views, but bone structures must be removed. After surgery, femoral bypass patency is well depicted as well as right iliac severe stenosis (*arrowhead*).

ADVANTAGES OF MSCT ANGIOGRAPHY IN CLINICAL APPLICATIONS

Inflow Vessels

One of the main principles of vascular surgery is to first consider proximal lesions and then the more distal ones, according to the blood flow. This surgical concept also applies to a noninvasive approach, since short iliac stenosis may be treated with angioplasty. Radiologists should be aware of this concept when reviewing lower limb examinations.

The iliac arteries seem to be easy to analyze because of their large diameter. However, they are oblique in the three planes. Consequently, we cannot have a good representation of these segments on strict axial images or on MIP views around the z-axis. In our opinion, additional postprocessing is always required at the iliac level (such as MPVR or automated analysis) to unfold the vessels and to allow a true axial study of the lumen or strict orthogonal reformatted views.[17] The challenge of MSCT angiography appears to be in small collateral or runoff vessel depiction, but demonstrating such distal arteries is useless if a proximal lesion is overlooked on axial images or on MIP angiogram (Figure 14-5).

The internal iliac artery is often calcified and runs very close to the iliac bone in the ischiatic region. It is therefore often removed with bone structures during postprocessing. However, its proximal portion always remains visible. Therefore, even in cases of gluteal claudication, MSCT angiography will likely provide enough information concerning this artery.

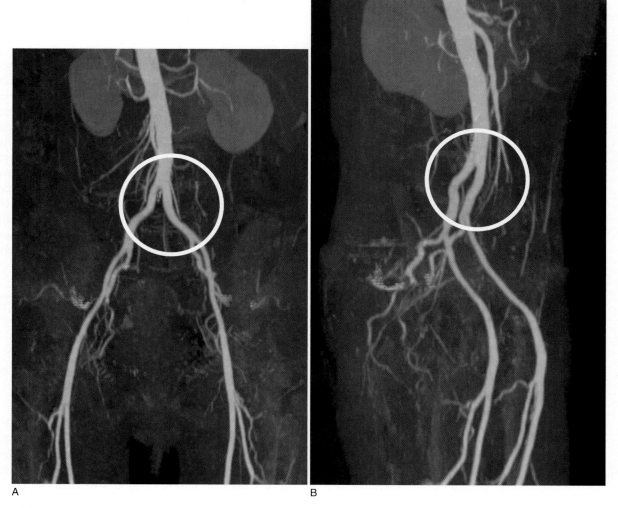

A   B

Fig. 14-5 Patient with left claudication. No stenosis is depicted on MIP views (**A, B**).

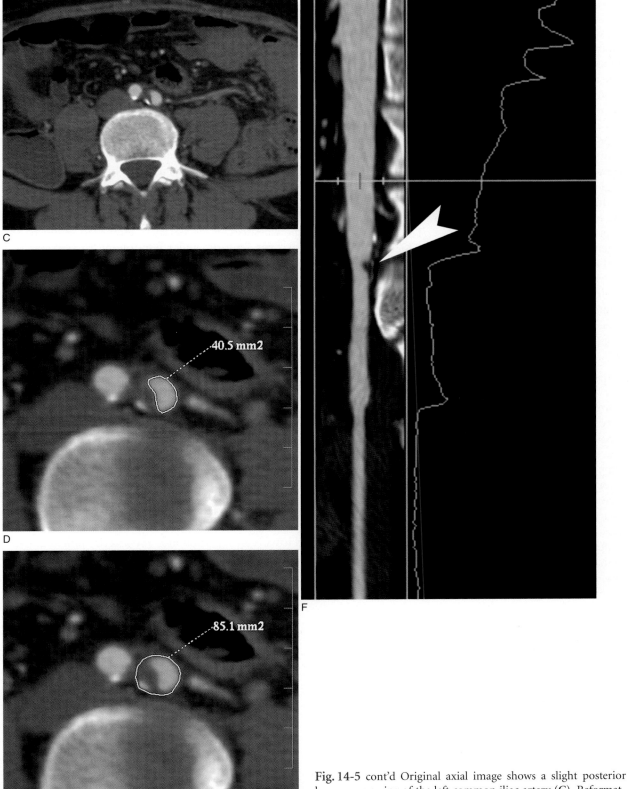

Fig. 14-5 cont'd Original axial image shows a slight posterior lumen narrowing of the left common iliac artery (**C**). Reformatted strict axial views depict a 50% stenosis (**D, E**) and automated analysis (**F**) (*arrowhead*).

Vascular Stents

As wall calcifications, CT angiography is able to show vascular stents and the underlying arterial lumen. Similarly, postprocessing of the calcifications can remove the stents and make the vessel lumen apparent on an angiography-like view. Even in cases of heavy artifacts caused by the stent, its patency can usually be evaluated, although discrete intimal hyperplasia may be difficult to depict. This point may be considered when a symptomatic patient is known to have been treated with a stent. Since MR angiography shows poor results in stent patency evaluation resulting from a signal void created by the metallic structure of the stent, CT angiography is prefered for these patients.[18-20] The best results when studying stent patency are achieved with a millimetric collimation and a low pitch value, which are inconsistent with an aortic and lower limb exploration using 4- or 8-row detector systems. Therefore, except for the most recent generation of CTs, stent patency evaluation may still require Doppler ultrasound (Figure 14-6).

Popliteal Aneurysms

Conventional and MR angiography techniques can only demonstrate the lumen of the arterial tree through the visualization of the contrast media or the blood flow. Since popliteal lumen narrowing may be caused by an aneurysm, adventicial cyst, or artery entrapment, these techniques may lead to an incomplete diagnosis, resulting in an inadequate treatment plan. In addition, depending on the thickness of the thrombus, popliteal aneurysms may appear on strict angiograms as an ectasic, regular, or narrowed arterial segment. With CT angiography, the vascular lumen can be identified as well as the arterial wall and perivascular spaces. Therefore, popliteal aneurysms cannot remain unnoticed if axial images are reviewed, whether a stenosis is present or not[21] (Figure 14-7).

Saphenous Vein

In the same way, when an arterial bypass is considered, it is beneficial to show the saphenous vein. CT angiography axial images provide information about the scarpa region, the position of the vein, its diameter, eventual varicose ectasias, the amount of collateral veins, and the anatomy of the popliteal region.[22] The contralateral vein is also visualized if a venous graft is required. This relevant information is not available when conventional or MR angiography is performed (Figure 14-8).

LIMITATIONS

Windowing

If MIP angiograms seem essential for illustrating reports, image reviewing must be realized on work stations. Because other pathologies may be discovered by chance, an overview in the cine view mode of the whole volume, or at least the abdominal and pelvic slices, is necessary.[23] However, study of the arteries requires wider windowing to separate soft tissues, iodinated contrast media, and wall calcifications. Because apparent blurring and vessel diameter are linked to the window settings, extra care must be taken when studying heavily calcified lumen narrowing.[24] Actually, preoccluded stenosis may be mistakenly considered as occluded because of inappropriate windowing and may therefore lead to surgery when angioplasty would have been sufficient.

Wall Calcifications

The visualization of wall calcifications seems to be a great advantage of MSCT. It is clear that heavily calcified segments may represent major difficulties if arterial bypass is considered. In the same way, their visualization may help determine an arterial puncture site when angioplasty is planned. However, they often hide the arterial lumen on MIP views. This may lead to a misdiagnosed stenosis under wall calcifications. In such circumstances, axial and MPVR views help to show the intraluminal iodinated contrast media, at least for larger vessels.

Additional postprocessing may remove these high-attenuation value voxels by thresholding and subtracting. Once the bone structures are removed, an additional thresholding step around 350 to 400 Hounsfields units isolates wall calcifications. This new volume with calcifications is subtracted from the bone-free volume to create a new angiography-like view without wall calcifications. A one-pixel dilation may be applied to the calcifications before the subtraction step (Figure 14-9).

With small arteries, such as runoff vessels, wall calcifications sometimes create such heavy artifacts

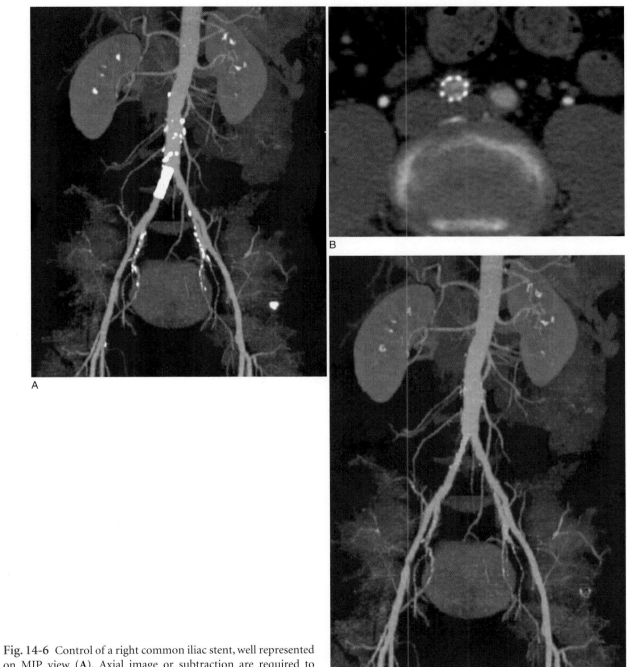

Fig. 14-6 Control of a right common iliac stent, well represented on MIP view (**A**). Axial image or subtraction are required to confirm patency (**B, C**).

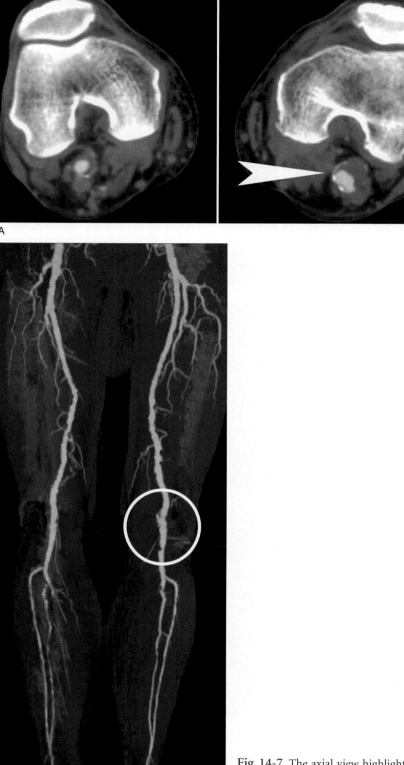

Fig. 14-7 The axial view highlights a left popliteal aneurysm (**A**) (*arrowhead*), overlooked on MIP angiogram (**B**).

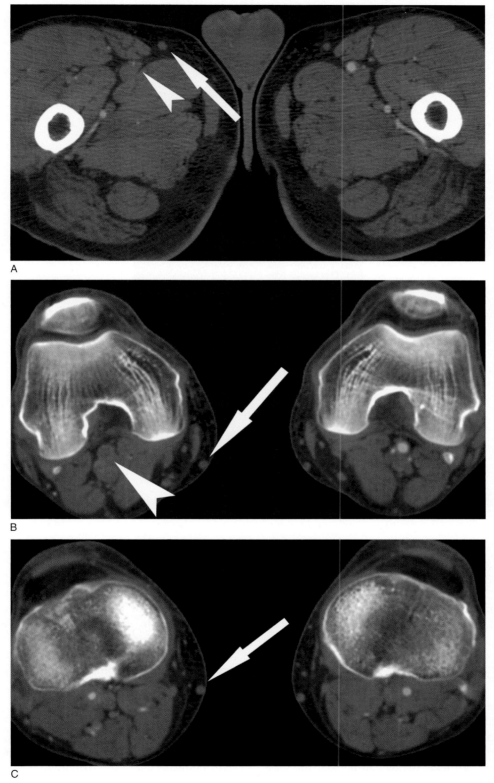

Fig. 14-8 Saphenous veins (*arrows*) are well shown on axial images in this patient with right superficial femoral and upper popliteal occlusion (*arrowheads*), which required bypass surgery (**A, B**). Lower popliteal artery patency is depicted (**C**).

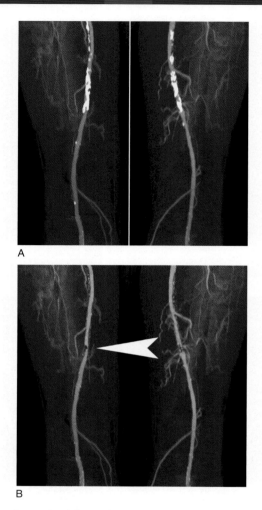

Fig. 14-9 Bilateral wall calcifications of superficial femoral arteries with MIP algorithm (**A**). An additional subtraction step is required to highlight the underlying arterial lumen and severe stenosis (**B**) (*arrowhead*).

that they prevent an accurate arterial patency diagnosis. This occurs particularly with diabetic patients.

Venous Pollution

A test bolus or automated detection of the bolus and a scanning duration less than 50 seconds are required to avoid venous pollution in the lower leg. When these conditions are fullfilled, venous opacification at the calf level is rare. Some patients with significant venous insufficiency may still show signs of an early venous opacification, making MIP view analysis difficult. Once again, reviewing axial images is helpful for diagnosis. Venous pollution can also occur with MR angiography. Unfortunately, reviewing native images usually does not help in such cases; however, the latest generation of software provides time-resolved imaging, which overcomes this obstacle.

Orthopedic Material

Hip and knee prostheses create strong beam-hardening artifacts and usually prevent the study of popliteal vessels in the knee. Because they also generate an important signal void in MR angiography, Doppler ultrasound examination is probably the most effective technique for patients with prostheses (Figure 14-10).

NONINVASIVE DIAGNOSTIC IMAGING: CT OR MR ANGIOGRAPHY

Although it is still considered the standard angiography technique, DSA may be replaced by MR angiography for lower limb arterial occlusive disease imaging.[25] Some studies point out that patent arteries under the knee could remain nonopacified when DSA is performed. Furthermore, one should consider that volumetric-imaging techniques such as MR angiography might provide more information about the arterial tree than 2D techniques like DSA, which is based on the projection of the x-ray beam on a plane.

The development of MSCT angiography emphasizes the interest of a noninvasive or minimally invasive diagnostic imaging for the aorta and lower limbs. In our opinion, the real issue is whether to use CT or MR angiography[26] (Figure 14-11).

CT and MR both yield 3D data, which enables imaging of arterial lesions from any angle. Both require contrast media infusion through a peripheral vein and last 10 to 30 minutes. Data must be postprocessed to create angiography-like views from the diaphragm to the ankle. Quality is reduced when venous pollution or metallic artifacts are present. MSCT angiography's main advantage is its ability to provide information about the arterial lumen as well as about the arterial wall and peri-vascular spaces. However, it remains slightly more invasive than MR angiography since it requires x-ray and iodinated contrast media (Table 14-1).

CONCLUSION

MSCT allows a large z-axis coverage. Imaging of the abdominal aorta and lower limb can be performed with a single infusion of iodinated contrast media. Despite time-consuming postprocessing, MSCT angiography remains easy to perform and is of significant clinical value, particularly when additional information is required other than just lumen patency (such as wall calcifications and presurgical anatomical data). MSCT angiography is also recommended when a venous-type arterial graft is considered or a popliteal aneurysm is suspected. Since modern MR angiography provides similar angiograms, the latter should be preferred when iodinated contrast media must be avoided, especially in cases of renal insufficiency, or with elderly or diabetic patients.

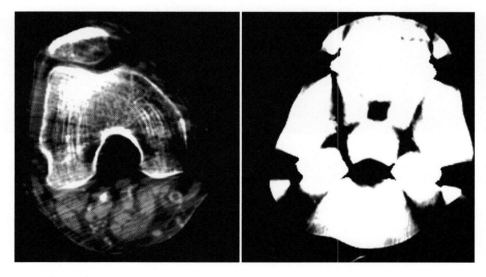

Fig. 14-10 Heavy metallic artifacts caused by prosthesis in the knee, preventing popliteal vessel depiction.

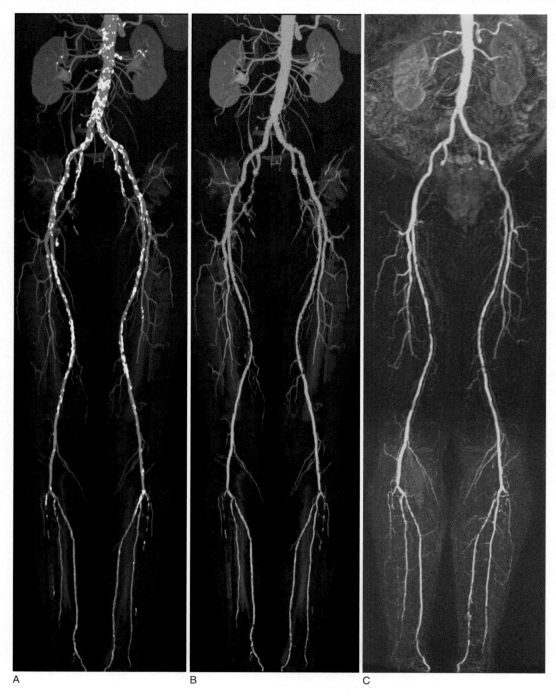

A   B   C

Fig. 14-11 CT angiogram before (**A**) and after wall calcification subtraction (**B**) and MR angiogram (**C**) with MIP algorithm in the same patient. Full-informative versus totally noninvasive imaging.

Table 14-1 Respective advantages and drawbacks of MSCT angiography (MDCTA), MR angiography (MRA), and digital subtraction angiography (DSA)

Advantages	MDCTA	MRA	DSA
Three-dimensional imaging	+	+	−
Short examination time	+	−	−
Short postprocessing time	−	+	+
Wall calcification visualization	+	−	−
Perivascular space visualization	+	−	−
Vascular stent patency evaluation	+	−	+
Calcified runoff vessels noninterference	−	+	+
Contrast media tolerance	−	+	−
Absence of irradiation	−	+	−

REFERENCES

1. Rieker O, Duber C, Schmiedt W, et al: Prospective comparison of CT angiography of the legs with intraarterial digital subtraction angiography, *Am J Roentgenol* 166:269-276, 1996.
2. Rieker O, Duber C, Neufang A, et al: CT angiography versus intraarterial digital subtraction angiography for assessment of aortoiliac occlusive disease, *Am J Roentgenol* 169:1133-1138, 1997.
3. Rankin SC: Spiral CT: vascular applications, *Eur J Radiol* 28:18-29, 1998.
4. Walter F, Leyder B, Fays J, et al: Value of arteriography scanning in lower limb artery evaluation: a preliminary study, *J Radiol* 82:473-479, 2001.
5. Rubin GD, Shiau MC, Schmidt AJ, et al: Computed tomographic angiography: historical perspective and new state-of-the-art using multidetector-row helical computed tomography, *J Comput Assist Tomogr* 23(suppl)1:S83-90, 1999.
6. Rubin GD, Shiau MC, Leung AN, et al: Aorta and iliac arteries: single versus multiple detector-row helical CT angiography, *Radiology* 215:670-676, 2000.
7. Prokop M: Multislice CT angiography, *Eur J Radiol* 36:86-96, 2000.
8. Katz DS, Hon M: CT angiography of the lower extremities and aortoiliac system with a multi-detector row helical CT scanner: promise of new opportunities fulfilled, *Radiology* 221:7-10, 2001.
9. Rubin GD, Schmidt AJ, Logan LJ, et al: Multi-detector row CT angiography of lower extremity arterial inflow and runoff: initial experience, *Radiology* 221:146-158, 2001.
10. Martin ML, Tay KH, Flak B, et al: Multidetector CT angiography of the aortoiliac system and lower extremities: a prospective comparison with digital subtraction angiography, *Am J Roentgenol* 180:1085-1091, 2003.
11. Ofer A, Nitecki SS, Linn S, et al: Multidetector CT angiography of peripheral vascular disease: a prospective comparison with intraarterial digital subtraction angiography, *Am J Roentgenol* 180:719-724, 2003.
12. Rubin GD: MSCT imaging of the aorta and peripheral vessels, *Eur J Radiol* 45(suppl)1:S42-49, 2003.
13. Fleischmann D, Rubin GD, Bankier AA, et al: Improved uniformity of aortic enhancement with customized contrast medium injection protocols at CT angiography, *Radiology* 214:363-371, 2000.
14. Cademartiri F, van Der Lugt A, Luccichenti G, et al: Parameters affecting bolus geometry in CTA: a review, *J Comput Assist Tomogr* 26:598-607, 2002.
15. Kasales CJ, Hopper KD, Ariola DN, et al: Reconstructed helical CT scans: improvement in z-axis resolution compared with overlapped and nonoverlapped conventional CT scans, *Am J Roentgenol* 164:1281-1284, 1995.
16. Sugahara T, Korogi Y, Hirai T, et al: CT angiography in vascular intervention for steno-occlusive diseases: role of multiplanar reconstruction and source images, *Br J Radiol* 71:601-611, 1998.
17. Ota H, Takase K, Igarashi K, et al: MSCT compared with digital subtraction angiography for assessment of lower extremity arterial occlusive disease: importance of reviewing cross-sectional images, *Am J Roentgenol* 182:201-209, 2004.
18. Maintz D, Fischbach R, Juergens KU, et al: Multislice CT angiography of the iliac arteries in the presence of various stents: in vitro evaluation of artifacts and lumen visibility, *Invest Radiol* 36:699-704, 2001.
19. Strotzer M, Lenhart M, Butz B, et al: Appearance of vascular stents in computed tomographic angiography: in vitro examination of 14 different stent types, *Invest Radiol* 36:652-658, 2001.
20. Maintz D, Tombach B, Juergens KU, et al: Revealing in-stent stenoses of the iliac arteries: comparison of multidetector CT with MR angiography and digital radiographic angiography in a phantom model, *Am J Roentgenol* 179:1319-1322, 2002.
21. Beregi JP, Djabbari M, Desmoucelle F, et al: Popliteal vascular disease: evaluation with spiral CT angiography, *Radiology* 203:477-483, 1997.
22. Wengerter KR, Veith FJ, Gupta SK, et al: Influence of vein size (diameter) on infrapopliteal reversed vein graft patency, *J Vasc Surg* 11:525-531, 1990.
23. Katz DS, Jorgensen MJ, Rubin GD: Detection and follow-up of important extra-arterial lesions with helical CT angiography, *Clin Radiol* 54:294-300, 1999.

24. Diederichs CG, Keating DP, Glatting G, et al: Blurring of vessels in spiral CT angiography: effects of collimation width, pitch, viewing plane, and windowing in maximum intensity projection, *J Comput Assist Tomogr* 20:965-974, 1996.

25. Koelemay MJ, Lijmer JG, Stoker J, et al: Magnetic resonance angiography for the evaluation of lower extremity arterial disease: a meta-analysis, *JAMA* 285:1338-1345, 2001.

26. Willmann JK, Wildermuth S, Pfammatter T, et al: Aortoiliac and renal arteries: prospective intraindividual comparison of contrast-enhanced three-dimensional MR angiography and multi-detector row CT angiography, *Radiology* 226:798-811, 2003.

APPLICATIONS

Preparation and hygienic requirements for biopsy with CT fluoroscopy are the same as for conventional or CT guidance interventions, except that sterile draping of the manual switch, or a separate control unit, is required. After the patient is positioned comfortably and local anesthesia is administered according to the puncture site and type of intervention, the needle is inserted into the skin. The needle position is controlled by moving the patient into the scanner so that the light marker matches the site at which the needle enters the skin. If the needle cannot be introduced parallel to the scan plane, the needle tip must be identified with a few "search" scans, depending on the examiner's experience.

Basically, two different applications of CT fluoroscopy have emerged[11]:

- Quick-check method: A single scan is acquired by briefly tapping on the foot switch. The scan is displayed and retained on the monitor in the scanner room after a short delay. This technique is very similar to conventional CT guidance, except that the examiner stands next to the patient during acquisition and is thus exposed to some radiation.

- Continuous method: Keeping the foot switch pressed for several seconds will provide nearly continuous image reconstruction at a frame rate of 6 to 12 images per second after an initial delay. During acquisition, the examiner can change the needle position or instruct the patient to continue breathing until the target lesion comes to lie exactly within the scanning plane.

According to two retrospective studies,[11,12] the quick-check method is used in 87% to 97% of the interventions performed in the CT scanner, which is also our experience. The continuous method is used rarely (2%), especially if access is difficult or if patients have a limited ability to cooperate. The two methods are combined in 3% to 11% of cases.

RADIATION DOSE TO THE PATIENT

During CT fluoroscopy, the patient is exposed to a radiation dose determined by the usual factors such as tube current, voltage, current modulation (where applicable), CT scanner geometry, x-ray beam filter, patient circumference, and volume. However, the mAs product (i.e., the linear relationship to the tube voltage chosen and the fluoroscopy time) is particularly important.

Typically, a very low value of 10 to 50 mA is used for CT fluoroscopy. This parameter is primarily chosen with respect to the image quality required for anatomical resolution and depiction of the needle tip (Figure 15-1). The lung, for instance, with its naturally high image contrast (air versus soft tissue), lends itself to scanning with very low doses (Figure 15-2). One manufacturer offers additional prefiltering (contour filtering) for greater beam hardening in the fluoroscopy mode, resulting in a dose reduction by a factor of 2.5.

Apart from these factors and with optimal parameter setting and positioning, the patient's radiation exposure is determined primarily by the total fluoroscopy time. The time given in the literature for biopsy and drain placement ranges from 1.2 to 407 sec (Table 15-1).[9,11,13,14] The resulting skin exposure to the patient can be calculated as 13 mGy to 4.5 Gy. A report describing a cumulative fluoroscopy time of 660 sec during drain placement with CT fluoroscopy guidance is noteworthy.[15] From the parameters given by the authors, a skin dose of up to 10 Gy can be estimated, which is above the threshold for deterministic radiation damage and is already in the range that occurs in radiation therapy. However, skin doses of over 3 Gy have also been reported in biopsies performed with conventional CT.[12]

At our department, the mean fluoroscopy time in CT-guided interventions, including all therapeutic measures such as injections and radiofrequency ablation, is 5.3 sec (1.5 to 40 sec). Based on this mean value and a tube current of 50 mA, a skin dose of about 90 mGy and an effective dose in the range of 0.7 mSv is calculated. This effective dose to the patient roughly corresponds to that of four conventional radiographs. Not taking into account the site of biopsy or therapy (the focus of fluoroscopy), an effective dose of about 0.1 mSv/sec can be assumed when the usual scanner parameters for CT fluoroscopy are used.

Longer CT fluoroscopy times potentially occur in therapeutic applications in which procedure monitoring is essential, such as in radiofrequency or laser ablation of the liver, kidney, lungs, or bone lesions, or in complex procedures such as percutaneous drainage of bile ducts. Data on mean fluoroscopy

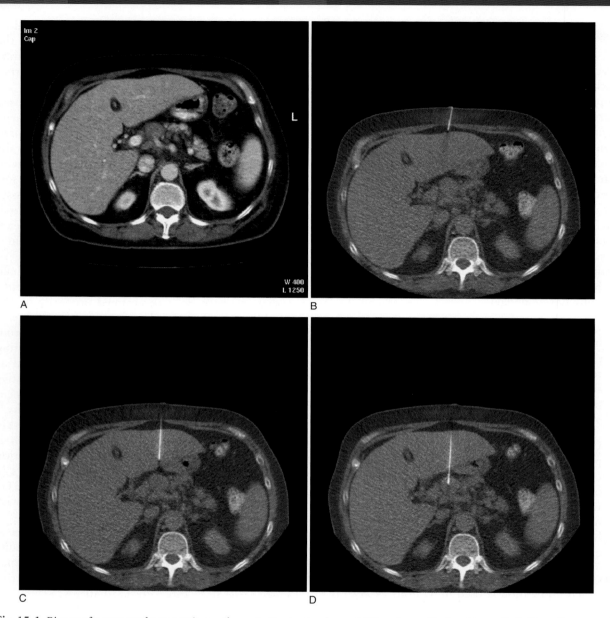

Fig. 15-1 Biopsy of a suspected pancreatic neoplasm. **A,** Contrast-enhanced CT performed before biopsy. **B-D,** Three fluoroscopic scans are obtained during the procedure. Because of the low-dose tube setting, the images contain increased image mottle, but the quality is sufficient for documenting the needle tip in relation to the target lesion.

times for such complex procedures are not available; however, it is likely that longer fluoroscopy times are necessary, not only for control of the therapeutic progress, but also for documentation of the results. Since patients undergoing this procedure typically have an underlying malignant tumor and a convincing indication, radiation protection is of minor importance as long as fluoroscopy times do not exceed several minutes.

RADIATION DOSE TO THE INTERVENTIONAL RADIOLOGIST

In CT fluoroscopy, the radiation exposure to the radiologist performing the intervention must also be considered since he or she is exposed to scattered radiation while standing next to the patient.

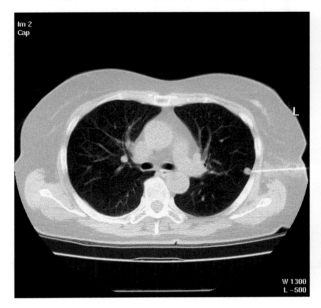

Fig. 15-2 Biopsy of a pulmonary nodule under CT fluoroscopy. This image was obtained with 25 mA at 120 kV during the biopsy. In addition, a contour filter was used for further dose reduction.

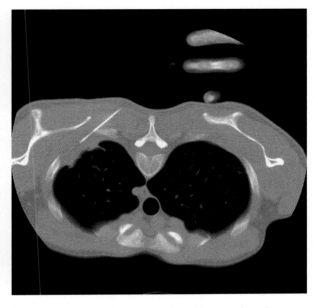

Fig. 15-3 Biopsy of a suspected malignant pleural tumor. Note the examiner's fingers in the primary beam, resulting in an exposure to the fingers of 3 to 4 mGy per second of fluoroscopy time.

Table 15-1 Radiation exposure in CT fluoroscopy

Author	Fluoroscopy times [sec]	Mean [sec]	Skin dose [mGy]*
Nickoloff et al.[13]	13-407	96.6	520-1600
Meyer et al.[9]	Not given	143	780-2360
Paulson et al.[11]	1.2-101.5	17.9	100-300
Sheafor et al.[18]	23-105	50	280-820
Carlson et al.[12]	1.2-187.6	Not given	—
Own group	1.5-40	5.3	45

*Calculated based on the mean values for axial doses free in air for CT scanners from GE, Philips, Siemens, and Toshiba (11 to 33 mGy/100 mAs). In cases where the scanner type is not available, the range is given for standardized scan parameters with 50 mA and 120 kV.

Although the average whole-body dose reported for the examiner is rather low at 0.025 mSv per intervention,[11] the cumulative annual dose will be 2.5 mSv for a radiologist performing 100 interventions per year (whole-body upper limit: 20 mSv/year).

The exposure of the examiner's hands, which move very close to the patient (a source of scattered radiation) should usually be considered separately. During fluoroscopy, exposing the fingers (e.g., holding the biopsy needle) to the primary beam should be avoided at all costs (Figure 15-3), which would involve an exposure of 3-4 mGy/sec. The annual acceptable dose for occupationally exposed persons would be reached after 125 sec of fluoroscopy. If the needle must be held to perform the intervention, needle holders can be used—either forceps or specially manufactured synthetic grips with openings for standardized needle heads (Figure 15-4). Performing biopsies with these needle holders requires accommodation time. However, such devices dramatically reduce the exposure of the fingers to 17 µGy/sec. Commercially available protective gloves reduce the dose by 11% to 49%.[13,16]

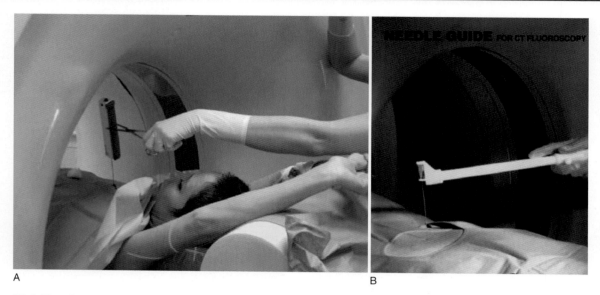

Fig. 15-4 Use of conventional metal forceps for holding the core biopsy needle (**A**), which causes metal artifacts if the forceps comes to lie in the scan plane. Needle holders made of synthetic material do not induce artifacts and can be used in combination with most puncture needles (**B**).

The following measures can be taken by examiners to reduce the amount of radiation to which they are exposed:

- Standing as far away from the source of scattered radiation as possible. The exposure can be significantly reduced by staying only slightly away from the patient, as long as this does not impair the interventional procedure.

- In addition to the mandatory lead apron, an additional thyroid protector and protective lead glasses are recommended.

- Use of a needle holder and a protective glove (see previous paragraph).

- Shielding the patient with a lead plate,[17] leaving only the skin region around the site of access uncovered, will reduce scattered radiation by 72%. This measure, combined with wearing protective gloves, will reduce the dose to the hands by 97%.[16]

- Lower kilovoltage. By using 120 kV instead of 135 kV, the radiation exposure to the physician is reduced by 40%.[17] Moreover, the effectiveness of protective gear (patient, apron, glove) also increases at a lower kV.

However, the most important measure of radiation protection for the patient and examiner is minimizing fluoroscopy time. Sensible use of CT fluoroscopy will even reduce the patient dose by 94% compared with biopsy performed with conventional CT guidance,[12] since search scans to identify the needle are not required. Finally, the overall procedural time is reduced by 32% using CT fluoroscopy.[12]

The radiation dose emitted by the scanner can be reduced by an additional form filter or by discontinuing emission of the tube during rotation between the 10 and 2 o'clock positions to minimize the effect of the tabletop tube (hands of the examiner). Both techniques are offered by different manufacturers.

CONCLUSION

CT fluoroscopy is a useful tool for the more rapid, and therefore less risky, performance of radiological interventions. The physician is in direct contact with the patient and can thus quickly react to movements and positional changes. Biopsies can be obtained faster than with conventional CT guidance.

Technical prerequisites are easy operation in the fluoroscopy mode to prevent inadvert activation of scanning. The risk of CT fluoroscopy lies in the radiation exposure involved, which can reach levels that can cause deterministic radiation damage if the technique is not used properly. Manufacturers should not only continue their efforts to reduce the radiation dose in the CT fluoroscopy mode but should also equip the scanners with a warning signal to indicate unduly long fluoroscopy times. However, dose reduction most crucially relies on the physician's experience, which is why proper training in this new technique is essential.

Many reports in the literature indicate that the use of CT fluoroscopy facilitates the biopsy procedure by shortening the time for needle placement, leading to an improved sensitivity and specificity. However, other factors such as lesion size, sampling techniques, and patient positioning may be more influential than how the needle position is visualized during the procedure. Nevertheless, in the hands of an experienced interventionalist, CT fluoroscopy is a useful tool that may shorten the overall time required to complete the biopsy procedure, which is particularly advantageous in uncooperative patients. Immediate identification of complications during a therapeutic intervention (e.g., radiofrequency or laser ablation of tumors) represents another strength of CT fluoroscopy. Overall, experience suggests that CT fluoroscopy helps to improve interventional procedures—both diagnostically and therapeutically.

REFERENCES

1. Krombach G, Schmitz-Rode T, Brabrand K, et al: Initial experiences with a new optical target system (SimpliCT) for CT-guided punctures, *RöFo* 172:557-560, 2000.
2. Holzknecht N, Helmberger T, Schoepf U, et al: Evaluation of an electromagnetic virtual target system (CT-guide) for CT-guided interventions, *RöFo* 173:612-618, 2001.
3. Muehlstaedt M, Bruening R, Diebold J, et al: CT/fluoroscopy-guided transthoracic needle biopsy: sensitivity and complication rate in 98 procedures, *JCAT* 26:191-196, 2002.
4. Gohari A, Haramati L: Complications of CT scan-guided lung biopsy: lesion size and depth matter, *Chest* 126:666-668, 2004.
5. Rogalla P, Mutze M: Process and device for computer tomography transillumination for treatment, Germany; 1996. US-Patent 5,835,556, 1996.
6. Froelich J, Ishaque N, Saar B, et al: Control of percutaneous biopsy with CT fluoroscopy, *RöFo* 170:191-197, 1999.
7. Spies V, Butz B, Altjohann C, et al: CT-guided biopsies, drainage and percutaneous gastrostomies: comparison of punctures with and without CT fluoroscopy, *RöFo* 172:374-380, 2000.
8. Yamagami T, Iida S, Kato T, et al: Combining fine-needle aspiration and core biopsy under CT fluoroscopy guidance: a better way to treat patients with lung nodules? *Am J Roentgenol* 180:811-815, 2003.
9. Meyer C, White C, Wu J, et al: Real-time CT fluoroscopy: usefulness in thoracic drainage, *Am J Roentgenol* 171:1097-1101, 1998.
10. Silverman S, Tuncali K, Adams D, et al: CT fluoroscopy-guided abdominal interventions: techniques, results, and radiation exposure, *Radiology* 212:673-681, 1999.
11. Paulson E, Sheafor D, Enterline D, et al: CT fluoroscopy–guided interventional procedures: techniques and radiation dose to radiologists, *Radiology* 220:161-167, 2001.
12. Carlson S, Bender C, Classic K, et al: Benefits and safety of CT fluoroscopy in interventional radiologic procedures, *Radiology* 219:515-520, 2001.
13. Nickoloff E, Khandji A, Dutta A: Radiation doses during CT fluoroscopy, *Health Phys* 79:675-681, 2000.
14. Kato R, Katada K, Anno H, et al: Radiation dosimetry at CT fluoroscopy: physician's hand dose and development of needle holders, *Radiology* 201:576-578, 1996.
15. Daly B, Krebs T, Wong-You-Cheong J, et al: Percutaneous abdominal and pelvic interventional procedures using CT fluoroscopy guidance, *Am J Roentgenol* 173:637-644, 1999.
16. Stoeckelhuber B, Schulz E, Melchert U, et al: Procedures, spectrum and radiation exposure in CT-fluoroscopy, *Röntgenpraxis* 55:51-57, 2003.
17. Irie T, Kajitani M, Itai Y: CT fluoroscopy-guided intervention: marked reduction of scattered radiation dose to the physician's hand by use of a lead plate and an improved I-I device, *J Vasc Interv Radiol* 12:1417-1421, 2001.
18. Sheafor D, Paulson E, Kliewer M, et al: Comparison of sonographic and CT guidance techniques: does CT fluoroscopy decrease procedure time? *Am J Roentgenol* 174:939-942, 2000.

16.

Dose in Multislice Computed Tomography

Michael Galanski
Georg Stamm

Because of a steady increase in the number of computed tomography (CT) examinations for diagnostic imaging, CT has become a significant source of x-ray exposure in many countries around the world. Today CT contributes to only 3% to 4% of all radiological examinations, but it leads to about one third of the radiation exposure of the population. An increased use of multiphase examinations and a tendency towards smaller slice collimations will undoubtedly result in a significant increase in radiation exposure.

Multislice CT (MSCT) suffers from a number of dose traps that can substantially increase patient dose if identical mAs settings are being used as in conventional spiral CT. However, higher doses are not inevitably necessary. Radiation exposure can be controlled if a few things are kept in mind.

The amount of radiation exposure arising from CT examinations depends on various factors, which can be divided into two main categories: scanner-related factors and application-related factors.

SCANNER-RELATED FACTORS

Radiation dose is influenced by the radiation quality, the geometry of the scanner, the detector type, and the current modulation of the tube.

Tube Voltage, Beam Filtration, and Beam Shaper

Dose increases nonlinearly with an increase in tube voltage. Typically, an increase in kVp from 120 to 140 kVp increases the dose by about 47%. However, at the same time, the penetration is improved, and an approximately 70% higher dose reaches the detector. By cutting down the mAs proportionally, patient exposure can be reduced by 15% to 20% while keeping the same noise level.

Radiation exposure depends on x-ray energy. Increasing the tube voltage from 120 kVp to 140 kVp increases the CT dose index (CTDI) by a factor of 1.4, but decreasing the tube voltage to 80 kVp lowers the CTDI by a factor of approximately 2.2. However, with a higher x-ray energy, absorption decreases significantly, resulting in a better dose utilization. This is particularly important in obese patients and in regions with high x-ray absorption (shoulders, pelvis), where the highest possible tube voltage is recommended.

The relative difference in x-ray attenuation (contrast) improves when the x-ray energy is reduced. This is especially important for all contrast-enhanced scans. The enhancement at a given concentration of iodine is about two times larger at 80 kVp than at 140 kVp. The effect can be used to optimize the contrast-to-noise ratio at a given radiation exposure.

Beam filtration is extremely effective for decreasing patient exposure, because x-rays of lower energy, which contribute to patient dose but not to the image, are reduced. Using good filtration also helps to minimize beam-hardening artifacts and thus improves image quality. The use of beam shaping or bowtie filters reduces the dose not only in the peripheral areas of the patient (which can be seen looking at peripheral CTDI values), but also in the central areas because of a decreased scattering of x-rays.

All CT scanners use a beam filtration of about 6 to 9 mm Al. Dedicated filters adapt the beam intensity to the reduced x-ray absorption in the peripheral areas of the fan beam, which depends on the configuration of the object. Accordingly, the ratio of the dose at the periphery and the dose at the center decreases, resulting in a more homogeneous distribution. The dynamic range requirements for the detector system can thus be reduced. Furthermore, beam-hardening effects are less likely to occur.

Scanner Geometry

Scanner geometry and focal spot scintillation are closely connected with rapid tube rotation in sub-second technology. Scanner geometry strongly influences the patient dose at a given mAs setting. The distance between focus and isocenter for most CT scanners is 60 cm. Shorter geometry reduces the centrifugal forces, allows faster rotation of the gantry, and thus provides a reduction in rotation time. In addition, the effective output of the x-ray source increases, so that lower mAs settings can be applied. This causes a potential dose trap because the reduced distance leads to an increase in patient dose. In particular, the skin entrance dose is higher if identical mAs settings are being used as in scanners with a greater focus-axis-distance. For this reason, the mAs settings must be adjusted in a way that $CTDI_{VOL}$ values remain more or less constant. However, when using scanners with a smaller gantry, the dose distribution becomes less homogeneous with an increased dose at the periphery in comparison to the dose at the center of the object.

Floating Focal Spot

Similar considerations apply for the focal spot scintillation. With fast rotational speed, the effect of centrifugal forces on the electron beam within the x-ray tube causes small alterations in the position of the focal spot during a spiral scan, especially if the anode is not supported on both ends. This can be compensated for by slightly widening the pre-patient collimation. However, this causes a substantial increase in patient dose, predominantly when thin collimations are required. Tracking the focal spot by slightly adjusting the collimator setting keeps the dose at the detector constant without having to raise patient dose. Such a technique is mandatory and is currently a standard procedure.

Geometric Efficiency

The overall dose efficiency of a CT system is more or less the product of the geometric efficiency of the detector, the sensitivity of the single detector elements, and the efficiency of the beam along the z-axis (Figure 16-1). Apart from the sensitivity of the detector elements—which depends on the detector's absorption and conversion properties—the geometric efficiency and the z-axis efficiency are of particular interest.

In MSCT, the single detector rows are separated by narrow stripes, which are not sensitive to radiation and therefore do not contribute to detector signal. Such septa are necessary to avoid cross-talk between neighboring detector elements and to absorb scattered radiation. The geometric efficiency can be calculated by dividing the active area of the detector array by the total radiated area of the detector. Typical values are 70% to 90% that decrease with additional slices.

Another point should be addressed in this context. By using cone beams in MSCT scanners instead of fan beams as in single-slice devices, scatter radiation is increased and requires either more dose or technical means associated with a decrease in geometric efficiency.

Z-axis Efficiency/Overbeaming

Z-axis efficiency is defined as the fraction of the dose profile that hits the detector elements in the z-direction. When a single detector row is being used,

not only the radiation from the ideal section profile, but also the penumbra of scattered and extrafocal radiation is used, and the z-axis efficiency is almost 100%. In MSCT, the detector is subdivided in four, eight, or more active detector rows. To ensure that each active detector row receives the same amount of radiation, it is necessary to widen the dose profile by opening the pre-patient collimation. In this situation—called *overbeaming*—the slope of the dose profile caused by the penumbra is not used (Figure 16-2). This results in reduced z-axis efficiency in MSCT compared with single-slice CT. However, with an increasing number of detector rows, the fraction of overbeamed area to total detector area decreases, and z-axis efficiency improves.

A dose increase may be seen when a post-patient collimation is used to improve the section sensitivity profile, and the pre-patient collimation is opened to compensate for the loss in detector dose.

Exclusion of the penumbra has the greatest relative effect if the total width of collimation ($n \times SC$) is small. It causes reduced geometric dose efficiency and thus increased CTDI. The effect is greatest for a 2- $\times$ 0.5-mm detector configuration and improves with a 4- $\times$ 0.5-mm collimation. With the introduction of scanners with 16 or more rows, the effect becomes almost negligible.

Overranging

With spiral scanning, radiation exposure is always slightly increased because of an additional rotation

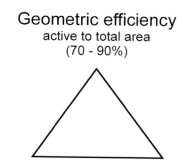

Geometric efficiency
active to total area
(70 - 90%)

Detector efficiency
absorption of scintillator
and conversion efficiency
(95 - 99%)

z-axis efficiency
overbeaming
(50 - 95%)

Fig. 16-1 Main components of total dose efficiency.

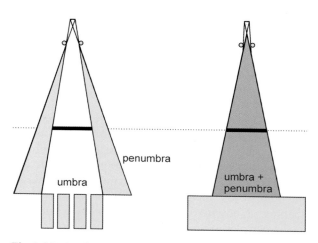

penumbra

umbra

umbra + penumbra

Fig. 16-2 Overbeaming caused by wider collimator settings to avoid penumbral effects in the outer portions of the multislice detector array (**A**). With single slice scanners, the radiation from the ideal section profile as well as from the penumbra is fully used (**B**).

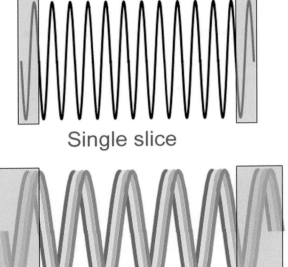

Fig. 16-3 Overranging. To reconstruct the first and last image of the nominal scan volume, extra rotations are required. With multislice scanners, the additional scan volume depends on various factors, especially collimation and pitch.

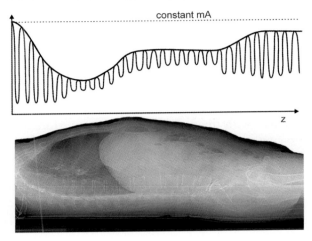

Fig. 16-4 Tube current modulation. The straight line corresponds to a scan with constant tube current. The curved line represents the dose level modulation adjusted to the patient size along the z-axis. This is calculated based on the AP and lateral tomogram before the scan. The second undulating line shows the real-time angular dose modulation according to the noncircular cross-section of the body.

at the beginning and end of the scan to provide data points required for interpolation (Figure 16-3). This increase is usually small in single-slice CT unless the spiral scan is very short. In multislice technology, this effect is always larger since the collimation can only be adjusted for all detector rows.

Tube Current Modulation

Automatic exposure control has been available on radiographic equipment for decades and is now becoming available on CT scanners.

The principal idea is to redistribute the dose for a 360-degree rotation according to the actual attenuation as a function of the projection angle instead of keeping the tube current constant. There are different ways to realize this. The basic ideas are illustrated in Figure 16-4. The earliest approach was a fixed (usually sinusoidal) modulation of the tube current based on attenuation measurements by two localizer scans: AP and lateral. The current approach is the online modulation of the tube current according to the actual course of attenuation from slice to slice, with a delay of only half a rotation and no fixation for a complete range. Spiral

CT is predestined for the use of tube current modulation, because the required reference data for modifying the tube current are available online. Dose reductions of about 20% may be reached with this approach, especially in regions with an elliptical cross-section. The next required step is the adaptation of the tube current to variations of the cross-section along the body's longitudinal axis.

Body scanning is characterized by large variations in attenuation, depending on the projection angle resulting from the noncircular cross-section of the body on one hand and the tissue composition on the other hand. In particular, this applies for continuous scans of the whole body, including the thorax, abdomen, and pelvis, in one step—a technique that is increasingly used in MSCT. Keeping the mAs constant throughout the scan inevitably leads to a dose that is too high for the thorax or too low for the abdomen. Modulating the tube current in these settings creates a dose reduction of 20% or more.

APPLICATION-RELATED FACTORS

Application-related factors have to be considered as a secondary category that may cause unnecessary high radiation exposure as a result of insufficient user experience. This category is tremendously important for the radiologist because with multi-slice technology, either larger volumes may be scanned, or the same volume is scanned with thinner slices without increasing the scan time. Indeed, in daily practice it is often observed that with MSCT, the user has a tendency to scan larger volumes with thinner slice collimations. Moreover, because of the very short scan time, MSCT allows multiphase studies where the same region is scanned two or more times.

With application-related factors, the following parameters that influence patient dose and cause potential dose traps need to be considered:

- Slice collimation, section width, and reconstructed sections

- Choice of filter kernel and window setting

- Repeated scanning of larger volumes

- A wider range of indications

Slice Collimation, Section Width, and Reconstructed Sections

Section width determines image noise in a similar manner as section collimation. Section width is directly dependent on section collimation in spiral CT, but it becomes an independent parameter in MSCT scanning and follows a more complex behavior with varying pitch. It ranges from 100% to 128% of the section collimation. Image noise shows a similarly complex behavior. At identical patient exposure, it is significantly higher if the section width is identical to the collimation and substantially reduced if the section width is increased by 28%.

Image noise increases with a thinner section collimation. This interrelationship parallels that of the mAs settings: reducing the collimation by a factor of 4 could be compensated for by an increase in mAs by the same factor. Without compensation, image noise increases by a factor of 2. Some manufacturers use z-filtering to keep noise independent of the pitch. They use a widened section width (e.g., 1.25 mm for 4- × 1-mm collimations or 3 mm for 4- × 2.5-mm collimations). In clinical practice, mAs settings are often chosen intuitively; however, there is a strong dependence on patient diameter. Tube current (mAs) can be cut in

half if the patient is 3 to 4 cm thinner in diameter. As a consequence, the mAs settings have to be markedly decreased in children and thin patients and may be increased in obese patients. However, it is not always necessary to increase dose. Reconstructing thicker sections from a thin-section raw data set reduces image noise similarly to using a thicker collimation to begin with (Figures 16-5 and 16-6).

The effect of reducing noise by reconstructing thicker sections is more efficient for multiplanar reconstruction (MPR) perpendicular to the scan plane. This is because image noise on consecutive axial sections correlates, although it is nearly independent for adjacent pixels within the scan plane. Because of the increased absorption in lateral projections, the noise on sagittal MPRs is higher than on coronal MPRs, especially for highly eccentric body regions like the shoulders or pelvis.

Considering these correlations, the optimum procedure using MSCT is as follows:
1. To scan with narrow collimation
2. To generate a secondary raw data set with thin axial slices and with a sufficient overlap of about 50%
3. To reconstruct thicker reformations from the secondary thin-section raw data for diagnostic evaluation

Reconstruction Filter Kernel and Window Setting

The filter kernel used for image reconstruction has a substantial influence on perceived image noise. A slightly smoothing kernel causes only minor reduction in spatial resolution but requires a significantly smaller dose while keeping image noise constant. Taking some impairment of spatial resolution into account, a dose reduction of up to 50% is possible. On the other hand, using a high-resolution kernel (edge-enhancing kernel) improves the spatial resolution, but the dose has to be at least doubled to keep image noise constant (Figure 16-7).

A similar effect applies for the window width (WW) setting. In clinical practice, WW is a more or less preset parameter that is chosen according to the displayed anatomical region. It is well known that window settings influence our perception of image noise. Increasing the window width can markedly reduce perceptible image noise. Doubling it from 200 to 400 or from 400 to 800 reduces the

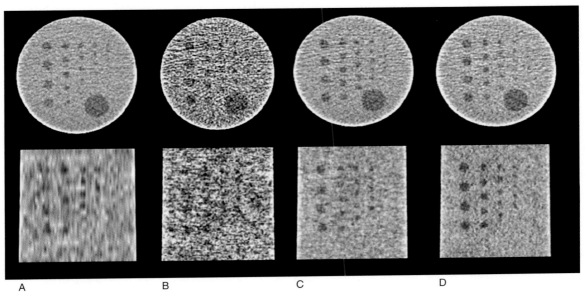

Fig. 16-5 Effect of slice thickness (slice collimation, or SC) and section width on image noise. Axial and coronal views of a low-contrast phantom (hypodense spheres measuring 3 to 8 mm) scanned with varying dose level and slice thickness. **A,** SC 5 mm (5 mGy). **B,** SC 1 mm (5 mGy). **C,** SC 1 mm (20 mGy). **D,** 5 × 1-mm slab (5 mGy). Thinner slice collimation at the same dose level results in increased noise (**B**). To achieve the same noise level as in **A,** a fourfold increase in dose is required (**C**). The same result can be attained using slabs without increasing dose (**D**). A further advantage of using slabs is the increased spatial resolution along the z-axis as seen on the coronal views (**D** versus **A**).

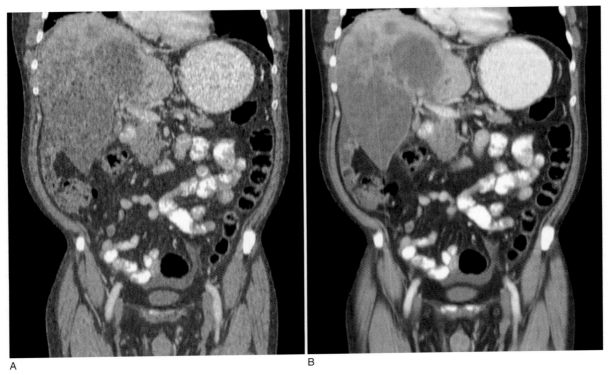

Fig. 16-6 Using a thin collimation guarantees high spatial resolution in all directions. However, to avoid disturbing image noise without excessive dose, a thin-slab technique is recommended. **A,** Coronal reformation of a thin-slice data set. **B,** 3-mm coronal slab of the same data set. Note the significant decrease in noise, resulting in improved visibility of contrast.

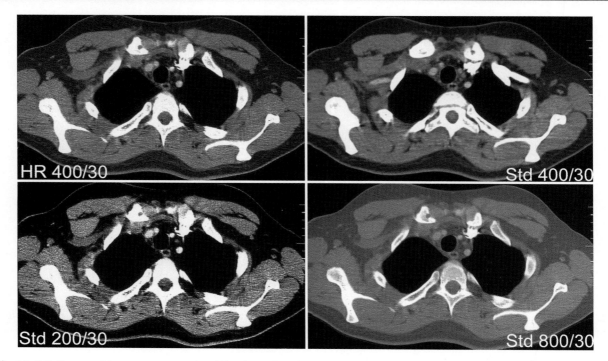

Fig. 16-7 Influence of image reconstruction (filter kernel) and window settings on perceived image noise. Higher spatial resolution and narrow window width result in increased noise. Therefore, standard or soft kernels and broader window width can be used to reduce image noise. However, either spatial or contrast resolution is decreased. *HR,* High resolution; *Std,* standard window width/window level.

perceived image noise by a factor of 2, but at the same time it reduces the image contrast by the same factor (see Figure 16-7). As a matter of fact, the choice of window width is a very important means for potential dose saving. Unfortunately, this factor is usually neglected, since it is merely regarded as a display tool that does not influence contrast-to-noise ratio.

As a result of these relationships regarding the filter kernel and window settings, high-resolution kernels should be used with window widths of more than 1000 only (e.g., in lung or bone studies). On the other hand, soft kernels should be used when narrow window widths are required for observing structures with low contrast, such as the soft tissue of parenchymal organs.

CONCLUSION

To reduce radiation exposure and to maintain diagnostic confidence in MSCT, the following factors are crucial for the radiologist:

1. Carrying out the scan with a narrow collimation
2. Reconstructing a secondary raw-data set of thin slices with a sufficient overlap of about 50%
3. Using thicker reformations from this secondary thin-section raw data to reduce image noise for diagnostic evaluation
4. Adjusting the mAs settings always to the patient diameter (note that the required doses can be reduced by 50% for every 4 cm decrease in the sagittal diameter of the patient—practically every 8-cm decrease should lead to a reduction of 50%)

The following mistakes should be avoided:

1. Overly high doses using thin slices
2. Overly high doses scanning high contrast objects, such as lung or bone
3. Incorrect reconstruction kernels or inadequate window settings
4. Multiphase studies that do not improve diagnosis
5. Incorrect indications

We should never forget that a strict indication is the best way to prevent unnecessary radiation exposure.

Table 16-1 Technical parameters influencing the patient dose

Parameter	Influence on patient dose
Tube voltage	Higher kVp values are advantageous for large patient diameter
Tube current	Linear increase in dose with mAs value
Scanning volume	Linear increase in dose with longer scan volume
Slice thickness	Increase in image noise
Scanning time	Linear increase in cases of constant tube current

Table 16-2 Dose-reduction possibilities

User-dependent possibilities	Manufacturer-dependent possibilities
Clear-cut indication–using MR or US instead of CT when appropriate	Pre-filtration of the x-ray beam beam shaper
Limitation of the scan volume according to the requirements	Attenuation-dependent tube current modulation (automatic exposure control)
Keeping multiple scans to a minimum	
Adjustment of the scanning parameters to the patient cross-section	Noise reducing image reconstruction advanced filtering techniques
Use of pitch-factors >1	
Adequate selection of image reconstruction parameters	
Reduction of kVp when using contrast media	

Tables 16-1 and 16-2 include technical parameters that influence patient dose.

REFERENCES

1. Nagel HD, editor: *Radiation exposure in computed tomography*, Hamburg, 2000, CTB Publications.
2. Kalender WA: *Computertomographie*, München, 2000, Publicis MCD Verlag.
3. Prokop M: Überblick über Strahlenrisiko und Bildqualität (Radiation dose and image quality in computed tomography), *Fortschr Röntgenstr* 174:631, 2002.
4. Kalender WA: Dose management in multi-slice spiral computed tomography, *Eur Radiol Syllabus* 14:40, 2004.

Index

Note: Page numbers followed by the letter f refer to figures; those followed by the letter t refer to tables.